UNDERSTANDING HEALTH POLICY

Other titles in the series

Understanding the finance of welfare

What welfare costs and how to pay for it

Howard Glennerster, Department of Social Administration, London School of Economics and Political Science

"... a brilliant and lively textbook that students will enjoy."
Ian Shaw, School of Sociology and Social Policy, University of Nottingham

PB £17.99 (US$26.95) ISBN-10 1 86134 405 8 ISBN-13 978 1 86134 405 2
HB £50.00 (US$59.95) ISBN-10 1 86134 406 6 ISBN-13 978 1 86134 406 9
240 x 172mm 256 pages May 2003

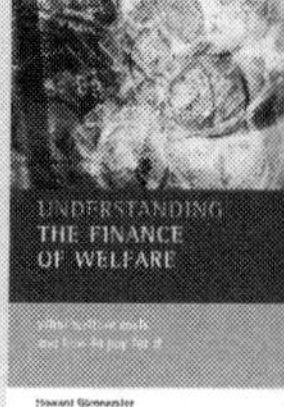

Understanding social security

Issues for policy and practice

Jane Millar, Department of Social and Policy Sciences, University of Bath

"This first-class text provides students with the most up-to-date review and analysis of social security issues. It will fast become the definitive guide to the subject." **Jonathan Bradshaw, Department of Social Policy and Social Work, University of York**

PB £17.99 (US$26.95) ISBN-10 1 86134 419 8 ISBN-13 978 1 86134 419 9
HB £50.00 (US$59.95) ISBN-10 1 86134 420 1 ISBN-13 978 1 86134 421 2
240 x 172mm 360 pages May 2003

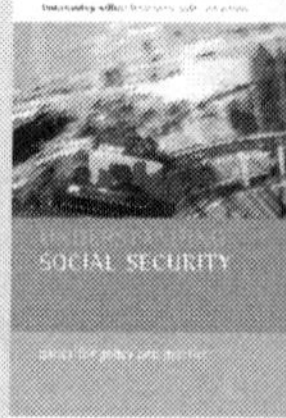

Understanding social citizenship

Themes and perspectives for policy and practice

Peter Dwyer, Department of Sociology and Social Policy, University of Leeds

"An excellent introduction to current debates about citizenship and the only general social policy text on the subject. Highly recommended. Students will certainly benefit from reading this book."
Nick Ellison, Department of Sociology and Social Policy, University of Durham

PB £17.99 (US$28.95) ISBN-10 1 86134 415 5 ISBN-13 978 1 86134 415 1
HB £50.00 (US$75.00) ISBN-10 1 86134 416 3 ISBN-13 978 1 86134 416 8
240 x 172mm 240 pages May 2004

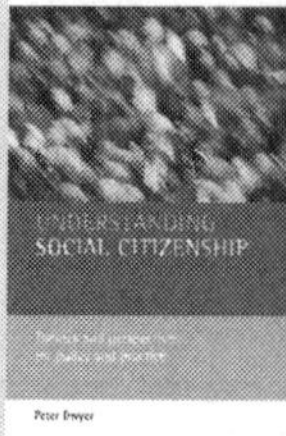

Understanding the policy process

Analysing welfare policy and practice

John Hudson and **Stuart Lowe**, Department of Social Policy and Social Work, University of York

"Hudson and Lowe's book provides an excellent review of the issues about the policy process in a changing society and a changing world." **Michael Hill, Visiting Professor in the Health and Social Policy Research Centre, University of Brighton**

PB £17.99 (US$28.95) ISBN-10 1 86134 540 2 ISBN-13 978 1 86134 540 0
HB £50.00 (US$75.00) ISBN-10 1 86134 539 9 ISBN-13 978 1 86134 539 4
240 x 172mm 304 pages June 2004

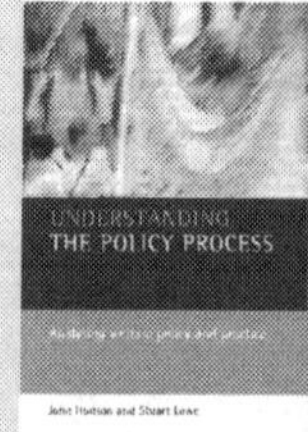

Forthcoming

Understanding health and social care
Jon Glasby
PB £18.99 (US$34.95) ISBN 978 1 86134 910 1
HB £60.00 (US$80.00) ISBN 978 1 86134 911 8
240 x 172mm 256 pages tbc June 2007 tbc

Understanding immigration and refugee policy
Rosemary Sales
PB £19.99 (US$34.95) ISBN 978 1 86134 451 9
HB £60.00 (US$80.00) ISBN 978 186134 452 6
240 x 172mm 240 pages tbc June 2007 tbc

If you are interested in submitting a proposal for the series, please contact Policy Press
e-mail pp-info@bristol.ac.uk
tel +44 (0)117 331 5020
fax +44 (0)117 331 5367

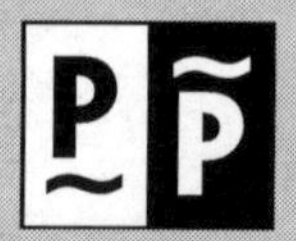

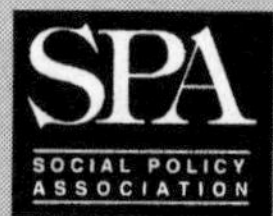

www.policypress.co.uk

INSPECTION COPIES AND ORDERS AVAILABLE FROM

Marston Book Services
PO Box 269 • Abingdon • Oxon
OX14 4YN UK
INSPECTION COPIES
Tel: +44 (0) 1235 465500
Fax: +44 (0) 1235 465556
Email: inspections@marston.co.uk
ORDERS
Tel: +44 (0) 1235 465500
Fax: +44 (0) 1235 465556
Email: direct.orders@marston.co.uk

UNDERSTANDING HEALTH POLICY

Rob Baggott

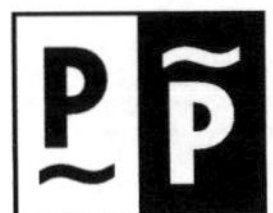

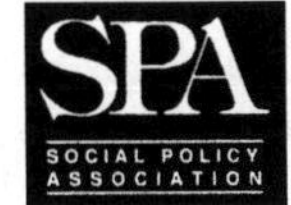

First published in Great Britain in 2007 by

Policy Press
University of Bristol
6th Floor
Howard House
Queen's Avenue
Bristol BS8 1SD
UK
t: +44 (0)117 331 5020
f: +44 (0)117 331 5367
pp-info@bristol.ac.uk
www.policypress.co.uk

North American office:
Policy Press
c/o The University of Chicago Press
1427 East 60th Street
Chicago, IL 60637, USA
t: +1 773 702 7700
f: +1 773-702-9756
sales@press.uchicago.edu
www.press.uchicago.edu

Reprinted 2011 twice, 2013

British Library Cataloguing in Publication Data
A catalogue record for this book is available from the British Library

Library of Congress Cataloging-in-Publication Data
A catalog record for this book has been requested

ISBN 978 1 86134 630 8 paperback
ISBN 978 1 86134 631 5 hardcover

Cover design by Qube Design Associates, Bristol.
Front cover: photograph kindly supplied by Getty Images.
Printed and bound in Great Britain by www.4edge.co.uk

Contents

Detailed contents

List of boxes, figures and tables

Boxes

Figures

Tables

List of abbreviations

ACHCEW	Association of Community Health Councils for England and Wales
APG	All Party subject group
ASH	Action on Smoking and Health
BMA	British Medical Association
CAG	Comptroller and Auditor General
CHC	community health council
CHI	Commission for Health Improvement
CHRE	Council for Healthcare Regulatory Excellence
CMO	Chief Medical Officer
Codex	Codex Alimentarius Commission
CPPIH	Commission for Patient and Public Involvement in Health
CSCI	Commission for Social Care Inspection
CSR	comprehensive spending review
DCCP	Devolution and Constitutional Change Programme
DCLG	Department for Communities and Local Government
DCMS	Department for Culture, Media and Sport
DEFRA	Department for Environment, Food and Rural Affairs
DfES	Department for Education and Skills
DfT	Department for Transport
DHSS	Department of Health and Social Security
DHSSPS	Department of Health, Social Services and Public Safety
DoH	Department of Health
DTI	Department of Trade and Industry
DWP	Department for Work and Pensions
ECJ	European Court of Justice
EDM	early day motion
EEC	European Economic Community
ESRC	Economic and Social Research Council
FAO	(UN) Food and Agriculture Organisation
FHSA	family health services authority
FPC	family practitioner committee
GLA	Greater London Authority
GMC	General Medical Council
GOR	government office for the region

HAS	Health Advisory Service (previously Hospital Advisory Service)
HAZ	health action zone
HMO	health maintenance organisation
HPRU	Health Policy Research Unit (De Montfort University)
HSM	health social movement
HSSB	Health Service Supervisory Board
IDG	interdepartmental group
IGC	Inter-government coordination
IHSM	Institute of Health Service Management (now Institute of Healthcare Management)
ILO	International Labour Organisation
IMF	International Monetary Fund
IPPR	Institute for Public Policy Research
ISTC	independent sector treatment centre
JASP	Joint Approach to Social Policy
JIP	joint investment plan
LAA	local area agreement
LHB	local health board
LIFT	local improvement finance trust
LSP	local strategic partnership
MAFF	Ministry of Agriculture, Fisheries and Food
MAT	modernisation action team
MEP	Member of the European Parliament
MMR	Measles, Mumps and Rubella
MOD	Ministry of Defence
NAO	National Audit Office
NCAA	National Clinical Assessment Authority
NCVO	National Council for Voluntary Organisations
NHS	National Health Service
NHSE	National Health Service Executive
NICE	National Institute for Health and Clinical Excellence (formerly National Institute for Clinical Excellence)
NPSA	National Patient Safety Agency
NRF	Neighbourhood Renewal Fund
NSF	national service framework
ODPM	Office of the Deputy Prime Minister
OECD	Organisation for Economic Cooperation and Development
Ofsted	Office for Standards in Education (now Office for Standards in Education, Children's Services and Skills)

OPSR	Office of Public Service Reform
OSC	overview and scrutiny committee
PAC	Public Accounts Committee
PCG	primary care group
PCT	primary care trust
PFI	private finance initiative
PMB	private member's Bill
PPI	patient and public involvement
PPIF	patient and public involvement forum
PPP	public–private partnership
PQ	parliamentary question
PSA	public service agreement
RCN	Royal College of Nursing
RDA	regional development agency
SAP	structural adjustment programme
SARS	Severe Acute Respiratory Syndrome
SEA	Single European Act
SHA	Strategic Heath Authority
SOLACE	Society of Local Authority Chief Executives and Senior Managers
SPS	sanitary and phytosanitary measures
SSI	Social Services Inspectorate
TBT	Technical Barriers to Trade
TRIPS	Trade-related Aspects of Intellectual Property Rights
UN	United Nations
UNCTAD	UN Conference on Trade and Development
UNDP	UN Development Programme
UNESCO	UN Educational, Scientific and Cultural Organisation
UNHCR	UN High Commission on Refugees
UNICEF	UN Children's Fund
WHO	World Health Organisation
WTO	World Trade Organisation

Preface

Health policy remains a topical and controversial area. If anything, the priority given to the NHS by the Blair government has heightened the political sensitivity of health policy. Most public attention has focused on policy issues rather than the processes that have produced policies. This book does not ignore important policy issues, but explores them through a much deeper examination of the contemporary policy process than is currently available.

The book is based on over 20 years of personal study. It is based heavily on secondary sources and previous research projects (in particular, an Economic and Social Research Council-funded project on health consumer groups and the policy process undertaken by myself, Professor Judith Allsop and Dr Kathryn Jones – grant number R000237888). Additional material was gathered through a series of interviews with participants in the policy process including representatives of professional organisations, health businesses, voluntary organisations and pressure groups as well as politicians, civil servants and journalists (see ***Box 1.2***). I would like to thank these participants, who cannot be identified for reasons of confidentiality, for their time and effort. Thanks also to De Montfort University for providing a small grant to cover the costs of these interviews.

I am extremely grateful to The Policy Press and series editor, Professor Saul Becker for the opportunity to write this book. I would like to thank the Press, and in particular Dawn Rushen, Emily Watt, Philip de Bary, Jo Morton and Dave Worth for their help. I would also like to thank several colleagues at De Montfort University, in particular Katherine Hooper, formerly Health Policy Research Unit (HPRU) administrator, who helped track down important documentary sources and assisted in the preparation of the final manuscript. Thanks too to Dr Kathryn Jones, Senior Research Fellow at the HPRU, who undertook some of the interviews on my behalf and provided valuable comments on the draft typescript. Thanks are also due to Dr Meri Koivusalo for providing additional information on global aspects of health policy and to Dr George Lambie for specific comments on Chapter Ten. I was also grateful for the helpful comments provided by an anonymous external reviewer. Nonetheless, as is customary, the responsibility for the work remains mine alone.

Finally, a big thanks to Debbie, Mark, Danny and Melissa, for their support during this project.

Rob Baggott
Leicester
December 2006

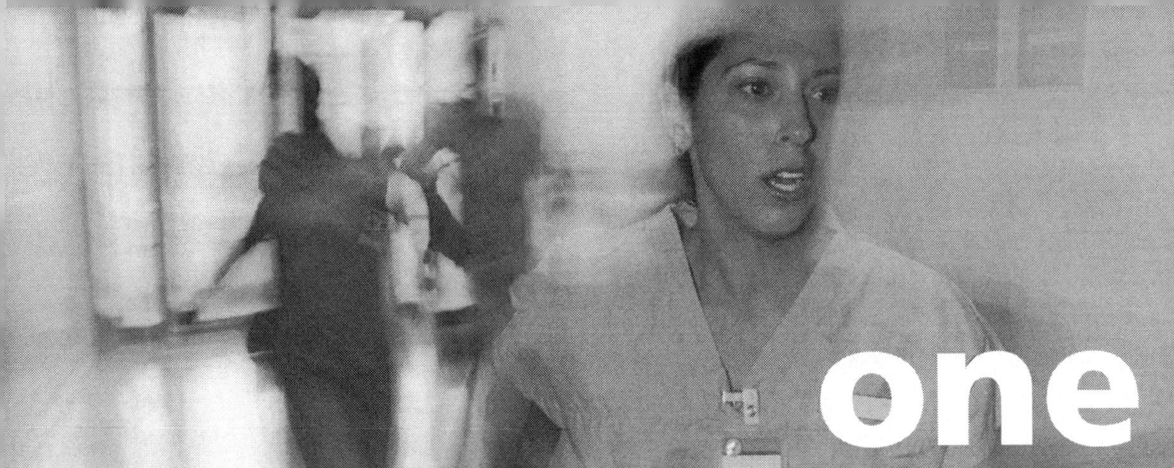

Analysing health policy

Overview

This chapter clarifies the meaning of health policy and reviews conceptual frameworks that are useful in the study of health policy.

Health policy

The task of defining health policy is actually very difficult, largely because both 'health' and 'policy' are contested terms, and therefore subject to a variety of different interpretations.

Health

Health can be interpreted in different ways (Aggleton, 1990; Blaxter, 2004). In a narrow, negative sense it can mean the absence of disease or illness. This approach, which conforms to the conventional biomedical model, interprets health as a state of normality disrupted by illness and disease. However, health can be defined in a positive sense, as in the World Health Organisation's definition as 'a state of complete physical, mental and social well-being and not merely the absence of disease or infirmity' (WHO, 1946, p 100). The distinction between positive and negative definitions has a bearing on the boundary of health policy. Adopting the negative approach marks out a much smaller territory for analysis. Here, policy analysis focuses on the provision of health services. However, if a positive approach is taken, health policy analysis becomes a much wider field of study, incorporating a huge range of social, economic, environmental and political processes affecting individual and community health and well-being.

Neither approach is really satisfactory. The first is too narrow, the other perhaps too broad. A more realistic approach is to retain a primary focus on policy processes that affect health and health services, while acknowledging that other policy sectors, such as housing, income support, social services, environment, the economy, taxation and trade, can impinge on health and health care.

Policy

Policy is also a contested term (see Ham and Hill, 1984; Hogwood and Gunn, 1984; Dye, 1992; Parsons, 1995; John, 1998; Marinetto, 1998; Colebatch, 2002; Hudson and Lowe, 2004). In broad terms, a policy is a position taken on an issue by an organisation or individual in a position of authority. More specifically, it might refer to a statement, a decision, a document, or a programme of action (see Hogwood and Gunn, 1984). Policy is not always a positive action: it may take the form of inaction or a deliberate attempt to block a decision. Colebatch (2002, pp 9-10) identified three central elements of policy. First, policy is concerned with order, implying a systematic and consistent approach. Second, it is legitimised by authority of individuals, offices or organisations. Third, policy implies expertise. Underlying policy debates are various bodies of expertise, including theories and findings relating to problems and how they might be resolved. Policy is often shorthand for 'public policy'. Public policy has been defined succinctly by Dye (1992, p 2) as '... whatever governments choose to do, or not to do'. But a key concern is how the authoritative positions of governing institutions are determined and how they are put into practice. This process involves non-governmental actors, such as the media, professional bodies, business and voluntary organisations. Therefore their activities also fall within the remit of public policy analysis.

Health policy

Several authors have attempted to define health policy. Blank and Burau (2004, p 16), while acknowledging the impact of broader social and economic policies on health, define health policy as 'those courses of action proposed or taken by a government that impact on the financing and/or provision of health services'. According to Buse et al (2005, p 6) '... health policy is assumed to embrace courses of action (and inaction) that affect the set of institutions, organisations, services and funding arrangements of the health system'. For Walt (1994, p 1) 'health policy is about process and power ... it is concerned with who influences whom in the making of policy, and how that happens'.

Meanwhile, Green and Thorogood (1998, p 9) define health policy analysis as 'the study of health policy concerns, the origins of that policy, its goals and its outcomes'.

Taking these various definitions into account, and bearing in mind the contested nature of both 'health' and 'policy', this book adopts the following perspective. It focuses upon the political processes that underlie the emergence of health issues, the formulation of policies and their implementation. It is mainly concerned with the institutions and processes of government, and this includes the activities of non-governmental organisations within the policy process.

Conceptual frameworks

When undertaking the study of any policy arena, one must be familiar with key concepts of policy analysis. The remainder of this chapter considers the main conceptual frameworks and their relevance to health policy.

Policy as a rational, hierarchical process

The rational model is neatly summarised by Marinetto (1998, p 7) as follows:

> According to the rational model, policy typically emanates from senior officials and ministers. Once a policy is set in motion by these central figures, it is seen to follow a linear course of development from implementation to completion.

This model owes much to Simon's (1945) work on administrative decision-making. He believed that even in a complex environment, rational decision-making was possible. Although decision makers lacked full information and knowledge, could not know all consequences of their decisions and operated within organisations that framed their choices, they should seek to identify the best possible options in terms of their values, based upon a comprehensive evaluation of the various alternatives (see Parsons, 1995; Bochel and Bochel, 2004). This meant identifying goals, listing alternative strategies, assessing the consequences of these options and choosing the strategy that achieved these goals. Simon recognised that in practice rationality was limited. Not all options and consequences could be fully explored. So decision makers should instead try to select alternatives that satisfy rather than maximise their values. Although this 'bounded rationality' was more realistic, Simon did believe, however, that the scope for rational decision-making could be improved through technology and new management techniques (Simon, 1960).

Others, such as Lindblom (1959), were more sceptical about human rationality within complex policy environments and the desirability of trying to improve rationality. He argued that by necessity decisions were made in an incremental fashion and that the analysis of options was limited, taking the form of a succession of comparisons rather than a comprehensive analysis. Moreover, for him, values and goals were inseparable from the evaluation of these options. Decisions emerged not from a rational analysis as described by Simon but by 'muddling through', interactions between various participants leading to mutual adjustment of competing objectives and ultimately compromise (Lindblom, 1965).

Nonetheless, the rational model has been influential. It underpins the 'stagist' approach to policy (see Rose, 1973; May and Wildavsky, 1978; Hogwood and Gunn, 1984; Dorey, 2005) which retains its appeal today. Basically, the stagist approach breaks the policy process down into various phases. Different authors adopt slightly different approaches, but the stages they identify are broadly similar. For example, in Hogwood and Gunn's (1984) model, the following stages are outlined:

- deciding to decide – including issue search and agenda setting
- deciding how to decide – deciding how decisions should be made
- issue definition
- forecasting
- setting objectives and priorities
- options analysis
- policy implementation, monitoring and control
- evaluation and review
- policy maintenance, succession or termination.

Although a useful way of thinking about the different aspects of policy, and a starting point for analysing factors that impinge on each stage, the model has been criticised for oversimplifying the multidimensional nature of the policy process and imposing an artificial rationality upon it (John, 1998). Defenders of the stagist approach have responded by emphasising the dynamics of the policy process and acknowledging 'feedback loops' between different stages (in particular, policy evaluation and agenda setting). For example, the notion of a 'policy cycle' linked the final stages of the policy process with the initiation of new policies (May and Wildavsky, 1978; Hogwood and Peters, 1983). Critics have also attacked the stagist approach for failing to provide explanations of policy development that can then be tested (Sabatier, 1999). However, its very simplicity has enabled it to remain attractive as a starting point for policy analysis and it retains considerable utility as a 'framework for organising our understanding of what happens' (Hogwood and Gunn, 1984, p 4).

There has been great emphasis on improving the rationality of policy making within government. Efforts have been made to improve policy analysis, with the creation of think tanks and policy research units (Gray and Jenkins, 1985). There has also been a drive towards improving the implementation of policy through 'managerialism' (see Clarke and Newman, 1997; Newman, 2001). This began with the efforts of Conservative and Labour governments in the 1960s and 1970s to improve policy and planning. This was followed through by reforms to impose stronger performance management on public sector organisations in the 1980s and 1990s. Subsequently, managerialism has been evident in the Blair government's approach to public services, heavily based on centralised targets, performance agreements and audit/inspection regimes to ensure compliance (Newman, 2001).

The top-down model of policy making has been particularly influential over how the process of implementation is understood (Hill, 1997; Hill and Hupe, 2002; Barrett, 2004). Traditionally, implementation was seen as an 'add on' to the process of policy making. The main focus of attention was upon explaining gaps or deficits between the intentions of policy makers and the outcomes of policy (see Pressman and Wildavsky, 1973; Hood, 1976; Dunsire, 1978; Hogwood and Gunn, 1984; Marsh and Rhodes, 1992a). An alternative 'bottom-up' perspective was also developed (Barrett and Fudge, 1981; Barrett, 2004) focusing on the processes of negotiation and mediation that could lead to modification of policy by agencies at the periphery, such as local government. Others highlighted the discretionary power of front-line professionals and workers or 'street level bureaucrats' (Lipsky, 1979) and the need to understand their actions in context (Ellmore, 1980). More recently, efforts have been made to transcend this 'top-down' or 'bottom-up' dichotomy. Elements from both have been synthesised in order to better understand the dynamics of policy implementation without the assumption that 'top-down' is necessarily the best way of operating (see Parsons, 1995; Hill and Hupe, 2002; Barrett, 2004).

Health policy does not necessarily follow a rational model. Indeed, attempts to centralise policy and strengthen top-down implementation may well be regarded as irrational and counterproductive. For example, crude performance targets have in some circumstances undermined the pursuit of good quality, accessible services in the National Health Service (NHS) and in other public services (Audit Commission, 2003; Select Committee on Public Administration, 2003). Nonetheless, the debates surrounding rational models of policy making and implementation are useful in helping to identify key features – such as the emergence of issues on to policy agendas, the role of central government in performance management and monitoring, the process of implementation – that no study of health policy should ignore.

Policy, ideology and political parties

Much attention has been paid to the role of ideologies, such as conservatism, socialism or economic liberalism in shaping policy. In short, conservatism emphasises the importance of tradition, hierarchy, private property, paternalism and social order. Economic liberalism, or more correctly 'neo-liberalism' in its modern formulation, stands for the primacy of markets, private property and freedom of the individual. Socialism emphasises equality, state ownership, collective action and social justice (Heywood, 1994). These ideologies have shaped policy in a number of ways, but a key channel of influence has been the political party system.

In the UK, the party system at national level is characterised by competition between two main political parties with very different ideological traditions (Conservative and Labour – see ***Box 1.1***). The 'first past the post' electoral system, has given these parties a disproportionate number of seats in Parliament. It has also produced 'majority governments', where the winning party can govern alone, without the support of others. Indeed, coalition governments are relatively rare in British government (although the story is different in the devolved assemblies of Wales, Scotland and Northern Ireland – see Chapter Nine). The swing of the political pendulum gives each of the two main parties an opportunity to bring its own ideology to bear on policy. According to Crossman (1972) parties are the 'battering rams of change' driving forward policy. This is perhaps enhanced by the tenure of each government (Webb, 2000). Since 1945 only one (the Conservative government of 1970–4) failed to secure at least a second period in office.

Box 1.1: The Conservative and Labour Parties

The Conservative Party

The modern Conservative Party emerged in the 1830s (Blake, 1985). It is the most successful party, having been in government more often than any of its rivals (Cocker and Jones, 2002, p 123). Since the Second World War the Conservative Party has been in government on the following occasions: 1951–64; 1970–4; 1979–97. The party encapsulates a range of standpoints, although certain principles have been fairly constant. These include an emphasis on individual responsibility, private property and enterprise, and a dislike of the state, public spending and taxation. However, this has been counterbalanced by a 'One Nation' tradition within the party that emphasises paternalism, social order and the protection of the weak and vulnerable. For most of the post-war period, despite its preference for private ownership and markets, the party accepted the need for state intervention in the economy and social welfare.

With specific regard to health policy, the Conservative Party was opposed to the NHS at the outset because it was a nationalised state system. However, the party acknowledged the need for a comprehensive system of health care. When in government, it reached an accommodation with the NHS largely for pragmatic reasons, not least of which was the popularity of the service. Under the leadership of Margaret Thatcher, the party shifted to the right and placed greater emphasis on neo-liberal ideas such as privatisation and the increased use of markets.

The Labour Party

The Labour Party was formed by socialist societies and trade unions in 1900. After a spell as the 'Third Party', it overtook the Liberal Party as one of the two major parties of government. Since the Second World War it has been in government during the following periods: 1945–51; 1964–70; 1974–9 and since 1997. Like the Conservative Party, the Labour Party is a broad church and its policies have shifted over time. Its fundamental principles are rooted in socialism, itself a very broad philosophy. In general terms, socialism seeks to use the state to improve social justice through redistribution of wealth and by regulation of capitalist enterprise. Although Labour established the NHS after the Second World War as a nationalised service, it did allow the continued provision of private health care. The party became more hostile to private medicine in the 1970s, attempting to phase out pay beds within the NHS.

Following General Election defeats in the 1980s and 1990s, the Labour Party rebranded itself as 'New Labour', under the leadership of Tony Blair. This involved a more pragmatic approach which led the party to embrace policies adopted by previous Conservative governments, such as the use of private finance to build and run health care facilities, greater use of private providers to supply care for NHS patients and the use of market forces to allocate resources within the NHS.

The Crossman thesis is related to the 'doctrine of the mandate', which states that a party victorious at a General Election is entitled to carry out its manifesto commitments (see Birch, 1964). Against this, it is argued that voters do not necessarily agree with each element of a manifesto. Moreover, manifesto commitments are often vague and give dubious legitimacy to a government's programme. Some argue that manifestos have fallen into disrepute. According to Hilder (2005) for example '... manifestos have slid towards marketing tools: undemocratic in their compilation, treated cavalierly after elections, they are anyway too general to determine every decision in the years that follow'. Indeed, circumstances can render some manifesto commitments redundant. They may be difficult or impossible to implement for political and technical reasons.

An alternative view to Crossman is provided by Rose (1984). He argues (and supports with empirical evidence – see Rose and Davies, 1994) that governing parties are constrained by the policies of their predecessors. Instead of sharp changes in policy following the replacement of one party in office by another, the outcome is in practice more stable and continuous, resulting in a 'moving consensus'. Rose argues that several factors constrain incoming governments. These include practical constraints (one cannot reverse all the previous government's legislation all at once) as well as political realities (some existing policies may be effective and/or popular). Other constraining factors include events and circumstances. According to Rose (p 141) 'much of a party's record will be stamped upon it by forces outside its control'.

In trying to assess the impact of party politics, one is concerned with much more than the formal positions of parties set out in manifestos and other policy documents. Party politics involves a great deal of posturing. What a party says it will do in government is not necessarily matched by its actions in office. Moreover, other intended policies may not be formally expounded or may be deliberately understated because of fears of creating internal party divisions or giving electoral opponents an advantage. Indeed, sometimes party positions are often deliberately vague in order to encompass the breadth of views and interests within the party. Once in office, the balance of power between these internal forces may change, leading to a different emphasis and possibly a change in policy direction.

Furthermore, party policy is influenced by competition and collaboration between parties (Webb, 2000). Parties often borrow ideas from each other in an effort to gain electoral advantage, or to solve a policy problem, although they rarely acknowledge this debt. In some circumstances, parties may have to depend on each other for support (for example, coalition governments, electoral pacts and other forms of collaboration) and may have to alter their policies as a result. These instances are relatively rare in national politics in the UK, but are an important feature of local government, devolved assemblies and the European Parliament.

In practice, the ideological breadth of the parties, coupled with the pragmatic nature of British government, has generated large areas of consensus on policy matters (Beer, 1965; Addison, 1975). This was certainly the case in the immediate post-war period, but has been true to some extent since, despite the polarisation of the parties during the 1980s. Nonetheless, the Conservative Party of Margaret Thatcher, strongly influenced by neo-liberalism, introduced radical policies such as the privatisation of nationalised industries and the introduction of markets in public services (Marsh and Rhodes, 1992a). However, tensions with traditional conservative values coupled with the unpopularity of some measures and the difficulties of implementation, diluted this radical programme. This was particularly the case in policy areas such as health where there was strong public and professional opposition. Thatcher's successor, John Major, proved more pragmatic, which meant that many policies formulated in the 1980s were implemented in much less ideological fashion than their original architects envisaged, including NHS reforms.

Under the New Labour government of Tony Blair since 1997, the role of ideology has been even less clear. During the 1990s the Labour Party adopted 'right-wing' policies in an effort to capture votes (Bara and Budge, 2001). Once in government, its policy incorporated elements of both neo-liberalism and socialism. This was heralded as the 'Third Way' (Giddens, 1998), drawing heavily on communitarian ideas that involved the rebalancing of individuals' rights and responsibilities and combining choice and enterprise with notions of social justice. The Blair government maintained key elements of policy from the Conservative years – the emphasis on markets to allocate resources, a growing role for the private sector, centralised performance management of public services and an emphasis on consumerism. The NHS was not exempt from these policy trends.

Health policy remains a key issue of party political contention. Health issues are emotive and attract considerable media attention. The NHS is a key area of public expenditure, employs a large workforce and provides services for the vast majority of the population. Politicians of all parties cannot ignore these factors and will always strive to gain electoral advantage in such a key area of policy.

An alternative approach sees ideological factors as transcending political parties, rather than operating through them. According to this perspective the 'worldview' of those within government is shaped by contextual factors, which in effect 'short-circuit' the system of party politics. Politicians and senior bureaucrats find themselves adopting similar positions irrespective of their ideological tendencies. This worldview is intimately connected to ideas about the role of the state, particularly with regard to the economy and social welfare. Indeed, several authors have noted how health policy is shaped by the paradigms of economic and social policy (Klein, 2000), by the context of the welfare state and capitalist economic arrangements (Moran, 1999, 2000) or by particular welfare state strategies. Indeed with regard to the latter point, Greener (2004b) argues that health policy reform can be understood in terms of a shift from a 'Keynesian Welfare National State' towards a 'Schumpeterian Workfare Post-national Regime' (see also Jessop, 1999). The former, characterised by full employment policies, mass consumption and production, paternalist welfare systems, national citizenship and state bureaucracy is believed to have given way to the latter, which emphasises a less state-controlled approach to welfare and greater emphasis on competition within a global context.

Policy as the interplay of interests

Policy can also be viewed as the product of interplay between different interests with particular goals and values (Baggott, 1995a; Grant, 2000). These interests may be organised or diffuse. However, most emphasis has been placed upon the participation of organised interests in the policy process, known as pressure groups, defined by Coxall (2001, p 3) as 'any organisation that aims to influence public policy by seeking to persuade decision-makers by lobbying rather than by standing for election and holding office'.

Pressure group theorists see interaction between such organisations and government as central to the policy process (Truman, 1951; Latham, 1965; Bentley, 1967). In their view, policy outcomes are determined by the relative influence of groups, which in turn have a range of resources. Groups that have financial resources, can mobilise their members and the wider public, and have good political contacts with decision makers, tend to have more influence over policy. Tactics and strategy also play an important part, and knowledge and understanding of the policy process is crucial. In the British system of government, where policy making is concentrated in the hands of central government, groups that have good contacts at this level – so-called insider groups (Grant, 2000) – are believed to be in a strong position to influence policy. Those which lack this status – outsider groups – are regarded as less influential. However, this simple model has been undermined by three factors: the growing impact of 'outsider' groups – such as the environmental lobby – on agendas and policy decisions (Ridley and Jordan, 1998); the decline in influence of some traditional insider groups – such as trade unions and some professional organisations; and a recognition that central government institutions are quite accessible, which means that relatively few organisations are refused contact if they seek it (Maloney et al, 1994).

The health policy process is host to a wide range of pressure groups: professional and labour organisations, commercial interests, and health consumer and patients' groups, as well as voluntary organisations and single issue groups. This makes it a particularly rich source of material for the study of pressure group politics. Indeed, one of the pioneering studies of pressure group politics was a study of the British Medical Association (BMA) (Eckstein, 1960). Health policy is also a haven for social movements. Social movements promote particular values among the population, often encourage direct action by groups and individuals, and seek to influence policy agendas and decisions (Habermas, 1976; Byrne 1997; Tarrow, 1998). In the health policy field, social movements have been identified in relation to women's health, mental health and patients' rights, for example.

Any consideration of pressure groups and social movements in health policy must also acknowledge the underlying structural interests relating to capital and labour. Marxists see these as setting the parameters within which issues and policies arise (see O'Connor, 1973; Doyal, 1979; Miliband, 1982; Offe, 1984). For example, with regard to health care, Navarro (1978) argued that the capitalist system forecloses certain policy options and facilitates others. Using a different approach, Alford (1975) identified three structural interests in the US health care system: the dominant professional interest, the challenging corporate and managerial interest, and the repressed community interest. According to his model, the professional interest maintains its supremacy through underlying power generated by the social structure and in particular by an ability to define the values of the health care system. His approach has been applied to the UK, with some modification (see North and Peckham, 2001; Baggott et al, 2005).

Another concept used in the analysis of pressure group politics and government-group relations is the 'policy network' (Richardson and Jordan, 1979; Marsh and Rhodes, 1992b; Smith, 1993). This focuses on relationships between government agencies and non-governmental organisations as the key to understanding policy formation and implementation. Marsh and Rhodes (1992b) identified two types of policy network: close-knit and stable 'policy communities', which exhibit a high degree of interdependence between government and non-government organisations, and 'issue networks', which are more open, less stable and exhibit low levels of interdependence. The policy networks approach has moved beyond describing and categorising different types of relationship towards an analysis of the impact of networks on policy (see Smith, 1993; Marsh and Smith, 2000). There has been an increasing interest in the dynamics of policy networks, and in particular how they change in response to external and internal pressures (see Baumgartner and Jones, 1993; Richardson, 2000). Of particular interest is how governments have applied different approaches to the 'management' of policy networks, how the membership of networks has changed, and how this has affected policy processes and outputs.

Applying the concept of policy networks to health policy facilitates a mapping of the range of government and non-government organisations involved in this policy arena (see ***Figure 1.1***). It is also useful in posing questions about how changing relationships between government and groups might affect policy formation, implementation and outcomes. Indeed, it appears that the tightly knit 'policy community' that characterised the immediate post-war period, exemplified by the close relationship between the BMA and the Ministry of Health, has given way to a looser and more inclusive 'issue network', involving groups representing patients and carers, for example (see Baggott et al, 2005).

Figure 1.1: *The health policy network in England*

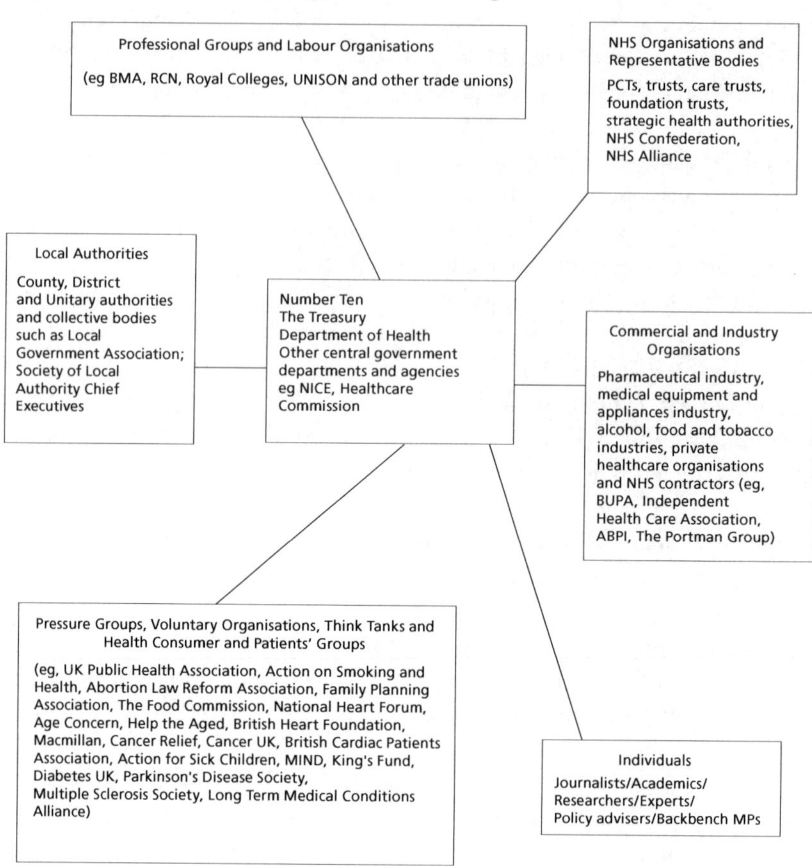

Policy, institutions and agendas

The so-called 'new institutionalism' revived interest in how political institutions can shape policy. As March and Olsen (1984, p 738) argued, 'the bureaucratic agency, the legislative committee, and the appellate court are arenas for contending social forces, but they are also collections of standard operating procedures and structures that define and defend interests. They are political actors in their own right.' The 'newness' of this approach has been disputed (Jordan, 1990; Rhodes, 1997; Hudson and Lowe, 2004). Critics maintain that institutions have always been part of policy analysis. Nonetheless, it is acknowledged that new institutionalism has reiterated the importance of institutions in the policy process, and in particular the way in which they structure interaction between policy actors.

A strand of new institutionalism focuses on the role of institutions in promoting stability and continuity. The path dependency model (David, 1985; Berman, 1998) is based on an assumption that institutions and previous decisions exert a strong influence over current policy making. The outcome is incremental rather than radical change. This model has been applied to health systems reform (see Wilsford, 1994; Immergut, 1992; Greener, 2004a), where the divergence in strategies between countries has been attributed to powerful institutional factors within each political system. This approach has been criticised for being too deterministic. Radical changes do happen, such as the creation of the NHS in 1948. Supporters of the path dependency approach, however, deny that today's decisions are automatically determined by past decisions. They believe that their model allows for deviation from the path which previous decisions and existing institutions have set, although only under exceptional circumstances. Wilsford, for example, argues that there are factors that can enable decision makers to break out of status quo, including the manipulation of incentives within institutions, the development of new technologies and 'conjecture' about future policy options. He also argues that centralised political systems – such as the UK – can be more effective in introducing 'big reform' and 'leveraging a wholly new policy path' (Wilsford, 1994, p 7). However, others argue that centralisation can prevent innovation and the emergence of new policies and practices from the bottom up (Greener, 2004a).

Policy change is closely connected with the setting of agendas and how issues are selected for debate and intervention. Downs (1972) identified an 'issue-attention' cycle, whereby issues attracted public attention, leading to pressure on government to intervene, only for the issue to subside as the costs of intervention became known. Others have since concluded that the emergence of an issue on the agenda does not necessarily reflect its importance in terms of social impact or cost (Cobb and Elder, 1972). Rather it is related to various 'triggers' attracting media attention and the efforts of those seeking to get issues on the agenda – including pressure groups and government. It should be noted that political actors vary in their ability to shape agendas (Schattschneider, 1960). Agenda setting is regarded as the 'second face of power' (Bachrach and Baratz, 1962) enabling powerful interests to prevent decisions that adversely affect their interests from being considered. There is also a 'third face' of power – the manipulation of values – that is also subject to influence by powerful interests and through the media (Lukes, 1974).

Related to this is the notion that policy is often a symbolic activity. There may be situations where government cannot solve a problem, or is perhaps reluctant to tackle it for fear of offending powerful interests. Here the government may devise a symbolic policy in order to maintain its legitimacy and authority. Government engages extensively in 'spin' and media manipulation of policy (see Fairclough, 2000; Jones, 2002), and is not afraid to use 'placebo policies' to convince people that action is taking place, even when it is not (Richardson and Moon, 1984). It is therefore vitally important that policy analysis should take into account the importance of language, discourse and symbolism. Several authors have considered this, notably Edelman (1964, 1971, 1977) who saw a tendency for government to adopt emotional symbols rather than tangible activities. Indeed, much government activity is concerned with appearing to do something rather than actually solving problems. Such an approach to policy analysis focuses on the role of the media and other policy actors in defining problems and policies. It takes a critical approach to methods used by government and by other participants in the policy process, and sees the underlying purpose of policy making as a means of reducing public power, avoiding dealing with serious public problems and benefiting powerful interests in society, in marked contrast to rational models of policy making which are based on normative assumptions of public good.

These concepts are highly relevant to health policy. Health issues are prominent on the political agenda, but some – such as mental health and chronic illness – tend to get less sympathetic coverage than others (such as breast cancer, for example). Furthermore, health policy is host to powerful commercial interests (such as the pharmaceutical, drink and tobacco industries) that seek to influence the perception of health issues. Meanwhile, government, which sees health as a highly political issue, is keen to influence the public perception of its management of the health system and its stewardship of public health. Moreover, the emotive nature of health issues, and their intractability, increases the scope for symbolic policy making.

Also relevant here is Kingdon's (1984) 'policy windows' model whereby policy is shaped by a complex interaction between three 'streams'. First, there is a *problem stream*, which comprises those problems that the government is considering. This is influenced by measures indicating such problems (such as NHS waiting-lists, for example), by events (such as outbreaks of infectious disease) and feedback (on current performance in meeting health service targets, for example). The second stream is a *policy stream*, where ideas about how to deal with problems circulate within policy networks and among 'political entrepreneurs' who play a crucial role in selling policy ideas. Finally, a there is a *political stream*, which consists of public opinion, organised political forces (such as parties, pressure groups), government and ways of building support and consensus. Kingdon argues that when these various streams come together – a problem gets on to the agenda, there is a perceived solution to this problem, and the political situation is supportive – a 'launch window' opens, enabling policy change to take place.

Policy as an adaptive, learning process

The policy process can be seen as an adaptive process that involves learning about the policy environment, the potential policy options and the political resources of supporters and opponents. One of the best known exponents of this approach is Sabatier (1987, 1999; also Jenkins-Smith and Sabatier, 1994), who argues that the key to understanding policy lies in the advocacy coalitions that inhabit 'policy subsystems'. These coalitions consist of pressure groups, politicians, policy advisers and experts, journalists and commentators as well as professionals, civil servants and service providers that endorse a particular set of ideas and beliefs about policy in a particular policy subsystem. Policy change occurs in two main ways. First of all, external factors, such as socio-economic conditions or changes in government, can affect fundamental policy positions (known as the 'policy core'). More commonly, however, 'secondary' changes in policy will occur and this results from policy-oriented learning within advocacy coalitions as well as between them. This policy-oriented learning takes the form of adaptation in the light of experience, as advocacy coalitions seek to refashion their strategies and policy ideas. Conflicting strategies are mediated by 'policy brokers' who aim to achieve a compromise that will reduce the intensity of conflict. The model is based on an assumption that policy change can only be understood over a long timespan – a decade or more.

Other models have emphasised the importance of learning within the policy environment. There is a growing body of literature on the role of experts in policy making, whether these be academics, scientist or professionals (see Collingridge and Reeve, 1986; Fischer, 1990; Barker and Peters, 1993). Although experts do not necessarily determine policy, they can exert influence over policy through legitimacy accorded to their scientific advice. Others may exert influence over the implementation of policy in view of their specialist knowledge. In the health field, government has relied heavily on medical experts to advise on policy, such as the Chief Medical Officer for example. It is also dependent on doctors to interpret and implement government policies and guidelines, giving the profession considerable leverage (Moran and Wood, 1992; Moran, 1999; Klein, 2000; Salter, 2004).

Another important aspect of policy-oriented learning is 'policy transfer' (Bennett, 1991; Rose, 1991; Dolowitz and Marsh, 1996). Policy transfer may involve, for example, the adaptation of policy instruments used in one health system to another. Indeed NHS reforms such as internal markets, privatisation and foundation trusts have been influenced by policies adopted in other countries (see for example, O'Neill, 2000). Policy-oriented learning is not confined to policy 'successes', real or apparent. Knowledge and understanding of policy failures and disasters (Bovens and t'Hart, 1996; Gray and t'Hart, 1998) can also have an impact on policy debates.

Policy learning is not exclusively a national-level phenomena. Policy learning can occur at the regional and local level (and between different states and territories of a country in federal and devolved systems of government). For example, locally devised policies may impact on a problem and this positive experience may be shared and taken up by other localities. Alternatively, local experiments and pilot projects may be established in a deliberate effort to inform and encourage future policy development elsewhere.

Health policy analysis

In this book, a 'multiple lens approach' has been adopted (Sabatier, 1999). It does not focus wholly on any single model of the policy process but is alive to the possibility that all may potentially contribute to our understanding of health policy. Most of the analytical approaches discussed so far are generic. They can be applied to policy processes in any field of domestic or international policy. However, context is important and any framework of analysis adopted must be sensitive to this. Moreover, it is not only the current context that is important. As Heinz et al (1993), in their study of the policy process in the US, observed, policy-making systems have historically situated social structures. Historical circumstance is important in shaping different policy domains such as health, education, criminal justice and so on, which often display different features and policy styles.

Health policy, as defined here, certainly has a number of distinctive features: it is an arena inhabited by high profile political issues, health issues are high on both government and public agendas, government is accountable for a national health service, there are powerful pressure groups involved as well as social movements. It is an area of considerable media interest, a significant chunk of public expenditure, and yet at the same time a field of substantial opportunities for business. Any approach must be able to capture these key features in a dynamic way, reflecting the weight of historical circumstances as well as contemporary political forces.

Box 1.2: Health policy: research methods

This book is based on over 20 years of research into health policy. Most of the sources used are secondary and include general studies of the health policy process as well as more specific analyses of policy issues. Further insights into the nature of contemporary health policy processes were generated by involvement in a major project that explored the role of health consumer groups and the policy process (see Baggott et al, 2005). A series of additional in-depth interviews with participants in the health policy process, undertaken in 2005, provided additional material. These informants were carefully chosen in order to cover a range of backgrounds and perspectives. They included politicians, senior NHS managers, civil servants, journalists, lobbyists, political advisers, and individuals representing charities, consumer groups, think tanks, professional organisations, trade unions and commercial interests, including the drugs industry. Comments made by these informants are used to illustrate points throughout the book.

The chapters that follow examine different aspects of the health policy process and are based on secondary sources and primary research (see Box 1.2). Chapter Two explores the impact of party politics and ideology in national policy. Chapter Three examines the role of central government, and Chapter Four, Parliament. Chapter Five analyses the role of the media in health policy, while Chapter Six looks at the activities of pressure groups. The following three chapters explore health policy at local and regional level, and in those parts of the UK that possess devolved powers and responsibilities. The penultimate chapter considers the international dimension and the role of global institutions. Finally, the analysis is brought together to draw conclusions about the nature of the contemporary health policy process in the UK.

Summary

- Health policy is a contested term, largely because both 'health' and 'policy' are contested.
- Health policy can be examined by using several different conceptual frameworks.

Key questions

1. What is health?
2. What is policy?
3. How is health policy defined?
4. What are the main conceptual frameworks for understanding health policy?

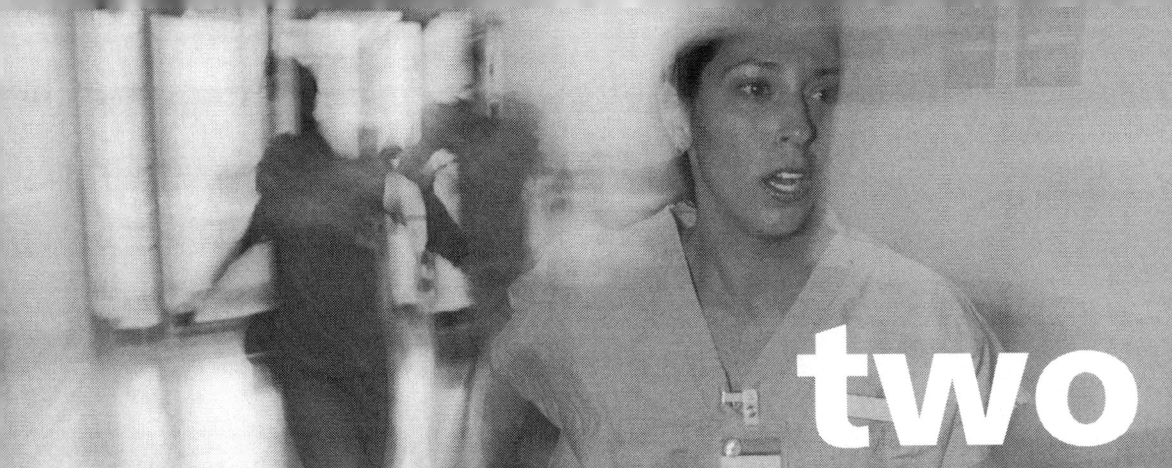

Party politics and health policy

Overview

This chapter explores the role of political parties in relation to health policy, focusing primarily on England (Chapter Nine considers party politics in other parts of the UK in the context of devolution). It explores the salience of health issues in party politics before examining the impact of party politics on health policy since the creation of the NHS.

As noted in Chapter One, parties are important political institutions that can shape policy. However, there is disagreement over the extent of their impact. This chapter explores the role of political parties in relation to health policy and assesses their influence in this field.

Health policy is often seen as a 'party political football'. It is a major issue of debate between the political parties. Health issues have also been prominent at election time (see ***Box 2.1***). One reason for this is that health is an important issue for the public. Health issues affect many people, often in a very intense and emotive way. Furthermore, the NHS affects many people in a significant way as an employer as well as a provider of services. Indeed, when people are asked which issues they feel are currently the most important, health and the NHS invariably appear among the most salient (see Mulligan and Appleby, 2001; You Gov/Sky News, 2005). Public interest is expressed and reinforced by media interest in health matters. This is explored more fully in Chapter Five. Suffice it to say at this stage that media coverage ensures that health issues remain a public concern and attract the attention of politicians.

Box 2.1: Health policies, parties and elections 1992-2005

Klein (2001) observed, that although the NHS has long been a prominent political issue, its emergence as an election issue is a more recent phenomenon. The turning point appears to have been the 1987 General Election where surveys of voters indicated that the NHS was the Conservatives' weakest issue but Labour's strongest. Labour focused heavily on health in this campaign, featuring cases of patients facing long delays for treatment. The Conservatives defended their record with statistics on NHS spending, increased levels of treatment and numbers of staff, and evidence of falling waiting-lists for operations. They also tried to accuse Labour of hypocrisy by identifying examples where senior party members or their relatives had used private health care.

At the 1992 General Election, health was again a key issue. Labour criticised the Conservative government for introducing a 'two-tier' system of health care and inappropriate commercial values into the NHS. During the campaign, a major row was sparked by a Labour political broadcast that portrayed the contrasting fate of two girls requiring the same ear operation. The first child was able to have the operation privately, the other remained on an NHS waiting-list. The resulting furore – which became known as the 'War of Jennifer's Ear' – initially put pressure on the Conservative government. However, ministers accused Labour of exploiting children and leaking the identity of the girl portrayed in the broadcast and her family. This was strenuously denied by Labour, but as the facts of the case were now in dispute, the government was able to sidestep the issue.

In 1997, health was a major issue in the General Election campaign. Labour campaigned strongly on the NHS, culminating in Tony Blair's declaration on the eve of the election that 'the very simple choice that people have in the next 24 hours is this. It is 24 hours to save our National Health Service' (www.labour-watch.com/health.htm). The strong public support for Labour's policies on the NHS was regarded as an important factor in the party's election victory.

Health was also a prominent issue at the 2001 election. Controversy surrounded the Labour Party's policy of increasing private provision of NHS services in the form of independent treatment centres, which indicated a shift towards Conservative policies rather than a division between the two parties. One tense moment for Labour campaigners occurred when Tony Blair, while visiting a Birmingham hospital, was ambushed by a woman who challenged him about the cancer care received by her partner (Rawnsley, 2001, pp 488-9). But the incident passed with no visible impact on the polls. An interesting twist, however, was the election of an independent MP, Dr Richard Taylor, who was elected on the basis of his opposition to plans to close down services at Kidderminster General Hospital.

Taylor was re-elected in 2005, where health was once again prominent. The main issues highlighted in this campaign were hospital cleanliness, NHS bureaucracy, the role of the private sector and the distorting effect of government targets. For the time being Labour retained its lead over the Conservatives as the public's favourite party to run the NHS. But, as public concerns about the NHS continued, this support could no longer be taken for granted.

Another reason why health has been a key issue in party politics is that it is the subject of ideological conflict between the two main political parties. The creation of the NHS fitted neatly with the Labour Party's traditional support for collective responses to social problems, but was at odds with the Conservative Party's traditional values of individual responsibility, private enterprise and market forces (see ***Box 1.1***). Although the Conservatives subsequently accepted the NHS, they continued to explore ways of increasing individual responsibility and curbing the rising costs of health care expenditure on the service. The 1970s brought conflict over pay beds and public expenditure, while attempts to privatise parts of the NHS and introduce market forces in the 1980s and 1990s exposed further ideological divisions between the parties. The differences have become less clear in recent years as Labour has endorsed individualist, market-based and private sector-oriented reforms. Nonetheless, the rhetorical elements of ideological debate remain strong. These trends will now be explored more closely.

Party politics and health policy

The creation of the NHS

By 1945 there was a broad consensus about the need for a comprehensive health service (Webster, 1988; Klein, 1995; Powell, 1997). This emerged out of dissatisfaction with the fragmented and inequitable health services of the inter-war period, the deliberations of the wartime coalition government about social reconstruction, and the experience of emergency health service planning. Following the collapse of the coalition and Labour's victory at the ensuing General Election, there was considerable scope for division. As Klein (1995, p 15) put it, 'the way was open for the politics of ideology to take over from the politics of compromise'.

The Conservative Party election manifesto of 1945 proposed 'a comprehensive health service covering the whole range of medical treatment from the general practitioner to the specialist ...' and that 'no one will be denied the attention, the treatment, or the appliances he requires because he cannot afford them' (Craig, 1975, p 118). Although recognising the role of the state, the Conservatives emphasised the importance of choice and individual enterprise. They wished to retain the voluntary hospital sector, working 'in friendly partnership with local authority hospitals'. Labour, on the other hand, was committed to public ownership of health service facilities – in 1945 its Party Conference declared an immediate takeover of voluntary hospitals (Webster, 1988, p 82). However, in its manifesto, there was little detail beyond a declaration that 'the best health services should be available to all' and that 'money must no longer be the passport to the best treatment' (Craig, 1975, p 129).

Once in office, and with the appointment of Aneurin Bevan as Minister of Health, Labour's plans developed in an unexpected way. Despite support within the party for a local government-run health service, Bevan decided to bring both voluntary and local authority hospitals into a nationalised health service. Local authorities remained responsible for administering community health services and public health functions, while separate bodies (Executive Councils) were established to administer the NHS contracts of general practitioners and other family practitioners.

The Conservative Party was fiercely critical of the government's proposals and opposed the legislation. Conservative MPs took the unconventional step of seeking to reject the government's NHS Bill at its Third Reading in the House of Commons (Foot, 1975, pp 155-6). The Conservatives were hostile to hospital nationalisation but the Labour government's large majority in the House of Commons (of 146) meant that it could achieve its legislative aims with relative ease. Only a number of minor concessions were given during the passage of the Bill. Further concessions were granted after the legislation had been passed in order to secure the cooperation of GPs with the new service (see Webster, 1988).

The partisan debates that surrounded the creation of the NHS were somewhat misleading, however. They reflected the restoration of peacetime adversarial politics and gave the parties an opportunity to attack each other. In reality, the creation of the NHS was more the product of a continuing and developing consensus rather than the clash of party ideologies. As Klein (1995, p 29) observed, 'the rhetoric of battle in the years between 1946 and 1948 served largely to conceal ... the very considerable degree of continuity and compromise involved in the creation of the NHS'.

It was intended that the new NHS would be free at the point of use. The Labour government did not want people to be discouraged from using the service because of inability to pay. However, the cost of the service was higher than expected and this created pressures for greater economy. In 1951, after narrowly winning a General Election in the previous year, the Labour government backed plans to introduce charges for prescriptions, as well as for dental and ophthalmic services. This caused internal conflict and led to the resignation of Bevan (who had by now moved to another department) and two junior ministers (including the future Prime Minister, Harold Wilson).

Later in that year, yet another General Election was called and the Conservative Party emerged victorious. Given that the creation of the NHS was seen as the post-war Labour government's 'most intrinsically socialist proposition' (Foot, 1975, p 104), one might expect it to have been a target for the incoming government. However, there was little overt threat. Although the 1951 Conservative manifesto barely mentioned health, the version prepared for the previous year's General Election pledged the party 'to maintain and improve the health service' (Craig, 1975, p 148).

The consensus years?

The NHS had become an issue on which there was much cross-party agreement. The Conservative minister Iain Macleod, writing in 1958, claimed that with the exception of charges, health was 'out of party politics' (quoted in Klein, 1995, p 29). However, the consensus was, at times, fragile. Soon after taking office the Conservative government established a review of the NHS, widely seen as an attempt to curb expenditure and restrict the scope of the service. This backfired when the report identified a shortfall in funding and strengthened the case for the NHS to continue in its present form (Cmd 9663, 1956). As Rivett (1998, p 114) observed, henceforth 'it became impossible for governments to attack the NHS'. Even so, later in the decade, the Conservative government considered proposals that could have undermined the consensus (Webster, 1988, 1996). These included extending charges to cover boarding costs for inpatients (a proposal later explored by Labour), scrapping free NHS dental services and imposing fees for GP consultations. Alternative ways of funding the NHS, through a compulsory insurance scheme, were also explored. During the Conservatives' long period in office between 1951-64, the NHS was not generously funded. Webster (1996) noted that as a result the health service did not develop the range and quality of services envisaged by its creators, but added that this should not be attributed to a partisan approach on the part of the government. Economic circumstances would have constrained a Labour government in a similar way.

The Conservatives' more radical plans to reform the NHS never materialised, however. There were two main reasons. First, the level of public support for the NHS kept ideological tendencies in check. The Conservatives were reluctant to introduce reforms that might be interpreted by the public as reducing entitlement to health services (Lowe, 1993). To have done so might have given the Labour Party an opportunity to win electoral support. Even fairly minor proposals, such as small increases in prescription charges, were highly sensitive. Indeed when Enoch Powell, as Conservative health minister during the early 1960s, decided to raise charges and cut some services, he faced fierce public criticism, giving the Labour opposition much political ammunition. According to Webster (1996, p 88), 'Powell handed to Labour a much needed opportunity to improve its performance as an opposition and regain its credibility as a party of government'.

The second reason why the Conservatives did little to disturb the consensus on the NHS was that many of its leading MPs in this period subscribed to 'One Nation' Conservatism. This emphasised the protection of the weak and vulnerable in society and stressed the importance of civic values and social responsibility (see ***Box 1.1***). In the 1950s many of the new Conservative MPs entering Parliament held these views (Webster, 1988, p 187). This affected the character of the Conservative Party in Parliament and provided some protection against any serious threat to the NHS.

The 1960s and 1970s: the reorganisation of the NHS and pay beds

The party political consensus surrounding the NHS was further revealed by the reorganisation of the service in 1974 (see Chapter Seven). Notably, party ideology had a marginal role in the development of proposals, first under a Labour government, in the late 1960s, and then under the Conservatives (Klein, 1995). Indeed, the most serious divisions were within rather than between the parties (Webster, 1996). For example, there was acrimony between the author of Labour's initial proposals on reorganisation (Ministry of Health, 1968), Kenneth Robinson, and his successor, Richard Crossman, who developed plans of his own (DHSS, 1970). Subsequently, under the Conservatives, Keith Joseph's reorganisation plans drew criticism from his Cabinet colleagues. Although the parliamentary debates on the NHS reorganisation Bill were characterised by adversarial rhetoric (Ingle and Tether, 1981), the posturing of the parties had little impact on the eventual outcome.

The 1974 NHS reorganisation was the high point of the post-war consensus. The years that followed brought more conflict and increasingly the rhetoric was matched by real policy differences. Starr and Immergut (1987, p 241) observed that, 'for decades, Labour and the Conservatives had moved closer together; now they moved farther apart, as each party went back to first principles'. The first signs emerged in the mid-1970s in the form of the pay beds controversy (see Klein, 1995; Webster, 1996) The Labour government had a manifesto commitment to phase out pay beds from the NHS. The existence of pay beds was opposed by the left of the Labour Party for corrupting the principle of treatment on the basis of need. Labour was seeking to attack, in the words of Klein (1995, p 109) 'the visible symbols of privilege'.

The medical profession sensed a broader threat to private practice and remained unconvinced by assurances from the minister responsible for the NHS, Barbara Castle, that she did not intend to outlaw private treatment altogether. Doctors' fears were confirmed by a Labour Party Conference vote to abolish private medicine. The profession protested and threatened industrial action. Meanwhile, fearful that the government would back down, trade unions representing ancillary workers took direct action, withdrawing services from some private wards. The government moved to placate the doctors, while seeking to reassure the trade unions and the left wing of the Labour Party. A compromise was reached that involved phasing out pay beds, a policy reversed subsequently by the incoming Conservative government.

According to Klein, the NHS emerged from the pay beds conflict 'battered and frayed, but still basically intact' (1995, p 112). In his view, the conflict was constrained by the underlying consensus. This consensus survived further challenges in the late 1970s, in the form of an economic crisis, public expenditure constraints and further industrial action. However, in the following decade, it faced a more severe test, with the election of a Conservative government whose ideology challenged the principles of the post-war welfare state upon which the NHS was based.

Thatcherism

The Thatcher government, elected in 1979, was strongly influenced by the philosophy of neo-liberalism. Neo-liberalism consisted of ideas drawn from liberal economists (such as Friedman, 1962; Olson, 1965) and libertarian political scientists and philosophers (such as Nozick, 1974; Hayek, 1976). Its adherents called for a much smaller state bureaucracy and less government intervention, a reduction in the power of organised labour, a bigger role for the private sector and market forces in the allocation of resources, greater individual responsibility and choice, more voluntary effort and self-reliance among individuals (Green, 1987). However, the 'new right' approach of the Thatcher government was not purely neo-liberal but involved a compromise with traditional conservative values such as strong government, hierarchy, maintenance of social order and paternalism, which created ideological tensions within the government itself (see Gamble, 1994).

Under Thatcher, the post-war settlement began to unravel. Industries such as gas, telecommunications and electricity were privatised and there was deregulation of industry and commerce. Meanwhile, in the welfare state, social security entitlements were cut and the long-standing commitment to full employment was dropped. Public services faced financial restraint in the light of the Thatcher government's aim to reduce public expenditure and taxes. The NHS could not escape these powerful trends. The Thatcher government encouraged private medicine (introducing tax relief for low-paid employees and elderly persons), introduced private sector management ideas into the NHS, allowed private companies to tender for NHS support services such as laundry, catering and cleaning and extended and increased charges for prescriptions and other NHS services.

However, compared with what happened to the nationalised industries and other areas of the welfare state, notably housing and social security, the impact of neo-liberal ideas on health policy was actually quite minimal. Thatcher (1993, p 606) herself declared that although she wanted to see a flourishing private sector of health, the NHS and its basic principles was always a 'fixed point' in her policies. It is certainly true that Thatcher, although more ideological than her post-war predecessors, was an astute politician. She realised that health policy raised sensitive political issues that could lose votes. Her instinct was to increase the use of private health insurance, particularly for the better-off (Ham, 2000, p 9), but she recognised that the NHS was popular and that the public needed reassurance. Indeed, early in Thatcher's premiership, a leaked report from a government think tank had outlined the scope for the privatisation of welfare, forcing the Prime Minister to declare that 'the NHS is safe with us' (Thatcher, 1982).

Public support for the NHS remained strong during the 1980s and this reduced the Thatcher government's room for manoeuvre (Fowler, 1991). But following a third electoral victory in 1987, Thatcher introduced her internal market reforms, a radical attempt to change health care in the UK. NHS bodies would in future become either purchasers or providers of specified health services. GPs would be given their own budgets to purchase care, while hospitals would be given a new self-governing status as NHS trusts. Resources would be allocated on the basis of contracts negotiated between purchasers and providers. In theory, hospitals that failed to derive sufficient income through contracts would go out of business. But this market ideal never fully materialised. Even before her resignation in 1990, Thatcher was apparently concerned about the impact of the internal market and had considered postponing implementation until after the next General Election (Timmins, 1995).

The Major government

Thatcher's successor, John Major, was regarded as a more genuine supporter of the NHS. In his first party conference speech after becoming Conservative Party leader, he reiterated his commitment to the NHS and ruled out further health service charges and privatisation of health care. Nonetheless, his government was still 'right wing' by post-war standards. It continued to implement Thatcher's legacy, the internal market, though in a much more regulated way than its original architects envisaged. The Major government also endorsed a greater role for the private sector in the NHS capital programme by extending its private finance initiative (PFI) to hospitals (see Chapter Seven). Although this did not necessarily lead to the privatisation of health care, it gave the private sector further opportunities to profit from the NHS. The Major government also extended competitive tendering to a wider range of NHS support services.

Major did not share the same ideological stance as Thatcher and was highly pragmatic. Although privatisation of support services and marketisation of the NHS continued under his stewardship, the expansion of private health care stalled (partly due to a prolonged economic recession). Major's pragmatism was also reinforced by political circumstances. The reformed Labour Party became more of an electoral threat. Moreover, after the 1992 General Election, Major's majority in Parliament was significantly reduced. As the 1992 Parliament went on, even this was eroded by by-election defeats and backbench rebellions.

The Major government also introduced *The Patient's Charter* (DoH, 1991). This represented an attempt to set out, albeit in a superficial way, what service users might expect from the NHS. It subsequently developed into a means of gauging the performance of health service providers. The idea of a patient's charter was promoted by other parties (Labour Party, 1990; Liberal Democrats, 1992). The opposition parties also called for a national health strategy, with clear health targets, something that the Thatcher government had resisted. This was subsequently introduced by the Major government in the form of the *Health of the Nation* strategy (Cm 1523, 1991; Cm 1986, 1992). Opposition parties, while welcoming the strategy, criticised its weakness on smoking and alcohol misuse and for ignoring health inequalities. These examples illustrate that the Major government was pragmatic enough to adapt policies advanced by its political opponents, while modifying them to be compatible with its own ideological stance. It was also careful not to foster excessive expectations. So while these policies were important symbolically in reassuring the public that the Conservative government cared about the NHS and the people's health, they were actually quite limited.

New Labour

After 1979, the Labour Party shifted further to the left, reflected in its 1983 election manifesto, which called for further nationalisation, state control of industry, withdrawal from the European Community, nuclear disarmament, and increased spending on welfare and public sector projects. With regard to health, it reiterated commitments to phase out charges and remove private practice from the NHS. But these were accompanied by more radical aims, to take a major public stake in the drugs industry, and to take over parts of the private health sector and prevent its expansion.

Labour's defeat at the 1983 and 1987 General Elections forced a rethink.

Under the leadership of Neil Kinnock (1983-92) and John Smith (1992-4), organisational changes were made to strengthen the party leadership's control of the policy process, accompanied by reviews of policy. Policy became less rooted in ideological considerations and more pragmatic, reflecting the party's desperate desire to win elections and gain office (Hughes and Wintour, 1990; Jones, 1995). This process was continued by Tony Blair, following Smith's sudden death in 1994. Blair rebranded the party as 'New Labour' and moderated its socialist principles. Notably, he secured amendment of the symbolic Clause Four of the Labour Party constitution, which had committed it to wholesale state ownership, replacing it with a general statement about the importance of the community, equity and social justice. Blair also further strengthened the leader's grip on the party's policy process (Webb, 2000).

In seeking to justify these changes, Blair appealed primarily to the overriding imperative to gain office. But ideas also played a part. Blair drew on communitarianism – which emphasises the importance of balancing community values with individual responsibilities (see Etzioni, 1993; Atkinson, 1994; Tam, 1998). Communitarianism is a rather imprecise philosophy and well-suited to those adopting a pragmatic approach. According to Driver and Martell (2002) there are several different types of communitarianism. They argue that New Labour's particular approach has promoted conservative values, is focused on individuals, is prescriptive and places emphasis on responsibilities as a condition for having rights.

A further key aspect of Blair's philosophy was the so-called Third Way (Giddens, 1998; Finlayson, 1999; Driver and Martell, 2002). The essence of the Third Way is a set of governing principles that are neither the property of socialism nor neo-liberalism, but incorporate elements of both. The Third Way endorses an inclusive and fair society with equality of opportunity, reflecting socialist principles. But it also incorporates neo-liberal ideas by encouraging the use of markets and the private sector. It also echoes neo-liberal values by highlighting the importance of individualism and the entrepreneurial role of the modern state in seeking solutions to social and economic problems. The state is seen as requiring modernisation to make it fit for purpose, which includes a pragmatic approach ('what counts is what works' in Blair's own phrase) and the break-up of traditional state bureaucracies. The goal is to 'modernise' state institutions and create new partnerships (with the private and voluntary sectors) that respond more effectively to the needs and preferences of the public.

These changes in party leadership, organisation and direction had ramifications for the Labour Party's policies on health. By 1987, it had already retreated from the most contentious statements contained in its previous manifesto. Subsequently, a new health strategy emerged in the form of *A Fresh Start for Health* (Labour Party, 1990), later developed as *Your Good Health: A*

White Paper for a Labour Government prior to the 1992 General Election (Labour Party, 1992). The Conservatives' internal market was heavily criticised in both documents and Labour pledged to abolish it, proposing that the newly created NHS provider trusts would be brought back under local NHS control and that the purchasing of services by 'fund-holding' GPs would end. However, there were signs that Labour was beginning to accept some aspects of government policy. Changes were proposed to the allocation of resources within the NHS to create incentives for providers that performed well and increased patient choice. The Labour Party was cautious about making spending commitments on the NHS and earlier pledges to phase out health service charges were not reiterated.

A further policy review in the mid-1990s reflected a growing acceptance of the Conservatives' reforms. In 1994, the Labour Party published *Health 2000*, a discussion document on health reform, followed in 1995 by *Renewing the NHS*, which stated that 'it is neither possible nor desirable to turn the clock back ... We do not intend to replace one dogmatic approach with another' (p 3). Labour had by now agreed to retain the division between purchasers and providers of health care established by the Conservatives. NHS trusts would be retained, but GP fund-holding would be replaced by a system of commissioning for all GPs. The existing contracts for health care established between purchasers and providers would be replaced by longer-term and more comprehensive health care agreements. However, hostility to the private sector remained. Labour was committed to abolishing tax relief for elderly people with private health insurance, for example. *Renewing the NHS* was seen by observers as a further retreat from ideology. Klein (1995, p 75), for example, saw it as 'a remarkably skilful document. It signals a retreat from dogmatism and an acceptance of the need for a pragmatic policy under a smokescreen of ideological rhetoric'.

The Labour government's 179-seat majority in Parliament in 1997, followed by a majority of 167 in 2001, certainly gave it both the legitimacy and ability to effect policy change. However, it would have been difficult to reverse 18 years of Conservative reform, even if the incoming government had wished to do this. During the period 1997-2000, the Blair government set about implementing its manifesto commitments on health, including a key pledge to reduce waiting-lists by 100,000 during the lifetime of the Parliament (Cm 3807, 1997). The internal market was reformed rather than dismantled. GP fund-holding was abolished and replaced by local primary care commissioning groups. The Labour government fulfilled its commitment to get rid of health insurance tax breaks for the elderly. This contrasted with its decision to expand the role of public–private partnerships (PPPs) in the financing, building and running of hospitals through PFI schemes (Ruane, 2000; Shaw, 2004). The Labour government adhered to the previous governments' spending plans

(Toynbee and Walker, 2001). This restricted health spending in the early years of the Blair government, probably by more so than if the Conservatives had been returned to office. In the event, financial pressures led to the allocation of further resources from contingency funds and subsequently to a review of health spending, an unprecedented expansion of resources for the NHS and a new blueprint for its future, in the form of the NHS Plan (see ***Box 3.3***).

During the 1980s and early 1990s, the Labour Party had been very critical of the Conservative government's record on public health and inequalities. It began to develop an alternative health strategy, which went further than the Major government's *Health of the Nation* strategy. Labour acknowledged the problem of health inequalities and proposed a range of social and economic interventions, including improved social security benefits and the building of more council houses. It also went further in proposing regulation to improve public health, including an independent Food Standards Agency, a ban on tobacco advertising, and random breath testing to deter drinking and driving. The public health agenda therefore represented an important battlefront between the two main parties. Once in office, the Blair government introduced a review of health inequalities (*Independent Inquiry into Inequalities in Health*, 1998) and a new White Paper on public health (Cm 4386, 1999), and appointed a minister for public health. It promised to ban tobacco advertisements (which after delays and controversy over exemptions was eventually introduced in 2003) and established an independent Food Standards Agency. The NHS was urged to give priority to public health and inequalities. Special health action zones were established, to coordinate efforts from a range of agencies in areas of high need. The government was prepared to use social and economic interventions to combat poverty (including a long-term commitment to abolish child poverty) and introduced new programmes aimed at reducing unemployment and regenerating economically deprived areas.

A further key aspect of health policy identified by the Blair government was health service quality. In opposition the Labour Party had expressed a desire to improve the regulation and monitoring of care. For example, in *A Fresh Start for Health* (Labour Party, 1990), a Quality Commission was proposed. By late 1997, this had developed into a proposal for a National Quality Audit Team (Smith, 1997). Labour did not have a monopoly of concern about service quality. Previously, the Conservatives had pursued a quality improvement agenda, through *The Patient's Charter*, performance indicators and league tables and by emphasising the value of quality assurance techniques imported from the business sector. Labour proposed a raft of new national bodies to set and monitor standards of health and social care (see Chapter Seven). In addition, new national service frameworks were introduced setting out standards and models of care for particular condition areas (coronary heart disease, diabetes) or patient/user groups (children, older people). Labour also introduced a new quality assurance system into the NHS – clinical governance – aimed at making NHS service providers more responsible for improving the quality of care provided.

In the period up to 2000, Labour Party policy closely reflected the proposals it developed in opposition. But following the review of the NHS initiated by the Prime Minister, government policy began to depart from this base in two main ways (see, for example, Baggott, 2004; Greener, 2004c). First, the government identified a greater role for the private sector in the NHS. PPPs were further extended through PFI and a new scheme for primary health care (see Chapter Eight). A concordat was agreed with the independent health care sector aimed at bringing about greater collaboration between this sector and the NHS. The sector was offered an opportunity to run 'failing' NHS services. A further opening was provided by the announcement of fast-track diagnostic and treatment centres. Although most were initially run by the NHS, they were supplemented by independent treatment centres run by private operators.

A second area of policy change was a new system of resource allocation in the NHS. Although retaining the division between purchaser and provider introduced by the Conservatives, Labour was committed 'to restore the NHS as a public service working cooperatively for patients, not a commercial business driven by competition' (Labour Party, 1997). However, it then decided to introduce 'payment by results' where health service providers would be paid on the basis of work done. This differed in detail from the Conservatives' internal market but nonetheless represented a shift back towards competition and the use of market forces. This was combined with policies to extend patient choice over where they would be treated. Meanwhile, foundation trusts were created, ostensibly to give providers more freedom to respond to market forces and patient choice. A further change occurred on the issue of budget holding by GPs. Initially, the Labour government replaced fund-holding with commissioning bodies constituted from all GP practices in a geographical area. Subsequently, it was decided to shift some responsibility for commissioning back to practices. In 2004, the Labour government declared its intention to implement 'practice-based commissioning' across the NHS. This was not exactly the same as GP fund-holding, but could produce similar inequalities as those attributed to the fund-holding scheme, where some practices benefited more than others.

The Blair government, although a Labour government, has not been afraid to adopt policy ideas from the right, despite, in the words of one interviewee from a professional organisation (see ***Box 1.2***), these policies being 'opposed by many Labour members, supporters and activists'. It was able to do this, largely because of the power of the party leadership over policy (Campbell and Zeichner, 2001; Hain, 2004). Meanwhile, at the time of writing, the Conservative Party is re-thinking its policies. Since 2005 it has committed to tax-based funding for the NHS and dropped proposals to supplement private health care spending. In some respects the stances of the two main parties on health policy have converged (see ***Box 2.2***), but there is still considerable divergence according to some commentators.

Box 2.2: Interviewees' comments on party politics

'There are still important differences between the parties' (peer)

'The two main parties are still very different in their health policies' (MP)

'Parties do matter. It makes a difference who's in power' (trade unionist)

'There is apparent convergence, but also important underlying differences' (former DoH civil servant)

'In England the gap between the parties has closed ... but there are still important differences' (voluntary organisation spokesperson)

'Parties do matter, even when policies converge. It is the interplay between the parties that is important' (former senior NHS manager)

'While there has been convergence between the two main parties on the supply side, differences in funding have if anything widened ... even if differences narrow, the dynamics of political debate between party platforms, especially at election time, means that you cannot ignore them' (policy adviser)

'Differences between the parties are not great' (spokesperson, think tank)

'The two main political parties have converged on policy. Labour has moved to the right but Conservatives may well move further to the right in future by championing social insurance and privatisation' (spokesperson, NHS management organisation)

'Parties do not matter as much as they used to' (MP)

'No one says anything terribly different. There is no huge philosophical debate.' (spokesperson, professional organisation)

'Do parties make a difference in health policy? Not a lot!' (former senior NHS manager)

Source: see **Box 1.2**

Conclusion

Parties are important vehicles of change in health policy. They play a crucial role in setting the terms of political debate and in shaping the policy agenda. Party ideologies can lead them to adopt certain policies, which can then become government policies if they gain office. In this sense they are important 'battering rams of change' as described by Crossman (see Chapter One).

However, the link between party ideology and government policy is not straightforward. For a start, party ideologies have themselves been subject to wider influences over the years, notably with regard to the permeation of neo-liberal ideas across the board. Furthermore, party policies are influenced by a range of other considerations, primarily the need to win elections, which may over-ride their ideological principles. Ideological factors may be thwarted by political and technical constraints of implementation, for example. Policy learning may also be relevant, as governments discard ideological party policies that are ineffective or impractical, and choose more pragmatic approaches. There is also a certain amount of 'path-dependency' in health, with governments retaining elements of their predecessors' policies, which limits the impact of party ideology. Governing parties may find themselves adopting policies introduced by their predecessors, or may borrow policy ideas from their rivals in order to address a policy problem. This is consistent with the moving consensus model of Rose (see Chapter One), which suggests greater policy continuity between governments irrespective of which party holds office.

Not only is there considerable continuity between governments of a different party political complexion, there is evidence of substantial policy changes under governments of the same party. This does not seem to fit well with either Rose's or Crossman's model, and is perhaps better explained by changing political circumstances (that is, where new problems arise or become more significant), electoral competition (where the party in office has to modify its policy because it fears losing votes) or internal party conflict (on either ideological or pragmatic grounds).

Summary

- Health is an important issue in party politics.
- There are significant political and technical constraints facing parties when in office, which limit their influence.
- Although parties can act as battering rams of change, there is evidence of a moving consensus in health policy.
- There is substantial evidence of policy change under governments of the same party.

Key questions

1. What are the main differences in health policy between the Conservative and Labour Parties today?
2. Have these differences stayed the same, narrowed or widened in recent years?
3. Why has health been a prominent issue in recent General Elections?
4. Can you give examples of where a political party has borrowed or adapted policies of its opponents?

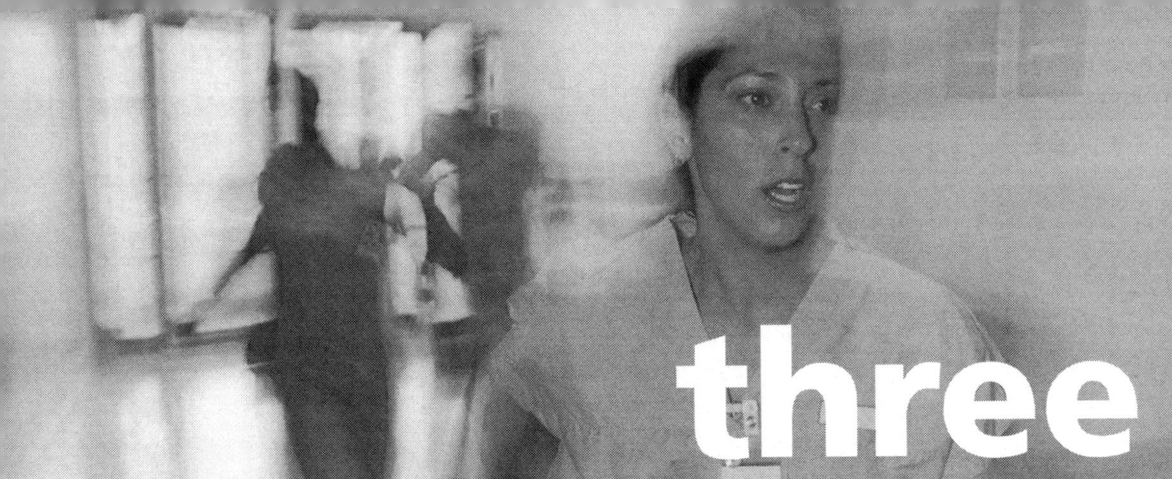

Central government and health policy

Overview

This chapter examines the role of central government institutions in health policy. It begins by looking at the functions, organisation and culture of the Department of Health (DoH). It examines the roles and responsibilities of ministers, civil servants and advisers within the department. The chapter also considers health and health-related responsibilities across government and examines how these are led and coordinated. In this context, the involvement of the Treasury and the Prime Minister's Office in health policy is explored. Finally, the chapter examines the interface between central government institutions and external organisations and experts in the formation and implementation of policy.

Central government (or 'the Executive') comprises government departments and agencies as well as the core institutions, the Treasury, the Cabinet Office and the Prime Minister's Office. Many of these organisations have an interest in health policy (see ***Box 3.1***). Nonetheless, the best place to begin is with the government department with overall responsibility for health and the NHS, the Department of Health (DoH).

The Department of Health

The history of the department

The Ministry of Health was created in 1919 (Gilbert, 1970; Honigsbaum, 1970). Its function, as laid down in the Ministry of Health Act, was 'to take all steps as may be desirable to secure the preparation, effective carrying out and coordination of measures conducive to the health of the people'. It should be noted that before the creation of the NHS, the new ministry did not have responsibility for securing the provision of comprehensive health services. Some services lay outside its remit, including school health services, which remained with the Board (and later the Ministry) of Education for another half century. However, the Ministry of Health did have important public health responsibilities, including environmental health, housing, water supply and sanitation.

The Ministry of Health acquired responsibility for the NHS, following its creation. But it lost control of important public health responsibilities when local government was ceded to the newly created Ministry of Housing and Local Government in 1951. According to Webster (1996), this 'adversely affected morale within the department' (p 4). It also focused the ministry's attention on health services, and in particular the hospital service, to the detriment of public and community health. The loss of functions also had an impact on the status of the Ministry of Health within government. Its senior minister was not guaranteed Cabinet rank, and between 1945 and 1970, this post was more often than not outside the Cabinet. As Webster (1996) observed, this had serious implications. Decisions affecting health were taken in the absence of its senior advocate. This compounded the ministry's lack of leverage in negotiating with powerful external interests and other departments of state, notably the Treasury. Furthermore, the Ministry of Health was regarded as a rather cautious, reactive and essentially non-interventionist department (Klein, 1995; Mohan, 1995; Webster, 1996), although it later adopted a more proactive stance, drawing up national plans for hospitals and community health services (see Chapter Seven).

The creation of the Department of Health and Social Security (DHSS) in 1968, from a merger between the Ministry of Health and the Ministry of Social Security, effectively guaranteed Cabinet status for its senior minister (the Secretary of State for Social Services). This was a big department employing large numbers of civil servants and deploying huge resources. It was responsible for a range of politically sensitive social welfare issues, including the NHS. The departments of health and social security were subsequently demerged in 1988, but by this time the health portfolio had expanded. Ever since, the post of Secretary of State for Health has been a Cabinet-level appointment.

Under the Blair government the status of the DoH has grown. Interviewees (see ***Box 1.2***) commented that the DoH was seen as exemplary in the way it embraced Blair's modernisation agenda. For example, a respondent from a health professional organisation observed that 'The DoH is regarded as a flagship or beacon within Whitehall in its efforts to slim down and rationalise'. A policy adviser similarly noted that 'The DoH has been on the rise. It has been reasonably well regarded because it has delivered on more areas than other departments.' A former DoH civil servant commented that the department '… is highly regarded by politicians in the government. They see the DoH as at the cutting edge of public services reform.' Subsequently, however, the reputation of the department was tarnished by a mounting financial crisis in the NHS, which led to the resignation of the permanent secretary of the department, Sir Nigel Crisp, in 2006.

The current responsibilities of the DoH can be summarised as follows. It is the principal government department for UK-wide health matters, and represents the UK government in international and European fora. The department is responsible for coordinating policy and action on matters affecting UK health as a whole, such as infectious diseases or biological threats. Otherwise, its remit is confined to England, where it supports ministers in fulfilling their statutory duties to improve the health and well-being of the people, to secure provision of high-quality health and social care, and to promote medical research. In other parts of the UK, other authorities are responsible for health and health care – the Welsh Assembly Government, the Scottish Executive Health Department and the Northern Ireland Department of Health, Social Services and Public Safety.

The internal politics of the Department of Health

As Ham (2004) observed, the DoH is not a monolith. It contains different personnel and cultures. Differences also arise from the internal structuring of work within the department. As one interviewee, from a professional organisation, put it 'there are competing ecosystems within the Department'. The Secretary of State for Health, as the most senior politician in the department, is formally accountable to Parliament for its activities. In theory, ministerial responsibility is extensive and reflects the principle, encapsulated in Bevan's phrase that 'when a bedpan is dropped on a hospital floor its noise should resound in the Palace of Westminster' (cited in Nairne, 1984). In practice, however, such comprehensive responsibility has long been regarded as a constitutional fiction (Cmnd 7615, 1979). Moreover, successive governments have attempted to devolve operational responsibility to NHS bodies (see Chapter Seven).

Nonetheless, ministers must answer parliamentary questions, carry legislation through Parliament, respond to debates and give evidence to select committees (see Chapter Four). The Secretary of State issues strategic statements and operational guidance on health and social care policy. As the department's policy must be consistent with the government's overall policies, the Secretary of State must engage in discussions with other ministers. He or she will also seek to ensure that the department's view is reflected in wider policy debates and strive to secure resources and powers needed to achieve policy objectives. This involves being a member of Cabinet committees and informal policy working groups. It also requires effective working relationships with the Treasury, the Cabinet Office and the Prime Minister's Office. The Secretary of State is also the public face of the department, appearing in the media, promoting the department's agenda and responding to issues of public concern.

The department's statutory powers are vested in the office of Secretary of State. In practice, however, the complexity of modern policy making means that there is considerable delegation, to junior ministers, policy advisers and civil servants. In addition, specific functions have been 'hived off' to special agencies, accountable to the Secretary of State for Health, which are discussed further below.

The Secretary of State is assisted by junior ministers. At the time of writing, there are five: four MPs and a member of the House of Lords (who acts as the spokesman for the DoH in the Upper House). Each minister has specific responsibilities for areas of policy and services (such as public health or social care). In practice, much of the burden of government business falls on their shoulders. Junior ministers are active in the policy process, negotiating with outside organisations, piloting legislation though Parliament, and implementing policy changes. In some cases, this provides a useful apprenticeship for future Secretaries of State (Ham, 2000). Since the 1980s four Secretaries of State of Health (Kenneth Clarke, Virginia Bottomley and Stephen Dorrell (Conservative) and Alan Milburn (Labour)) previously served as junior ministers in the department.

The particular style of the Secretary of State can make a crucial difference to the department's approach to policy making (see Ham, 2000). Interviewees pointed out key differences between the four Health Secretaries holding office under the Blair government (see also Edwards and Fall, 2005). Frank Dobson, who held the health portfolio until 1999, was said to be a collegial and consensual policy maker who sought to establish a good working relationship with the health professional groups and who listened carefully to advice from civil servants. His successor, Alan Milburn, was described as a more driven character with clear objectives. It was said that he preferred to work with individual professionals who shared his vision rather than the professional groups as a whole. John Reid was described as a tough and uncompromising policy implementer who demonstrated little enthusiasm for the health brief. His successor, Patricia Hewitt, was described as a more emollient character, who was trying to build bridges with the professional organisations while attempting to set a new agenda that emphasised primary care and community-based models of care, although she had struggled to do so in the context of financial deficits and growing criticism of NHS privatisation.

Civil servants

Traditionally, senior civil servants have been able to influence policy by providing advice to ministers. Even middle-ranking civil servants have contributed to policy formation – by briefing their superiors on specific issues, liaising with outside interests and garnering expert advice (Johnstone, 1984; Miller, 1990; Baggott et al, 2005). Furthermore, civil servants' role in implementing decisions involves considerable discretion, enabling them to shape policies on the ground.

However, there is evidence that civil service influence over policy has diminished in recent years. Several interviewees, including former DoH civil servants and senior NHS managers, detected a decline in the traditional channels of civil service influence, a trend accentuated by the Blair government. Some observed a distrust of the traditional civil service based on suspicion of its principles of 'neutrality'. This was reflected in ministers deciding to look elsewhere for policy advice – to individual experts and special advisers (see also Dorey, 2005; Edwards and Fall, 2005, p 201; Sheard and Donaldson, 2006). Also, the performance of civil servants has been more closely monitored, reducing their discretion in the implementation process. Linked to this, a new breed of 'managerialist' civil servant has emerged, whose rise is discussed later.

Another trend identified has been the declining influence of DoH civil servants with a professional background, such as doctors, nurses and others who are professionally qualified in health or social care. The distinction between these health professionals and other civil servants is long standing and at one time was clearly reflected in the structure of the department. Formerly, professionals had their own divisions that were accountable to their professional head, and ultimately, the Chief Medical Officer (CMO). Professional staff would supply their expertise within a system of multidisciplinary units that brought together lay, professional and technical staff on specific areas of policy. This system has been superseded by a more integrated approach. Although these specialist civil servants remain 'professionally' accountable to their respective professional leader, they are now employed within a single structure.

Some observers believe that professional power has been diminished as a result, compounded by a weakening of the post of CMO within the department. The CMO (who also acts as the medical adviser for the government as a whole) has been seen as a check on the power of Secretaries of State for Health, and as an important source of policy influence (Edward and Fall, 2005; Sheard and Donaldson, 2006). CMOs have also acted as important 'go-betweens' in dealings between government and the medical profession (Ham, 2000). However, staff cuts, increased management responsibilities and internal restructuring seem to have undermined the CMO's traditional role and influence (BSE Inquiry, 2000; see also Sheard and Donaldson, 2006).

Under the Blair government, senior clinicians were brought in as national clinical directors (also known as 'czars') for priority areas such as cancer, heart disease, mental health, diabetes, older people, children, emergency services, and primary care (Cox, 2001; Burns, 2004). The incorporation of senior clinicians in this way has created new opportunities for professional influence over policy (see also Chapter Six). The czars have the ear of health ministers, and, in some cases, access to the Prime Minister. Interviewees certainly believed they were influential. One former civil servant, for example, described them as having 'enormous influence'. They are regarded as an important channel for medical influence and a target for other lobby groups, such as the drug industry and patients' groups. Some interviewees noted that the appointment of czars narrowed the channels of clinical influence, bypassing traditional forms of lobbying and expert advice. Several also suggested that czars could provide a useful scapegoat for ministers if policies ultimately proved unsuccessful. Elsewhere, others pointed out the risk that czars could become 'creatures of the civil service' and be drawn into defending government policy on political grounds (Burns, 2004).

Another development, already mentioned, has been the rise of 'managerialist' civil servants. Even before the Blair government came to office, Day and Klein (1997) found a degree of cultural change had occurred as a result of bringing NHS managers into the department. They distinguished between the traditional civil service approach – which emphasised risk avoidance and written communication, was process-oriented, collegial and minister-centred – and the managerialist approach – which emphasised risk taking, was NHS-centred, outcome-oriented, individual rather than collegial and emphasised verbal communication. The authors noted that interaction between these stereotypes, coupled with pressures towards managerialism within Whitehall, had tended to blur the boundaries leading, in their words, to a certain amount of 'cultural cross-dressing'.

Interviewees from within the policy process also acknowledged these changes. One former civil servant stated that 'the culture of the department has changed. The Oxbridge traditional civil servant has been replaced to a considerable extent by managerialists – "hands-on" people recruited into the civil service.' Another added that 'the DoH is now dominated by civil servants with an NHS background'. The result is a hybrid culture. Civil servants are more focused on performance management and delivery, and more accepting of business models. But at the same time elements of the traditional civil service ethos – in particular the over-riding goal of protecting ministers and the wider government from criticism – remains strong.

Special advisers

Special advisers are not a new phenomenon. Indeed both the DoH and its predecessor, the DHSS, employed special advisers in the past (Ham, 2004, pp 124-5). Even so, the numbers of special advisers has increased across government in recent years. They also appear to have exerted more influence over policy recently than in the past. Those interviewed for this study identified special advisers as key players in the policy process. They also commented on the crucial role of the Prime Minister's special adviser on health, considered in a later section of this chapter.

Several functions of special advisers have been identified. First, they provide and develop ideas for ministers. One interviewee, a peer, described them as 'brain power for ministers'. All interviewees identified special advisers as key figures of influence over policy (see also Edwards and Fall, 2005). One, from a health professional organisation, commented that the 'ideas that have driven health policy have come from special advisors'. Another, a former DoH civil servant, stated that 'special advisors are seriously influential', while an official from a national health charity described them as 'hugely influential'. However, some respondents noted that some advisers were more effective than others. A slight decline in their influence of late was detected by some. Also, the DoH advisers were generally seen as less influential than those advising the Prime Minister.

Advisers play an important part in defending government policy. One interviewee noted that they acted as a counterweight to ideas and arguments opposed to government policy coming from the media and Parliament: in short, 'they supply the counterarguments'. Some advisers act as 'spin doctors', influencing the media and the public perception of issues (see also Chapter Five). Special advisers are also central to the process of monitoring the implementation of policies within the department and in the NHS. They act as the eyes and ears of ministers and feed implementation problems back to them.

Advisers mediate between pressure groups and the department. They can be seen as a valuable political contact for lobbying organisations (Sheard and Donaldson, 2006). Indeed, one interviewee stated that 'Whenever we try to speak to a minister we would try to get to the special adviser first to prepare the ground or to try and find how they were likely to approach the subject'. Interviewees also noted that some special advisers were more accessible than others, and this reflected different ministerial styles (see above) and their willingness to work with outside interests.

The structure of the department

Following the Griffiths management report (see Chapter Seven) structural changes were undertaken in an effort to separate health policy from management (see Edwards and Fall, 2005). This led to the creation of a Health Services Supervisory Board (HSSB) and an NHS Management Board. In 1989 these bodies were replaced by a Policy Board and an NHS Management Executive, respectively. The latter, although officially still part of the DoH, was moved to Leeds. This physical separation of policy and management matters is now widely regarded as a mistake (Edwards and Fall, 2005). Indeed, as various authors have shown, NHS policy and management are intimately linked (Harrison et al, 1992; Day and Klein, 1997; Edwards and Fall, 2005). This was acknowledged by government when the by now renamed NHS Executive (NHSE) acquired policy-making functions in the mid-1990s (see Day and Klein, 1997). Subsequently, the Blair government showed little confidence in the NHSE and it was marginalised, particularly after the appointment of Alan Milburn as Secretary of State in 1999 (Edwards and Fall, 2005). In 2000, the posts of Permanent Secretary at the DoH and Chief Executive of the NHS were combined (only to be separated again in 2006) and the NHSE's functions reintegrated back into the main body of the DoH.

Another feature of restructuring has been the establishment of separate executive agencies to undertake areas of DoH work. These include the Medicines and Healthcare Products Regulatory Agency and the NHS Purchasing and Supply Agency. There are also a number of non-departmental public bodies in the health field, which have a degree of independence from the DoH, including regulatory bodies such as the Healthcare Commission and the Commission for Healthcare Regulatory Excellence (see Chapter Seven). In addition, special health authorities under the DoH have been established to manage specific areas of activity, such as prescriptions and blood transfusion. The National Institute for Health and Clinical Excellence (NICE), which gives guidance to the NHS on the cost-effectiveness of treatments, is also a special health authority. Taken together these various 'arm's-length' bodies employed 22,000 staff and had a combined annual budget of £2.5 billion in 2004. However, as part of a broader programme across government to cut bureaucracy, a process of rationalisation is now underway. This is expected to lead to a halving of their number, a 25% reduction in staffing and savings of £500m by 2008 (DoH, 2004a).

The establishment of separate agencies and authorities at national level was partly responsible for the substantial reduction in DoH staffing levels in recent years. Staff numbers also fell as a result of shifting responsibilities for strategy and operational matters to local NHS bodies, discussed further in Chapter Seven. The department was reorganised into three groups: a

Strategy and Business Development Group (dealing with strategy, corporate development communication and cross-cutting issues); a Health and Social Care Standards and Quality Group headed by the CMO (dealing with health protection, international health, research and development, quality standards, health improvement, care services and regional public health); and a Health and Social Care Delivery Group (dealing with issues such as access, finance, workforce, information systems and performance). At the time of writing, a further reorganisation of the department is being implemented, with new directorates in policy and strategy, finance, and commissioning and service development (see DoH, 2006c).

Other departments and the core executive

Although most health policy activity takes place within the DoH, key decisions affecting health and health care are also made by other departments and agencies (see ***Box 3.1***). In recent years there has been a redoubling of efforts to overcome what Butcher (1995, p 59) called the 'notorious departmentalism of Whitehall' and to promote 'joined-up approaches' to government. This has been a particularly strong theme of the Blair government's modernisation project (Newman, 2001), characterised by a concentration of power within the Prime Minister's Office, the Cabinet Office and the Treasury.

Box 3.1: Departmental responsibilities and health-related issues*

Department for Communities and Local Government (DCLG)
Environmental health, fire safety, housing, homelessness, community cohesion, diversity and equality, urban regeneration, planning, neighbourhood renewal, and regional and local government.

Department for Education and Skills (DfES)
Children, young people and families. School-based education for drugs, alcohol and smoking, sex education in schools, school sport, school health and safety, school transport, further and higher education (including college and university-based education of health workers and professionals, and research and innovation in universities).

Department for Work and Pensions (DWP)
Income support for people in poverty, unemployed people, people with disabilities and their informal carers. Rights and opportunities for disabled people. Workplace issues including health and safety.

Home Office
Community safety, policing, crime and disorder and community cohesion. Prisoners and offenders. The voluntary sector. Drugs strategy. (Note: prison health services, formerly a Home Office role, is now the responsibility of the NHS.)

Department for Culture, Media and Sport (DCMS)
The media (coverage of health issues and advertising of products harmful to health). The National Lottery and the Big Lottery Fund (funding of voluntary health projects and some NHS services). Regulation of alcohol sales and gambling. Promotion of arts and sport (with implications for health and well-being).

Department of Trade and Industry (DTI)
Sponsors many industries that have adverse implications for environmental health, such as chemicals, the motor industry and the energy industries. Policy on science and innovation (specific responsibility for the pharmaceutical and health care equipment industries, except electronic medical equipment, resides with the DoH). Consumer safety matters, including accidents in the home.

Department for Environment, Food and Rural Affairs (DEFRA)
The environment, sustainable development, farming, food and drink, rural affairs.

Department for Transport (DfT)
Transport safety and accidents. Transport policy and planning. Socially inclusive transport.

Ministry of Defence (MOD)
Health and safety of armed forces personnel. Funding and provision of health services for men and women serving in the armed forces via the Defence Medical and Dental Services. (Note: the MOD contracts with the NHS and other providers for supplementary and specialist health care and other services when necessary.)

HM Treasury
Public expenditure on health services. Other costs of ill health that fall on taxpayers (for example, unemployment, disability benefits). Taxation of alcohol, drink and other products and services that have implications for health.

*Note: some departmental functions are exercised through government agencies accountable to departments, such as the Food Standards Agency, the Health and Safety Commission, Sport England and the Arts Council.

Other government departments

The DoH and its precursors have had a mixed experience of interdepartmental relationships. At one end of the spectrum there has been mutual distrust and hostility. This was evident in the relationship between the department and the former Ministry of Agriculture, Fisheries and Food (MAFF) on issues of food safety (BSE Inquiry, 2000). The relationship between health and education departments has also been poor in the past, marked by disputes over health education in schools in the 1980s and prior to this, battles over school health services (Webster, 1996). It remains to be seen whether the increased emphasis on integrated services for children, the location of a designated Minister for Children in the DfES and the appointment of the DoH children's health czar as the Children's Commissioner will improve coordination between these departments. Relationships between health and social security departments have also been poor. Between 1968 and 1988 these functions were actually contained in the same department, the DHSS, with little improvement in cooperation on matters affecting the key client groups. Indeed, this was demonstrated by the lack of coordination between the social security arm of the department and the community health and social care divisions during the 1980s (Butcher, 1995).

Some interdepartmental relationships have worked well. For example, interdepartmental cooperation led to an action plan on accident prevention (DoH, 2002). In the late 1990s, government departments agreed a strategy for the prevention of drug abuse. Joint working across departments has also occurred on measures to reduce health inequalities (see ***Box 3.2***). More generally, there is good cooperation between departments on technical or low-profile issues, where interdepartment conflict tends to be low.

Coordinating policy

Disputes over policy are managed within the Cabinet system. The Cabinet itself is not a forum for extensive policy debate, except perhaps in times of crisis (James, 1992; Burch and Holliday, 1996; Smith, 1999). Nonetheless, its subcommittees, known as Cabinet committees, have an important role in agenda-setting and decision making. Cabinet committees consist of ministers drawn from several departments with an interest in the policy areas covered. They also include others who have a coordinating or strategic role within the government. An example is the Public Health Cabinet Committee (known as MISC 27) established in 2004. The committee's members include: Secretaries of State from DoH, DCMS and DfES as well as the Chief Secretary of the Treasury, Ministers of State from DCLG and DTI, and junior ministers from the Home Office, DfT, DWP, DEFRA, Department of Constitutional Affairs,

Northern Ireland Office, Scotland Office, Wales Office, and the Minister of Public Health from the DoH. The CMO also attends the committee.

One suggestion, which has resurfaced from time to time, has been to create a 'Super Department' to coordinate all aspects of social policy, including health. For example, Webster (1996, pp 40–1) discusses the debates within government in the post-war period about the creation of an overarching Ministry of Welfare and Pensions, a move supported by both major parties at one time. Although this ambitious amalgamation did not take place, health and social security departments were merged in the 1960s. The late 1960s and early 1970s also saw attempts to join up government in the form of a Joint Approach to Social Policy (JASP), cross-departmental policy analyses by the Central Policy Review Staff (Blackstone and Plowden, 1988; Challis et al, 1988), and efforts to get departments to consider the wider impact of their spending programmes (see Deakin and Parry, 2000). None of these initiatives was regarded as effective.

Another approach has been to identify a key minister as the coordinator of a particular cross-government policy. The creation of a Minister for the Disabled in the 1970s was regarded as a moderate success in raising disability issues across government (Ashley, 1992). A Minister for Community Care was appointed in the late 1980s (DHSS, 1988), but the post-holder lacked a cross-governmental remit and powers to coordinate departments. A Minister for Public Health was appointed by the Blair government in 1997 to coordinate policy across government. After a promising start, the post was effectively downgraded when its incumbent was replaced by a less senior minister. Following increased attention on public health issues, it has now been upgraded. Another example was the appointment of a Minister for Children within the DfES, mentioned earlier, taking responsibility for children's services, childcare and under-fives provision, teenage pregnancy and family policy. Although this was accompanied by the transfer of some functions (teenage pregnancy from the DoH, family policy from the Home Office and family law from the Lord Chancellor's Office), others (DWP for child support, the Treasury for tax credits, DoH for children's health and social care) remained with their host departments.

The core Executive

Coordination of policies across government also falls within the remit of the core Executive institutions. These consist of the most powerful central government institutions. This comprises the Prime Minister's Office (also known as Number Ten), the Cabinet Office (which supports the Prime Minister and has a coordinating role across government) and the Treasury (which holds the government's 'purse strings'). Although these institutions play an important role in leading and coordinating policy, there is significant tension between them (Hennessy, 1998; Richards and Smith, 2002; Burch and Holliday, 2004). In recent times this has been given a further twist by the often-fraught political relationship between Prime Minister Tony Blair and Chancellor Gordon Brown (Rawnsley, 2001; Naughtie, 2002; Peston, 2005). In the health arena, tensions were clearly evident in the internal battles over foundation trusts, for example (supported by Number Ten but opposed by the Treasury). Most interviewees believed that it was Number Ten rather than the Treasury that called the shots on health policy, although the latter provided an important counterweight.

The intervention of the Prime Minister in health policy is not new. In the 1970s, Harold Wilson intervened in the escalating dispute over pay beds and established a Royal Commission on the NHS to look into its problems. In the late 1980s, Margaret Thatcher took control of health policy by initiating the internal market reforms in the NHS. Under Blair, however, the intervention in health policy has been more sustained and systematic. There are several reasons for this. First, health and the NHS has been a key government priority. Second, this policy area has been a 'test bed' for the government's public service modernisation programme. Third, Blair's style of government has been 'presidential', allowing much more direct intervention in departmental affairs than hitherto (see Driver and Martell, 2002; Short, 2005). Finally, and related to this, important changes in the machinery and processes of central government have facilitated prime ministerial intervention.

Those involved in health policy are in no doubt that Number Ten is now more involved than in the past. One informant, from a health charity, stated that 'since 1997 the PM has become even more powerful than Thatcher and Major'. Another, a former DoH civil servant, stated that 'I have never seen a more powerful Prime Minister than Blair. Number Ten has been the dominant force in government.' A respondent from a health professional organisation stated that 'health policy reflected a more presidential style of government with the main decisions coming from Number Ten'. An MP commented that 'the main driver of health policy has been Number Ten' and linked this to the high profile of health on the government's reform agenda.

Interviewees gave examples of prime ministerial intervention in health policy. Many of the key policies of recent years – foundation trusts, payment by results, patient choice and the increased use of the private sector by the NHS – were attributed to Number Ten. The national service frameworks (NSFs), which set out plans and service models for specific condition areas and population groups (such as cancer, heart disease, people with mental illness and the elderly), and the NHS Plan were closely scrutinised and influenced by the Prime Minister's Office (see also Hogg, 2002; Baggott et al, 2005, p 207).

The increased influence of Number Ten has been linked to the rise of special advisers (see Richards and Smith, 2004; Dorey, 2005; Short, 2005). The

Prime Minister's health policy adviser is regarded as a highly influential person who can effectively set the health policy agenda within central government (Society Guardian, 2000; Baggott et al, 2005). Prime Ministers have often retained health policy advisers. Margaret Thatcher, for example, appointed Sir Roy Griffiths as her health adviser and he exerted considerable influence over health policy, including NHS management and community care reforms (Wistow and Harrison, 1998).

Interviewees agreed that the Prime Minister's health policy advisers were extremely influential. They were regarded as having more influence than the DoH special advisers, mentioned earlier. Comments included: 'the PM's special adviser is in a particularly powerful position' (MP), 'the Number Ten advisers were not merely messengers. They are "ideas men" who really do shape policy' (former civil servant); 'the PM's adviser is very, very strong' (trade union spokesperson). For example, Simon Stevens, who was Blair's policy adviser between 2001 and 2004, after performing a similar role for the Secretary of State for Health, was closely associated with many of the health policies introduced after 2000 (including patient choice, the NHS market reforms, foundation trusts and the increased use of the private sector). Interviewees saw Stevens as a key figure. One noted that: 'the movement of Stevens to Number Ten as Blair's adviser increased the centralising tendency within government on health policy' (former senior NHS manager). Another commented that 'Simon Stevens was a key individual, initially as Milburn's adviser and then as the Number Ten adviser on health' (former DoH civil servant).

Another important figure identified by interviewees was Professor Paul Corrigan. Like Stevens, Corrigan was an adviser to the Secretary of State for Health before moving on to Number Ten. Corrigan has been credited with initiating a number of key policies, including reforms in primary care and public health. He is said to have written the White Paper *Choosing Health* (Cm 6374, 2004) and had a strong influence over the *Our Health, Our Care, Our Say* White Paper of 2006 (*Health Service Journal*, 2006).

The increased intervention of Number Ten in policy matters has been reflected in the reorganisation of institutions at the heart of government. The Prime Minister's Office was restructured, with the creation of a policy directorate to monitor the implementation of policies across government. There have also been changes in the Cabinet Office, which coordinates policy across government (Kavanagh and Seldon, 2000; Burch and Holliday, 2004). These placed greater emphasis on supporting the Prime Minister and his 'government-wide' initiatives. They included the creation of a Prime Minister's Strategy Unit, a Delivery Unit, and an Office of Public Service Reform (OPSR, which has since been abolished).

According to interviewees, the Prime Minister's Strategy Unit has been heavily involved in policy development. An interviewee from an NHS management organisation commented that 'the Strategy Unit is very powerful and virtually instructs departments to do things'. For example, when the Strategy Unit undertook a review of alcohol strategy (Prime Minister's Strategy Unit, 2003, 2004), its final report was endorsed as government policy. The Strategy Unit has explored other health-related issues such as drugs, global health, GM crops, sport and the voluntary sector. Meanwhile the Delivery Unit monitors the implementation of policies and reforms, particularly with regard to the government's public services modernisation programme (see Cm 4310, 1999).

Despite the increase in the Prime Minister's resources, he cannot control all policy, all of the time. Indeed, as some commentators have noted more generally, '... policy-making, most of the time, goes on regardless of the Prime Minister. The impact of the Prime Minister is highly variable, depending on the policy, the departmental minister and the particular circumstances' (Smith et al, 2000, pp 161-2). Indeed, departmental ministers have their own resources and the Prime Minister's approach is generally one of alliance-building with departments rather than dictatorship (Richards and Smith, 2002). In recent times, Prime Ministers have adopted an informal approach when dealing with policy issues. Informal bilateral discussions with senior ministers and other advisers have been a key feature of the Blair era (Seldon, 2001), a technique also used extensively by Margaret Thatcher (Kavanagh and Seldon, 2000) and less so by John Major, who had a more collegial style (Seldon, 1994). Blair also introduced bi-monthly 'stocktaking' meetings with senior departmental ministers and their officials as a further opportunity for bilateral discussions. Interviewees commented on the 'bilateral axis' between Number Ten and the DoH, and argued that although the former often drove policy in a particular direction, the department was able to exercise more influence over policy detail. They also noted that the appointment of 'Blairite' ministers to the DoH from 1999 onwards ensured a consensual dialogue between the department and Number Ten, as health ministers were keen to implement the Prime Minister's policies.

The Treasury

As noted earlier, the Treasury has provided a counterweight to the policies driven by Number Ten. It is a small but powerful department that derives its influence from its control of the budget (see Likierman, 1988). It negotiates with the major spending departments on the overall size of their budget. It also monitors public spending. Designated Treasury civil servants 'shadow' the spending departments, meet with departmental civil servants and also observe how services operate. In recent years the Treasury has moved beyond the control of public spending and the monitoring of expenditure, towards matters of policy and management (Deakin and Parry, 2000; Treasury Committee, 2001; Richards and Smith, 2002). Its concern with value for money has led it to focus more strongly on policy outcomes.

In the realm of health policy, the Treasury has attempted to encourage prevention as a means of reducing health care costs in the long term (see Webster, 1996). More recently, its concern with the long-term growth of the NHS budget led it to establish an inquiry that made recommendations about health care reform (Wanless, 2002) and, subsequently, public health policies (Wanless, 2004). In addition, the Treasury has introduced new systems of budgeting and performance assessment to push departments, including the DoH, in a particular direction. In 1998, the Blair government introduced comprehensive spending reviews (CSRs), which involved closer scrutiny of each departmental budget.

Public service agreements (PSAs), introduced by the Treasury in the late 1990s, are also used to promoted departmental action. Each department must agree a PSA with the Treasury, which includes policy objectives and targets. The Treasury reviews the progress of the department concerned against its PSA. The current PSA targets for the DoH include an increase in life expectancy, reductions in health inequalities, improvements in health outcomes for people with long-term conditions, better access to services and improvements in patient and user experience. More specifically key targets include: that by 2008 no patient will wait more than 18 weeks for treatment from GP referral to hospital treatment; and a reduction in heart disease and stroke mortality by at least 40 per cent in people under 75 by 2010. The DoH is not alone in facing closer scrutiny of its policies from the Treasury. As Deakin and Parry (2000) have shown, others such as the DTI and the DWP have been strongly influenced by Treasury policies. The Treasury has had a significant impact on health policy and the DoH in recent years, in some cases by supporting policies and in others by opposition. For example with regard to NSFs, the Treasury was able to exert a major influence on the final versions of these documents (Hogg, 2002).

The Treasury also established cross-cutting reviews and performance agreements in an endeavour to promote joined-up working. The DoH and DfES now share a target to reduce teenage pregnancies, while the DCMS, DfES and DoH have a joint target to reduce childhood obesity. Government policy on health inequalities has also been subjected to this kind of cross-cutting approach (see ***Box 3.2***).

Box 3.2: Cross-cutting review on health inequalities

One example of how central government organisations can work together to tackle a particular health problem was the cross-cutting review of health inequalities, undertaken by the Blair government in 2001/2. The review was prompted by the decision to adopt national health inequalities targets aimed at narrowing the gap in life expectancy between different areas and reducing the variation in infant mortality rates between different social classes by 2010. The cross-cutting review was one of several established by the Treasury that explored policy issues spanning across several departments, and which fed into the 2002 Comprehensive Spending Review.

At ministerial level, the review was led by the Minister for Public Health. An interdepartmental group (IDG) of officials was also formed, drawn from the following: the Audit Commission, the Cabinet Office, DCMS, DEFRA, DfES, DoH, DCLG, DfT, DWP, the Home Office, the Local Government Association, the Neighbourhood Renewal Unit, the Number Ten Policy Unit, the Social Exclusion Unit, the Teenage Pregnancy Unit, the Sure Start Unit, and the Women and Equality Unit.

Its terms of reference were to develop the evidence base about health inequalities and their relationship with patterns of resourcing and service provision, and to develop a cross-government strategy for tackling the causes of health inequalities. This led to a programme of action (DoH, 2003a), which set out a range of actions in four areas: (1) supporting families, mothers and children, (2) engaging communities and individuals, (3) preventing illness and providing effective treatment and care, and (4) addressing the underlying determinants of health and the long-term causes of health inequalities. The programme also identified a number of specific commitments including an expansion of Sure Start (a scheme for supporting families with pre-school children), child care and support centres for children, improved mental health services for children and initiatives to improve health in schools. Targets were set out in a number of areas including improvements in housing, diet and exercise and reductions in fuel, poverty, smoking, drug abuse and child poverty. The responsibilities of all the departments concerned were identified and their progress toward these targets was monitored by the Treasury.

Subsequently, further efforts have been made to integrate action on health inequalities at the local level. Local authorities are expected to focus on reducing health inequalities in local area agreements (LAAs), formulated with local partners, including NHS organisations (see Chapter Eight).

Sources: see DoH (2003a) *Tackling Health Inequalities: A Programme for Action*, London: DoH; HM Treasury/DoH (2002) *Tackling Health Inequalities: Summary of the 2002 Cross-Cutting Review*, London: DoH.

Interviewees from the health arena believed that the Treasury had influenced health policy. Its control of expenditure and the use of PSAs were seen as the principal mechanisms of influence. However, there was wide agreement that although providing an important counterweight to Number Ten, the Treasury usually played a secondary role in policy development. Indeed, some commented that the longer-term financial settlements had weakened the influence of the Treasury in recent years. It was further pointed out that the Treasury had failed to prevent key reforms with which it disagreed, notably foundation trusts, although it had limited the impact of this policy (see also ***Box 4.3***).

Relationships between central government and outside organisations

Central government is bound to the outside world by many relationships. It has links with individual experts, voluntary organisations, local authorities, the NHS, professional bodies, trade unions, educational institutions and business organisations, among others. These relationships are important in the formulation and implementation of policy. Groups and individuals supply expertise and information that is useful in the policy-making process. They also provide political support for policies and can help implementation through their cooperation.

Government consults with such bodies in a variety of ways. It may issue proposals (in the form of a Green Paper, or a consultative document) for comment. Or it may establish an inquiry – such as a Royal Commission, a committee of inquiry or even a public inquiry – to take evidence from interested parties. Government also consults through a system of advisory committees. Groups and experts are co-opted onto these bodies, which make policy recommendations. Outside organisations and individuals also meet directly with ministers, civil servants and special advisers to put their case on a particular issue.

Post-war governments adopted a consultative style, and engaged closely with groups and individual experts (Stewart, 1958). This approach began to break down during the 1970s, a time of growing social conflict marked by a decline in consensus on key social and economic issues (Baggott, 1995a,

1995b). During the 1980s the Thatcher government adopted a hostile approach to some producer groups that had formerly enjoyed a close relationship with government, such as the BMA, for example. Important reforms were introduced with little or no prior consultation, illustrated starkly by the NHS internal market reforms of the late 1980s. These plans emerged out of a small working group appointed by the Prime Minister to formulate policy ideas (Butler, 1992; Timmins, 1995; Ham, 2000). This 'top-down' approach proved problematic. In particular, reforms failed to account for practical and technical barriers to implementation. Subsequently, government had to rebuild relationships with producer groups in order to secure their cooperation in implementing policy (Baggott, 1995a, 1995b).

The Major government was portrayed as more consensual and appeared to herald a re-emphasis on consultation and building effective working relationships with outside organisations (Baggott, 1995a, 1995b; Baggott and McGregor-Riley, 1999). This led to slight improvement in relationships, although prior consultation remained patchy and lacking on some key policy issues. The Major government was not afraid to confront organised interests, although with less overt hostility than its predecessor. Because the Major government lacked the resources of Thatcher – notably a smaller parliamentary majority coupled with an increasingly hostile media and a resurgent Labour opposition – it was forced to compromise on policy issues, particularly at the implementation stage.

On taking office, the Blair government called for an inclusive approach to policy making. The government argued that by consulting outside experts, those who implement policy and those affected by it, early in the policy-making process it would be possible to develop policies that were deliverable (Cm 4310, 1999). In this period the Blair government's inclusive style was reflected in a host of task forces appointed to explore a range of policy issues, including health (Platt, 1998). The formulation of the NHS Plan in 2000 was an example of this style of policy making (see ***Box 3.3***).

Box 3.3: The NHS Plan for England

The NHS Plan was published in 2000. It was formulated with the help of six task forces known as modernisation action teams (MATs). In addition to government personnel, these contained people drawn from NHS management, the professions, the voluntary sector, and health consumer and patients' groups, social services, trade unions, the Local Government Association and the Audit Commission. Each MAT proposed reforms in a particular area of the NHS. One looked at partnership between different parts of the health and social care system. Another explored how to improve clinical performance and health service productivity. A third examined the professions and workforce, and in particular how to increase the flexibility of training and working practices. The fourth MAT looked at how to tackle health inequalities and to focus the health system on preventing avoidable illness. The two remaining MATs focused on patients: one examined how to ensure fast and convenient access to services, the other explored patient empowerment and information. Five of the MATs were chaired by a minister, with the prevention and inequalities group chaired by the CMO. Civil servants from the DoH, the Treasury and the Prime Minister's Office (including the Prime Minister's adviser on health) were involved as members of MATs.

Research has shown that MAT discussions were wide-ranging (Baggott et al, 2005). One informant noted that discussion was open with 'no holds barred'. Another confirmed that the government was 'looking for radical ideas'. There were examples of the MATs having an impact on policy, most notably with regard to the health inequalities targets (see ***Box 3.1***). Previously the government had decided not to adopt such targets (Cm 4386,1999) but was persuaded by the Prevention MAT to introduce them.

Some participants interviewed commented that there was a lack of time to consider possible reforms in any depth. As one noted 'to rewrite the plans for the NHS for the next fifty years in a couple of months seems to pushing it'. There was concern about how the members of MATs were appointed, with insufficient consultation with organisations on this matter beforehand. Patients' representatives were represented on the MATs, but felt that they were still outweighed by professional interests.

Once the MATs had reported, the NHS Plan was developed as a result of discussions between the Treasury, the DoH and the Prime Minister's Office. A public consultation exercise was also undertaken (which supported action on issues such as hospital food, hygiene and clearer responsibilities for these standards in the form of a 'matron' style figure), which also fed into the Plan. A Cabinet Committee chaired by the Prime Minister was established to oversee the reforms.

The NHS Plan was launched in July 2000. It outlined a range of targets and initiatives, including new hospital schemes and additional staff. New targets were set for the reduction of waiting times (see Chapter Seven). Other commitments included an expansion of intermediate care, an increase in diagnostic and treatment centres, and the creation of care trusts to integrate health and social care services (see Chapter Eight). The NHS Plan also heralded an expanded role for the private sector as a partner in health service provision. In addition, it introduced a new performance management regime for the NHS (see Chapter Seven). The Plan also heralded reforms in patient and public involvement (see ***Box 4.4***).

Source: Cm 4818 (2000) *The NHS Plan: A Plan for Investment, A Plan for Reform*, London: TSO

Notwithstanding its declared intentions, the Blair government attracted increasing criticism for its autocratic style and for failing to consult adequately. Relationships with producer groups, notably the BMA, deteriorated (see Chapter Six). After 2000, reforms tended to emanate from special advisers, business organisations and think tanks, rather than from pressure groups representing professionals, health workers, patients and the public. Indeed, some reforms, notably foundation trusts, were strongly opposed by organised interests in the NHS (notably trade unions and professional groups).

Interviewees from within the policy process commented on the Blair government's approach to consultation. Most believed that the government had initially placed a lot of emphasis on consultation, and that in the years immediately following the 1997 election victory, much of this was a genuine attempt to build consensus. One informant commented that 'the government has made an effort to consult with groups. It has been successful at the "Big Tent" approach' (think tank spokesperson). Another stated that 'the Blair government has been extremely inclusive ... it has a pretty good record on consultation' (former senior NHS manager). However, some voices were more critical. A former DoH civil servant commented that 'although there has been more consultation, much less notice is being taken of it'. Another respondent, from a national charity, stated that 'government has been ... very keen to consult with outside health bodies ... our concern is that these consultations are a process of window dressing and that decisions have already been made'. A health professional body spokesperson observed that although consultation was extensive, it often did not reflect the importance of issues: 'some minor issues are heavily consulted on, while some big issues are not ...'.

Some policy actors complained that consultation periods were often short and offered insufficient time to produce a meaningful response. As one peer noted, 'consultation is not very productive. The time limits for consultation are often short and there is little obvious change to policy.' The government's guidelines on consultation, setting a minimum 12-week deadline for comments (Cabinet Office, 2004), were regarded as too short. As a respondent from a Royal College stated: 'Even 12-13 weeks is not really sufficient time for consultation when you are a member-based organisation'. This view is shared by health consumer groups (Baggott et al, 2005), which also felt that they received insufficient feedback from government on comments they had made in consultations.

Interviewees believed that consultation practices were shaped by ministerial styles. Among recent health ministers, Dobson and Hewitt were regarded as more consultative than Reid and Milburn. Another factor was the government's agenda. In the late 1990s, the government was keen to bring all stakeholders on board and adopted a strong consensual approach. In contrast after 2000, policies such as choice, privatisation and foundation trusts were driven by Number

Ten in the face of direct opposition from some stakeholders, especially trade unions and professional organisations. As one interviewee, a former government insider, commented, 'consultation depends much on what the government wants to do. If stakeholders are committed to oppose the government's agenda then engagement is not as important.'

Conclusion

This chapter has explored the institutions at the heart of health policy making. It has shown that health policy is not the sole preserve of the DoH, but involves other central government institutions. The important roles of core Executive institutions such as Number Ten and the Treasury have been identified. Although there appears to have been a centralisation of health policy in recent years, intervention is not unprecedented. Prime Ministers have previously intervened in health policy and the NHS, but under the Blair administration these centralising tendencies have become more overt and systematic.

This appears to have been part of an attempt to impose a more rational policy-making style within central government. The clarification of goals, centralisation, target-setting, public service agreements, monitoring and the joining-up of central government activities all reflect this. The shift in the balance of power between ministers and their advisers and civil servants is also an indicator of this approach. The rational approach is, however, at odds with a more inclusive and negotiated style of policy making. Although the Blair government initially tried to work constructively with stakeholders and sought to generate policy ideas from discussions with them, it proved difficult to sustain given the dominance of the top-down model, which brought confrontation with key interests.

Summary

- Although the DoH is the main focus for health policy, other government departments have health-related responsibilities.
- Health is a key policy area for the Prime Minister, the Cabinet Office and the Treasury.
- There has been an increase in the intervention of the core institutions of central government in health policy, particularly since the Blair government came to office in 1997. The Prime Minister has exerted a strong influence over the direction of health policy, with the Treasury providing a counterweight to this.
- Special advisers have become very influential over health policy, particularly those working for the Prime Minister. Civil servants appear to have become

less influential over policy formation but still retain an important role in relation to implementation.

- Government interacts with a wide range of outside experts and organisations. These are consulted on policy. Recent governments have faced criticism that these consultation processes are not inclusive and do not contribute effectively to policy formation.

Key questions

1. Why has Number Ten intervened in health policy to a greater extent than previously?
2. Many believe that the influence of civil servants within the DoH has been weakened in recent years. Is this the case and, if so, why has this occurred?
3. What are the main functions of special advisers?
4. How is health policy coordinated across government departments?
5. Why is it important for government to consult outside experts and interest groups on policy?

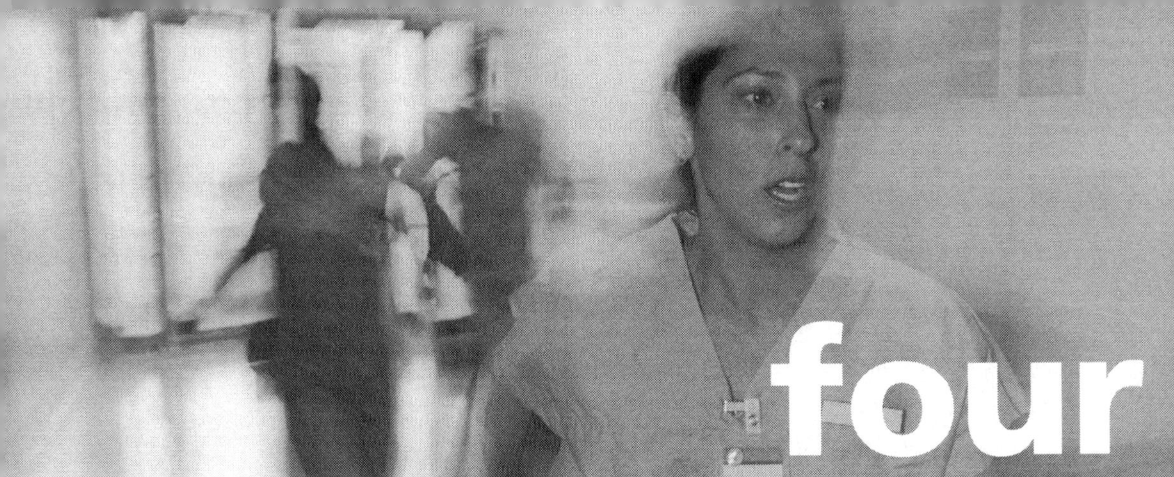

Parliament and health policy

Overview

This chapter looks at the impact of Parliament on health policy. It begins with a discussion of the health interests of MPs. The chapter then moves on to analyse the role and function of the House of Commons in health policy. This is followed by an examination of the role of the House of Lords.

Ingle and Tether (1981) found that Parliament had minimal influence over health policy. They argued that Parliament was largely powerless when faced with a majority government and that the House of Commons did not scrutinise health policy and administration effectively. More positively, scrutiny by the House of Lords was acknowledged as 'of a high order', but counterbalanced by an observation that the House 'simply lacks clout' (Ingle and Tether, 1981, p 47). The ability and commitment of MPs to raise issues of concern to their constituents was acknowledged, but the tools of trade (debates and questions) found wanting. Twenty-five years have passed since Ingle and Tether's study. This chapter examines whether or not their findings are still relevant today.

The health policy interests of MPs

Individual background and personal factors

MPs' interests are shaped by a range of background and personal factors (Richards, 1972). Some MPs have worked in health care, including, for example, Dr Richard Taylor, the independent MP for Wyre Forest, who is a former

NHS consultant (see ***Box 2.1***). Some have an interest in health arising from personal or family experience of illness. Others have health policy interests as a result of working with health charities, while some sit on NHS boards as non-executive directors. Finally, an MP may have an interest as a result of undertaking a parliamentary, party or government role in relation to health, such as having held a relevant committee chair or ministerial post.

Constituency interests

MPs' interests are shaped by constituency factors. Local NHS staff and patients may approach them to raise issues. Responding to such concerns is part of an MP's 'welfare officer' role, discussed further later. Involvement in local health matters is undertaken partly out of civic duty and partly by political calculation. MPs are keenly aware of the importance of health issues to their constituents. Moreover, local press, radio and television take a close interest in health issues and this offers opportunities for MPs to maintain and raise their profile.

Economic interests and other affiliations

MPs have a range of health-related economic interests and other affiliations, which they are required to declare. Some have a stake in health care businesses. For example, in the 2005 Register of Member's Interests, Tim Boswell (the MP for Daventry) declared shareholdings in the pharmaceutical company, Glaxo Smith Kline. Some MPs advise outside organisations, such as Dr Andrew Murrison, MP for Westbury, who declared his interest as an adviser to the Wessex Pharmaceutical Group. Others receive funds towards their constituency costs, including Martin Salter, MP for Reading West, whose constituency party has received donations from the public services trade union, UNISON. Some MPs also work for public relations or lobbying companies that lobby on behalf of business or other interests in the health field.

Collective interests

MPs and peers (members of the House of Lords) may develop health policy interests by participating in various parliamentary events and activities. They often attend parliamentary receptions, hosted by outside organisations, where they receive information from business interests, professional organisations and other pressure groups. This might involve highlighting new research, raising awareness about particular conditions, identifying problems and possible solutions (Baggott et al, 2005).

All Party subject groups (APGs) are also useful in enabling MPs and peers to develop health interests. APGs are not official committees, but can perform several useful functions, notably as a source of information for parliamentarians (see Jones, 1990). They are mainly fora for backbench MPs, but ministers do attend them. In 2005, 249 APGs were approved and listed by the House of Commons. Of these 56 covered health-related subjects (for example, drugs misuse, food and health, integrated and complementary medicine), and 26 APGs focused on specific conditions (for example, asthma, diabetes, breast cancer).

Interviewees from within the health policy process saw APGs as a useful way of informing MPs and peers and as a means of persuading them to raise issues. They were regarded as a useful channel of communication between outside groups and Parliament, and as a means of building cross-party support (see also Baggott et al, 2005). They were seen as a useful forum where MPs and peers could put their views to ministers, and where the latter could explain their policies. However, their shortcomings include duplication and overlap, lack of focus and, more commonly, limited resources. Health APGs appear to be most effective when they have a clear focus to their work and assistance from external organisations, which includes administrative and sometimes financial support. For example, the British Heart Foundation provides the secretariat for the APG on heart disease; the Association of British Pharmaceutical Industry provides administrative support for the APG on the pharmaceutical industry, while the APG on breast cancer receives administrative assistance from the charity, Breakthrough Breast Cancer.

In addition, each parliamentary party contains health subject committees, which consider policy issues. There is uncertainty about their exact role (see Jones, 1990). Although they are primarily a means by which party leaders can manage dissent among backbench MPs, examples of such committees exerting policy influence can be found (see Silk and Walters, 1998). They are regarded as 'valuable forums' by some (Norton, 1981 cited in Jones, 1990), facilitating communication between party leaders and their MPs. Outside interests also seek to influence party subject committees, but generally regard them as less important than APGs and select committees (discussed later) (see Rush, 1990, p 292).

Nonetheless, the health subject committee of the governing party can be influential, as several interviewees noted. The parliamentary Labour Party Health Committee chair has access to ministers. Ministers appear before the committee to explain their policies. On controversial issues the committee has been used to secure concessions (for example, on the issue of foundation trusts – see ***Box 4.3***) from ministers. Ministers also use the committee to gauge party backbench opinion and to 'firefight' backbench discontent. Under the Conservative governments of the 1980s and 1990s, the party's health subject committee had a similar role. For example, it helped secure concessions from the government on some issues, including exemptions for new charges on eye and dental checks.

Scrutiny, accountability and policy influence

Parliamentary questions, debates and early day motions

Parliamentarians have several instruments to question government, to obtain information or to put a case or argument (see Silk and Walters, 1998; Rush, 2005). MPs can table questions, initiate or contribute to debates, and initiate or support early day motions (EDMs).

Parliamentary questions (PQs) are directed at ministers (including the Prime Minister) and receive a written or oral response. Each department faces 'oral questions' at least once a month (and the Prime Minister, once a week), providing an opportunity for MPs to challenge ministers in front of the House. As can be seen from ***Table 4.1***, more than one in ten PQs is now answered by the DoH. The number and proportion of health questions has risen substantially since the 1960s. MPs and outside organisations interviewed commented that PQs are useful to obtain information on health issues that is not in the public domain and to raise concerns. One respondent noted that 'parliamentary questions can set alarm bells ringing in Whitehall'. On a negative note, ministers and their departments were seen as giving unhelpful or evasive responses. Ministers can refuse to answer questions if the cost is too high, the information is not available centrally, the matter is commercially sensitive, or it is not in the public interest to divulge it (see Select Committee on Public Administration, 2002). As one interviewee, an MP, observed 'Any minister half worth their salt can slip out of a corner on a question'. Notably, the DoH was singled out for criticism by the House of Commons' Public Administration Committee in 2002 for failing to give adequate answers to PQs, and in some cases, falsifying answers.

In the health domain, as in other policy areas, ministers have been able to limit the impact of PQs. The establishment of arm's-length institutions (see Chapter Three), has enabled ministers to refuse to answer questions about operational matters. Following the creation of foundation trusts (see ***Box 4.3***), the DoH informed MPs that questions should be directed to these new institutions. Furthermore, PQs have also been restricted as a result of NHS privatisation. The involvement of private contractors in running NHS services and capital schemes has enabled ministers to draw a cloak of commercial secrecy over what would normally be a legitimate subject for MPs' questions.

Table 4.1 Parliamentary questions (Department of Health)

Year/Session	Number of health questions	Total number of parliamentary questions	Health as per cent of total
1960-1	971	13, 778	7.0
1970-1	1,820	33,946	5.3
1980-1	2,169	30, 863	7.0
1999-2000	4,206	41,410	10.2
2000-1*	2,102	19,278	10.9
2001-2	9,349	74,073	12.6
2002-3	8,036	57,886	13.9
2003-4	6,687	55,853	12.0
2004-5**	2,693	23,552	11.4

* (December to May)
**(November to May)
Source: House of Commons

Parliamentary debates provide an opportunity to scrutinise government policy. Those launched by opposition parties can put pressure on government. Such 'set-pieces' are usually reserved for high-profile issues. Backbenchers may initiate short adjournment debates on specific issues. Although adjournment debates are poorly attended and attract little media coverage, they do guarantee a response from the minister responsible (Baggott et al, 2005). As ***Box 4.1*** indicates, health is a popular topic for adjournment debates in the House of Commons.

Box 4.1: Adjournment debate topics January-April 2005*

18 January 2005 Medical Services Northumberland *Alan Beith* (Berwick, Lib Dem)

25 January 2005 Suicide Promotion on the Internet *Mark Hendrick* (Preston, Lab)

27 January 2005 Childhood Anaemia *Bob Laxton* (Derby North, Lab)

10 February 2005 Hospital Services Paddington *Karen Buck* (Regent's Park and North Kensington, Lab)

25 February 2005 Manchester Health Finances *Graham Stringer* (Manchester, Blackley, Lab)

28 February 2005 Mental Hospitals NE Cambridgeshire *Malcolm Moss* (NE Cambridgeshire, Con)

2 March 2005 Mechanised Wheelchairs *Bob Russell* (Colchester, Lib Dem)

7 March 2005 Stem Cell Research *Ian Gibson* (Norwich North, Lab)

16 March 2005 Brighton and Sussex University Hospitals NHS Trust *Sir Nicholas Soames* (Mid Sussex, Con)

22 March 2005 Saneline (mental health) Funding *Sir Nicholas Winterton* (Macclesfield, Con)

15 March 2005 Cholesterol and Disease Prevention *Howard Stoate* (Dartford, Lab)

23 March 2005 Children's Hospices *Jeff Ennis* (Barnsley East and Mexborough, Lab)

5 April 2005 HIV/AIDS in Africa *Sally Keeble* (Northampton North, Lab)

6 April 2005 Acute Hospital Funding *Andrew George* (St Ives, Lib Dem)

*10 January-7 April 2005

Note: There was also an Opposition Debate during this period on Hospital Acquired Infections (2 March 2005)

Source: House of Commons *Hansard* Debates, 2004/05 session

Another instrument is the EDM. These are statements about an issue, institution or policy, which MPs may initiate or support. EDMs provide a useful barometer of opinion. When supported by a large number of backbench MPs, particularly from the governing party, they can capture the attention of government. According to Lord Ashley (1992, p 193), 'over 100 signatures on a motion is usually regarded as significant'. Health issues are popular topics for EDMs. In the 2004/5 session 122 out of 1,033 EDMs (11.8%) were on health-related topics. Subjects included: 'Carers in the UK' (supported by 144 MPs); Macmillan Cancer Relief's 'Better Deal' Campaign (supported by 126); and 'cystic fibrosis and prescription charges' (supported by 89). In comparison, 153 of the 1,201 (12.7%) EDMs tabled in the 2000-1 session of Parliament were on health-related subjects, a slightly higher proportion than four years later.

Those involved in the health policy arena argue that these various instruments are relatively weak when used in isolation. However, they can be effective when deployed in a coordinated manner and coupled with external pressure from the media and pressure groups. One interviewee, a peer, pointed out that they 'are useful as part of a broader campaign or strategy'. They can be used by outside organisations to mobilise MPs and get them to raise the profile of an issue. The value of PQs, debates and EDMs is that they indicate parliamentary opinion on a particular health issue. If this opinion is strong, the government may give concessions. Parliamentary opinion expressed in this way (and through other channels such as party committees, APGs and select committees) can attract the attention of health ministers and civil servants to an issue currently low on the political agenda, or may indicate opposition to a policy currently being pursued. For example, between June 2001 and March 2003, a parliamentary campaign to raise the profile of prostate cancer involved four EDMs (attracting support from 26, 114, 146 and 59 MPs respectively), 46 PQs and an adjournment debate.

Select committees

Select committees are official committees of the House of Commons that inquire into policy, administration and expenditure (Dorey, 2005). They take written and oral evidence from individuals and organisations and publish a report with recommendations. Government usually publishes a response to each report. Select committees consist of backbench MPs. Although they have an in-built majority of MPs drawn from the governing party, some are chaired by MPs from other parties. Some select committees have a wide-ranging brief across government, such as the Public Accounts Committee and the Select Committee on Public Administration, and include health issues as part of their remit. Others focus on the work of particular departments, such as the Health Committee, which focuses on the DoH, health policy, the NHS and public health issues such as obesity (see ***Box 4.2***). Several other committees cover health and safety issues, including the Transport Committee (road safety), and the Environment, Food and Rural Affairs Committee (environmental health and food safety).

Box 4.2: The Health Committee and obesity

The Health Committee inquiry into obesity in 2003 took evidence from a range of organisations including the Automatic Vending Association, the DoH, the DCMS, the Snack, Nut and Crisp Manufacturers' Association, Cancer Research UK, the National Heart Forum, The Sugar Bureau, the British Heart Foundation, the Central Council of Physical Recreation, the Food Commission, the Royal College of General Practitioners, Sport England, the Food and Drink Federation, Diabetes UK, the Medical Research Council, Weightwatchers, the Royal College of Nursing, the British Retail Consortium, PepsiCo UK, McDonald's Restaurants, Asda, the Consumers' Association, Cadbury Schweppes and the Royal College of Psychiatrists. The committee also received evidence from individuals with expertise in clinical, health and education matters relevant to diet, obesity, child health and public health. The Health Committee made many recommendations including:

- a wide-ranging and long-term programme to reduce obesity
- a traffic-light system of labelling
- a new council on nutrition and physical activity
- a health promotion campaign on obesity
- a higher priority for obesity on school agendas, including the development of school nutrition policies and replacement of vending machines selling unhealthy products
- the development of a food technology curriculum inspected by the Office for Standards in Education (Ofsted)
- a minimum of three hours of physical activity per week for schoolchildren (also an extension of Ofsted's remit in this area)
- a review of advertising regulation
- public health targets for food companies
- coordinated efforts to promote the use of pedometers in schools, the workplace and the wider community
- more resources to fund obesity services and treatment.

Source: House of Commons, Health Committee (2004) *Obesity*, London: TSO

The Health Committee was perceived by most interviewees as a useful scrutiny body. However, it operates within constraints facing all such committees (see Hansard Society Commission on Parliamentary Scrutiny, 2001). These include: limited resources to conduct inquiries; a lack of publicity for reports; insufficient time for debating reports; and limited opportunities to follow up recommendations in a systematic way. But perhaps the most serious constraint is the influence of the party whips, whose job is to ensure that their colleagues do not embarrass the party leadership. Although select committees are expected to be non-partisan, the whips can influence the composition of select committees and the appointment of chairs. They have been able to remove select committee chairs who are critical of party policy. For example, in 1992, the Conservative Party whips prevented Nicholas Winterton from continuing as chair of the Health Committee by introducing a new rule limiting chairs' terms of office. Whips have also been accused of interfering with the work of committees, as in 1991, when a Conservative MP on the Health Committee admitted that his office had been involved in leaking a draft report to ministers.

The Health Committee, like all select committees, has the potential to influence policy. Interviewees noted that the committee could be influential, particularly in highlighting neglected issues and helping to get 'less fashionable' issues (such as mental health and sexual health) on to the agenda. One informant, from a health charity, argued that one of the key roles of the committee was 'to get government to reflect and rethink'. Several interviewees noted that pressure groups are keen to have their recommendations endorsed by the Health Committee (see also Baggott et al, 2005) as they believed this added weight and credibility to their case. Some argued that by revisiting issues, the committee has a cumulative impact (particularly on issues such as mental health, public health and private medicine) enabling it to have a more subtle and longer-term influence over policy. However, other interviewees pointed out that the committee's influence over policy was marginal, particularly when it went against the grain of current government policy.

Legislation

A key role of Parliament is to scrutinise legislation. MPs get an opportunity to debate and vote on various stages of a Bill as it passes through Parliament. Select committees may also undertake pre-legislative scrutiny of draft Bills before their formal introduction. The detailed task of legislative scrutiny, however, falls to standing committees, appointed in proportion to the party strengths in the House of Commons. The government's in-built majority on these committees (assuming it has a majority in the House as a whole), coupled with the system of party discipline, enables government to exert considerable control over the legislation process.

Those interviewed commentated on the weakness of Parliament in shaping health legislation. The large majorities enjoyed by the Blair governments (and the Thatcher governments of the 1980s) were crucial to the success of their legislative programme. In the 1980s, the Thatcher government was able to create an internal market in the NHS, despite opposition from many of its own backbench MPs. More recently, in 2003, the Blair government introduced foundation trusts despite having many opponents to this policy on its own backbenches (see ***Box 4.3***). In both these cases, some concessions were given to ensure that the measures became law, but these did not undermine the purpose of the legislation.

Box 4.3: Foundation trusts and the 2003 Health and Social Care (Community Health and Standards) Act

The passage of the 2003 Health and Social Care (Community Health and Standards) Act, which provided the statutory basis for NHS foundation trusts, illustrated both the strengths and weaknesses of Parliament. Although making no manifesto commitment at the 2001 General Election, the Labour government introduced plans to establish foundation trusts as 'not for profit' public benefit corporations, accountable to a local governing body comprising members of the public, staff and other stakeholders (such as primary care trusts (PCTs)). Foundation trusts were promised freedom from ministerial directives, and greater autonomy over the retention of surpluses, borrowing and investment decisions, asset sales, and ways of incentivising staff. However, as a safeguard, government proposed an independent regulator (known as Monitor) to approve applications for foundation status and with powers to intervene if trusts failed to comply with the terms agreed (relating to financial matters, governance and services provided). Foundation trusts would also remain subject to other regulators, such as the Healthcare Commission, for example.

The policy was vociferously opposed by many backbench Labour MPs, who believed that foundation trusts would destabilise local health systems, exacerbate inequalities in service provision and lead to further privatisation of the NHS. These sentiments produced several rebellions as the legislation went through Parliament. In the House of Commons, the government's majority was almost overturned on several occasions. In July 2003, 62 Labour MPs voted against the second reading of the Bill and over 50 abstained, leaving it with a much-reduced majority of 35. During the final stages of the Bill in November, the government's majority fell to only 17 (the lowest since Labour returned to office in 1997). Meanwhile, the House of Lords voted against the principle of foundation trusts on several occasions. Eventually, acknowledging the constitutional supremacy of the elected chamber, the House of Lords conceded.

The failure to prevent foundation trusts illustrates the weakness of Parliament in the face of a highly committed government with a large majority in the House of Commons. But when one examines the detail of this legislation, it is clear that Parliament had some impact. The government accepted 90 amendments to the Bill. Many were technical and from the government's view strengthened the legislation by closing loopholes, providing clarification and addressing drafting errors. But others reflected compromise, influenced by the government's desire to see the legislation on the statute book before the end of the parliamentary session.

This was a long and complex piece of legislation and it is not possible to give a detailed account of its passage. However, concessions achieved by the government's opponents included the following:

- The composition of foundation trust governing bodies was amended to include at least one local authority nominee. Other 'partner' organisations could also be represented.
- The number of governing body members elected by staff was increased from one to three.
- Staff employed by subcontractors on 'rolling contracts' were permitted to become members of the foundation trust.
- The requirements for including certain executive directors on the board of directors were amended to include a doctor and a nurse/midwife.
- The government's original intention was to allow foundation trusts complete freedom to choose auditors. It was persuaded to allow Audit Commission auditors to perform this task (although foundation trusts would not be compelled to use these auditors).
- Initially the government stated that it would not compel foundation trusts to have patient and public involvement forums (PPIFs – statutory bodies representing the public, patients and carers recently established in all trusts). This was fiercely contested and the government offered several compromises (including a requirement that foundation trusts retain their forums for at least a year). Eventually, the government acknowledged that PPIFs should be retained by foundation trusts (although subsequently proposals were brought forward to abolish PPIFS).
- The government accepted that minimum requirements should be imposed on applicants wishing to become foundation trusts to consult with local people, patients, staff and local stakeholders such as local authorities.
- An amendment established the foundation trust regulator as a public board rather than as an individual office.
- In an effort to strengthen accountability to Parliament the regulator was required to lay a copy of his/her annual report before Parliament directly (and subsequently to send a copy to the Secretary of State).
- The government also promised an independent review of foundation trusts, to assess their impact and that these bodies would have to abide by the

minimum requirements of *Agenda for Change* (a national agreement on pay and conditions) and other national level staff agreements.

Source: House of Commons *Hansard* Debates, 2002/03 session

Although the size of the government's majority is important, other factors are also relevant to its power over Parliament. One interviewee, a peer, spoke of a 'cultural mindset of executive domination' common to all recent British governments. Others noted that the Blair government's large majorities since 1997 had weakened parliamentary influence over policy and legislation. Blair's 'presidential style' (see Chapter Three) was also held responsible. For example, according to one informant (a former DoH civil servant), 'Blair is not a Parliamentarian. He does not have much regard for Parliament.'

Nonetheless, as several interviewees observed, Parliament does have some residual influence. When the government needs Parliament to enact legislation, MPs (and peers) can have significant leverage. Parliamentary opposition can bring delays and media criticism. As the end of a parliamentary session nears, these pressures strengthen and there is a greater willingness of government to compromise in order to get measures onto the statute book. However, amendments proposed by backbenchers must be broadly consistent with the government policy in order to succeed, as both the foundation trust legislation (***Box 4.3***) and the abolition of the community health councils (CHCs) (***Box 4.4***) illustrate.

Box 4.4: The abolition of community health councils in England

In 2001 the Labour government faced opposition in Parliament to its plans to reform patient and public involvement in the NHS (see Baggott, 2005). The controversial decision to abolish CHCs and their national body (Association of Community Health Councils for England and Wales (ACHCEW)) and replace them with a network of PPIFs based in trusts was criticised by many Labour MPs, who, along with colleagues from other parties, mounted vigorous opposition. Over a hundred MPs signed an EDM opposing the decision. As the 2001 General Election loomed, the government accepted an amendment from David Hinchliffe – the then Labour chair of the Health Select Committee – to establish bodies called Patients' Councils that would organise patient and public involvement over a larger geographical area (rather than being focused on trusts as the government planned). It also made other concessions (such as the creation of a national patients' organisation) to ensure the passage of its legislation. A further amendment made in the House of Lords reinstated CHCs. The government refused to countenance this and dropped this part of its legislation. After its General Election victory, the Labour government returned with new legislation (the NHS and Health Care Professions Bill), which established PPIFs in NHS trusts and PCTs, along similar lines to the original proposal. An attempt by MPs and peers to revive the Patients' Councils amendment was opposed by the government. Although 26 Labour MPs rebelled against their party on this amendment, the government won the day. However, it did retain provisions for a national patients' body (the Commission for Patient and Public Involvement in Health (CPPIH)) – which was given a brief to advise health ministers, represent PPIFs at national level, and provide consistency, support and guidance to these local forums. It also amended the Bill in an effort to address concerns that the new system of patient and public involvement would be fragmented: it introduced a statutory duty on PPIFs to cooperate with each other; extended the role of PCT fora to provide an overview across various services used by patients, including social care and public health; and provided for a proportion of PCT forum members to be drawn from trust forums within their area. Subsequently, the government introduced plans to abolish CPPIH and replace PPIFs with local network organisations established by local authorities.

Some issues cut across party lines, including matters of conscience such as embryo research, abortion, and genetic testing. Here, MPs are usually permitted to debate and vote in a non-partisan way. MPs may also bring forward Bills (known as private member's Bills (PMBs)) on these or other matters. However, the government's control of the parliamentary timetable means that its support is necessary in order for them to have any chance of success (see ***Table 4.2***). An example was the Human Fertilisation and Embryology (Deceased Fathers) Bill, which became law in 2003. It was introduced by a backbench MP and a peer, with the government's support and encouragement. This clarified the

Table 4.2: *Parliamentary Bills on health topics (2000-5)*

Year/Session	Number of government Bills introduced (number passed)	Number of private member's Bills introduced (number passed)
2000-1	2 (1)	9 (0)
2001-2	3 (3)	19 (0)
2002-3	3 (3)	18 (2)
2003-4	3 (2)	12 (1)
2004-5	4 (4)	11 (0)
Total	15 (13)	69 (3)

law on registering deceased fathers on birth certificates where the child is conceived with the assistance of fertility treatment. Notably, in this case, the government wanted to change the law, but did not have sufficient space in its legislative programme. Indeed, government departments are often proactive in discussing with backbench MPs the possibility of introducing legislation that is important to government, but not a major priority.

Parliament can influence policy indirectly by using legislative procedures to raise issues and concerns. MPs can intervene in debates on government Bills to plant ideas for future legislation. PMBs are also useful in raising matters. Indeed, there are several cases where an Act of Parliament has been preceded by PMBs in previous sessions. Bills to ban tobacco advertising were introduced almost perennially by MPs until eventually the government initiated its own legislation. From the government's perspective PMBs are a useful way of testing the strength of opinion on controversial issues.

The ability of MPs to scrutinise legislation has been adversely affected by the rise in 'secondary legislation' (see Silk and Walters, 1998, pp 146-151; Parliament First, 2003; Rush, 2005). Primary legislation (Acts of Parliament) grants 'secondary' powers that enable ministers to make further legal provisions. The number of such regulations (also known as statutory instruments) has increased over the last 20 years. Although an efficient way of dealing with routine and uncontroversial matters, they enable government to avoid scrutiny on important matters. There are few opportunities to debate secondary legislation, and most become law without a debate or vote. Even when they are debated, the instruments cannot be amended and are rarely rejected. There is a special committee (established jointly with the House of Lords) that scrutinises secondary legislation, but it is overworked, confines itself to technical matters (that is, consistency with the relevant primary legislation) and has no powers to amend secondary legislation or prevent it from coming into force. However, government does withdraw a small number of statutory instruments each year that attract the most intense criticism from this committee. Another body, the House of Lords Committee on the Merits of Statutory Instruments, was recently created to examine the policy implications of statutory instruments.

A huge amount of secondary legislation is produced on health matters. Although statutory instruments are mainly technical they do have an impact on the way in which health policy is implemented. Examples (from 2004) include the Care Standards Act 2000 (Extension of Protection of Vulnerable Adults Scheme) Regulations; the Health Act 1999 (Consequential Amendments) (Nursing and Midwifery) Order; the Medicines for Human Use (Clinical Trials) Regulations; the Primary Medical Services (Sale of Goodwill and Restrictions on Subcontracting Regulations); NHS Direct Regulations; and the NHS (Personal Medical Services Agreements) Regulations.

Finance

Parliament's scrutiny of government expenditure is, historically, a key function. Again because of party discipline, there is little opportunity for MPs to challenge the government's public spending decisions in advance or to refuse to approve spending plans (see Hansard Society Commission on Parliamentary Scrutiny, 2001; Parliament First, 2003). However, there are procedures for reviewing expenditure plans and to examine how money has been spent. Departmental select committees can scrutinise and comment on expenditure plans. Their activities are useful in probing and deriving information about government priorities. Each year, the Health Committee examines health spending and receives a response to its written questions from the DoH. The committee may also call in ministers and senior officials to give further evidence on particular issues.

A number of specialist offices and committees also monitor expenditure. The National Audit Office (NAO), headed by the Comptroller and Auditor General (CAG), audits the government's accounts and issues reports on specific topics. The NAO has undertaken inquiries in the following areas of health policy and service provision, for example: the refinancing of the Norfolk and Norwich Hospital PFI scheme; clinical governance; the management of suspensions of clinical staff in the NHS; and the NHS Cancer Plan. The CAG/NAO undertakes an initial investigation and produces a report, which can be followed up by a special select committee, the Public Accounts Committee (PAC). PAC has 16 members (currently 10 Labour, four Conservative and two others – in proportion to party strengths in the House of Commons). It is chaired by an opposition MP. PAC follows up key issues and takes evidence from the relevant departments and agencies. It then publishes its own report, which adds to pressure on government to deal with the issues raised. It should be noted that although these investigations are inspired by concerns about overspending, inefficiency and value for money, they also often raise issues about public health and the quality of health services. For example, the 2003-4 inquiry into the management of suspensions of clinical staff found that trusts failed to undertake specified employment checks when recruiting staff. Another report in 2005 found that several important recommendations made earlier with regard to preventing hospital-acquired infections had not been implemented. Like the Health Committee, PAC is also able to revisit issues if it believes insufficient steps have been taken to address them.

Another body, the Audit Commission, also has an important role in financial scrutiny. It seeks to ensure that public money is spent economically, efficiently and effectively. It is responsible for auditing the finances of the NHS. The Audit Commission also issues reports on the management of resources in health and social care, corporate governance in health and social care organisations, and on cross-cutting issues across public services. It formerly produced national 'value for money' studies into different aspects of NHS services. However, this is now a function of the Healthcare Commission, whose role is explored further in Chapter Seven.

Redress of grievances

MPs have a 'welfare officer' role (Richards, 1972, p 164), which involves helping constituents who are facing problems with government and public bodies, including the NHS.These include maladministration (see below), delay, unfair decisions and incompetence. MPs engage in many activities for their constituents. This includes contacting authorities on their behalf, and raising PQs, EDMs or debates to gain attention for their plight. Another option is to raise the matter with the relevant ombudsmen whose role is discussed in a moment. MPs' actions can lead to a case becoming the subject of national debate. For example, in 2000, Mavis Skeet was found to have inoperable throat cancer after having her exploratory operation cancelled several times. Her MP (David Hinchliffe) raised concerns in the House of Commons and her case attracted widespread media interest. Subsequently, the government was forced into a wide-ranging review of the NHS. A similar sequence of events occurred in 1987, when cancelled operations were raised by MPs and highlighted by the media, leading to pressure on government to initiate reform. The welfare officer role is not, strictly speaking, a policy-making activity, nor is it formally part of the scrutiny function, although it is important to both. By highlighting cases of maladministration and injustice, issues can be raised thereby providing impetus for policy change. Such cases also illustrate general problems of policy implementation and public sector management, leading to closer scrutiny of these activities by Parliament and the media.

The Ombudsmen

The Parliamentary Ombudsman (full title, the Parliamentary Commissioner for Administration) was established in 1967 (Gregory and Giddings, 2002). The Ombudsman's remit is to investigate complaints about maladministration by government departments and other public bodies. Maladministration includes bias, neglect, rudeness, unresponsiveness, faulty procedures, delay, perverse decisions, partiality, arbitrariness and inequitable treatment. The Ombudsman is not permitted to look at policy matters, but investigations inevitably raise policy issues.

The Ombudsman can only respond to a complaint through an MP. He or she cannot initiate investigations and cannot force authorities to comply with his or her recommendations (which can include financial redress).

However, media interest can raise awareness of cases. A Select Committee on Public Administration reviews the Ombudsman's reports and may follow up particular issues. The Committee (and its predecessor, the Select Committee on the Parliamentary Commissioner for Administration) have often pressed for an extended remit for the Ombudsman and increased powers, notably with regard to health services.

Complaints about the DoH and other public bodies in health, such as the Human Fertilisation and Embryology Authority, Food Standards Agency and the Healthcare Commission, are within the remit of the Ombudsman. The NHS was initially excluded from the Ombudsman's remit. However, a series of scandals in the NHS in the late 1960s, coupled with pressure from the Parliamentary Commissioner's Select Committee, led the government to establish Health Service Ombudsmen posts in each part of the UK in 1973. As initially constituted, the Health Service Ombudsmen's remit excluded clinical matters. This was addressed in the mid-1990s when a single complaints process for administrative and clinical matters extended the Health Ombudsmen's role into this realm.

The Health Ombudsmen's powers differ from those of the Parliamentary Ombudsman. Health service complaints are not subject to being channelled through MPs, although most complainants are expected to take up the matter initially with the relevant health service body or clinician. The right to complain about health services extends to individuals (including staff) acting on behalf of a patient incapable of voicing a complaint. Nonetheless, the Health Service Ombudsmen cannot look at policy matters, investigate issues that are not identified through specific complaints, nor enforce compliance with recommendations. However, an additional power was granted to produce special thematic reports, based on earlier investigations. This has been used to highlight areas where many complaints have been upheld, notably with regard to long-term care and NHS complaints procedures.

The reports of the Health Service Ombudsman for England are examined by the Select Committee on Public Administration. This provides an opportunity to pursue issues further, and to call to account NHS bodies and individuals who have not responded to previous recommendations, and who may be subjected to further criticism and possibly adverse media coverage. There are similar accountability arrangements in other parts of the UK, although it should be noted that in Northern Ireland, Scotland and Wales, there is now a single Public Services Ombudsman covering government departments and agencies as well as the NHS and local government.

The House of Lords

The House of Lords has a significant scrutiny role and can make matters uncomfortable for government. In some situations, it may persuade government to amend legislative proposals. However, unlike the House of Commons, it is not elected by the public. Until this happens – and various reforms have been proposed to introduce elections for the Upper House – it will continue to lack democratic legitimacy. Moreover, its power to delay and oppose legislation is limited by statute.

Interests

Although peers do not currently have a public constituency, they are not isolated from concerns of the public and of special interests. Individuals and groups frequently bring matters to the attention of peers, who, in turn, are active in raising these issues in the House of Lords. Peers have a wide range of health interests. Some have commercial and financial interests, as directors or shareholders of companies in the health policy field (such private health care organisations, drugs companies, and alcohol, tobacco and food companies). Others have an interest arising out of a professional career in the health service, have led trade unions in this field, or been involved in professional bodies at a senior level. Examples include Lords Winston, Turnberg and Walton, all prominent members of the medical profession. Others have served as non-executive directors or in some other lay capacity on NHS bodies (for example, Lord Chan, a non-executive director of a PCT; Lord Harris of Haringey, a non-executive director of an ambulance trust).

A large number of peers are ex-MPs, many of who have taken an interest in health matters while in the House of Commons, such as Lord Ashley, an active campaigner on behalf of disabled people (Ashley, 1992). Some are former health ministers, and maintain an active interest in health issues. For example, Baroness Cumberlege, a minister in the Major government, has a long-standing interest in health issues, particularly with regard to maternity and childbirth issues, has served on NHS bodies and has been involved with several health organisations. She is a patron of the National Childbirth Trust, a trustee of Cancer Research UK and vice-president of both the Royal College of Nursing and the Royal College of Midwives.

In addition, other peers take a keen interest in health policy as a result of their former or current occupations in academia, the civil service, science and the voluntary sector. Examples include Baroness Pitkeathley (former director and now vice-president of Carers' National Association); Lord Allen (member, MENCAP), Lord Clement-Jones (trustee, CancerBACUP), Baroness Greengross (former director, Age Concern), Lord Bragg (President,

MIND), Baroness Finlay (a professor of palliative medicine), Baroness Gould (President, British Epilepsy Association), Lord Joffe (member of the Voluntary Euthanasia Society), Lord Smith of Clifton (trustee and director of the Stroke Association), and Baroness Morgan of Drefelin (chief executive, Breakthrough Breast Cancer).

Scrutiny, legislation and influence

The House of Lords uses similar instruments to the House of Commons when scrutinising government. Peers can table questions to ministers (each department, including the DoH, has a member of its ministerial team drawn from the House of Lords) and raise debates. Select committees also exist in the House of Lords, although these are not focused on specific departments. Health falls within the remit of several committees – including the Science and Technology Committee and the European Union subcommittee on social policy and consumer affairs. Peers use these to hold government to account, to highlight problems with policies and services and to propose changes to policy. For example, the Science and Technology Committee in recent years has explored several important health issues such as stem cell research, infection control and antibiotic resistance.

One the key functions of the House of Lords is legislative scrutiny. The government and the House of Commons need the House of Lords to undertake the routine task of examining proposed legislation to identify loopholes and inconsistencies. This function gives the House of Lords a certain amount of leverage. Failure to secure cooperation can delay important legislation, although it rarely rejects it. Because of the relative weakness of party discipline in the House of Lords, it can defeat the government more easily forcing a reconsideration of legislative proposals. One interviewee, a former government adviser, stated that 'the House of Lords can be influential on some issues as a result of its revising role. It can block legislation and force government to compromise and amend its legislation.' It is often argued that debates in the House of Lords can be more persuasive because they are not conducted in such an adversarial atmosphere as in the House of Commons. Peers can be persuasive because of their expertise, understanding and knowledge of health policy and the NHS. They are believed to be particularly influential on issues that cut across controversial party lines, such as stem cell research, alternative therapies and euthanasia.

Between 1979 and 1997 the Conservative government was defeated in the Lords on an average of 14 occasions in each parliamentary session. Between 1997 and 2001, there was an average of 24 defeats per session for the Labour government. This increased sharply in 2002-3 with 56 defeats. Because, ultimately, the will of the House of Commons tends to prevail, these defeats are usually reversed (as occurred in both the foundation trust and the public involvement legislation – see ***Boxes 4.3*** and ***4.4***). But the government may offer a compromise to avoid delaying the legislation or to head off further rebellion among backbenchers in the House of Commons. Indeed, sometimes the matter will not be put to a vote, following informal agreement between the government and its opponents in the House of Lords, enabling the government to move its own amendment to a Bill.

In summary, the House of Lords has a useful function in relation to health policy. It can influence the details of legislation, help to get issues on the agenda and can contribute to important debates, particularly those cutting across party lines. The effectiveness of the House of Lords is to some extent undermined by its currently undemocratic composition. But this is counterbalanced by the greater independence of peers from the system of party discipline and the repository of knowledge and experience in the House of Lords. It is vitally important that future reforms to democratise the House of Lords do not remove these important attributes.

Conclusion

Little has changed since Ingle and Tether's analysis. Health remains an issue of considerable importance to MPs and peers, and, if anything, is higher on their agenda than it was thirty years ago. But parliamentary scrutiny, of public policy generally and health in particular, remains limited and influence over policy is marginal. Parliamentary accountability has been described by David Hinchliffe, former chair of the Health Select Committee as 'a nonsense' and 'largely mythical' (Edwards and Fall, 2005, p 189). Reforms such as the introduction of departmental select committees – such as the Health Committee – appear to have little impact. Longer-term factors associated with the decline of Parliament, such as 'strong government', the 'presidential style' of recent Prime Ministers, the growth of secondary legislation and the rise of alternative mechanisms of accountability, such as the media and new regulatory bodies, have outweighed any positive effects of reform (Riddell, 2000). Indeed, many now believe that only a comprehensive programme aimed at strengthening the powers of Parliament will enable MPs and peers to hold government more closely to account and exert greater influence over policy (Commission to Strengthen Parliament, 2000; Hansard Society Commission on Parliamentary Scrutiny, 2001; Parliament First, 2003).

However, Parliament is not irrelevant. In certain circumstances, notably with regard to conscience issues, when government is in a minority, or if it faces serious divisions within its own ranks, some influence over policy can occur. When they combine with other political actors, such as pressure groups and the media, MPs and peers can provide a counterbalance to government and may help to shape agendas and contribute to policy changes, particularly in the longer term. Parliament is still an important arena where outside individuals and organisations can advocate or oppose policy ideas. Moreover, its scrutiny powers, although currently weak, can be used to shed light on government policy and administration and thus generate wider pressures for change.

Summary

- Health is an important issue for MPs and peers.
- A variety of factors shape MPs' interests including background and personal factors, constituency interests, membership of groups or committees in Parliament, economic interests and affiliations.
- MPs have a variety of activities in which they may engage to raise issues and scrutinise government in the health policy arena, although these are relatively weak in promoting policy and ensuring effective scrutiny of government.
- Select committees have an important potential role in health policy and in strengthening accountability. However, they have had only a limited impact on policy and face obstacles in holding government to account.
- Government dominates the process of legislation. Parliament can exert some influence over primary legislation, in particular circumstances. Yet as long as government has a large parliamentary majority and party discipline remains strong, there are few opportunities to change government policy.
- Parliament's powers over finance are relatively weak. However, by highlighting waste and inefficiency, it can cause the government considerable embarrassment.
- Parliament helps to secure redress for those who have faced problems at the hands of government and the NHS. There is scope for increasing the powers of ombudsmen in this field.
- The House of Lords has played a useful role in scrutinising health policy. It can influence the details of legislation in particular circumstances.
- Only a comprehensive programme of reform will strengthen Parliament and enable it to exercise influence over health policy and hold government more closely to account.

Key questions

1. What factors shape MPs' and peers' interests in health policy?
2. Which parliamentary committees have an interest in health policy?
3. What are the main parliamentary activities used by MPs and peers to raise issues and scrutinise the government's health policies?
4. How effective are select committees in influencing health policy and scrutinising government in this field?
5. Has Parliament become weaker in its ability to influence and scrutinise health policy? If so, why? What can be done to address this?

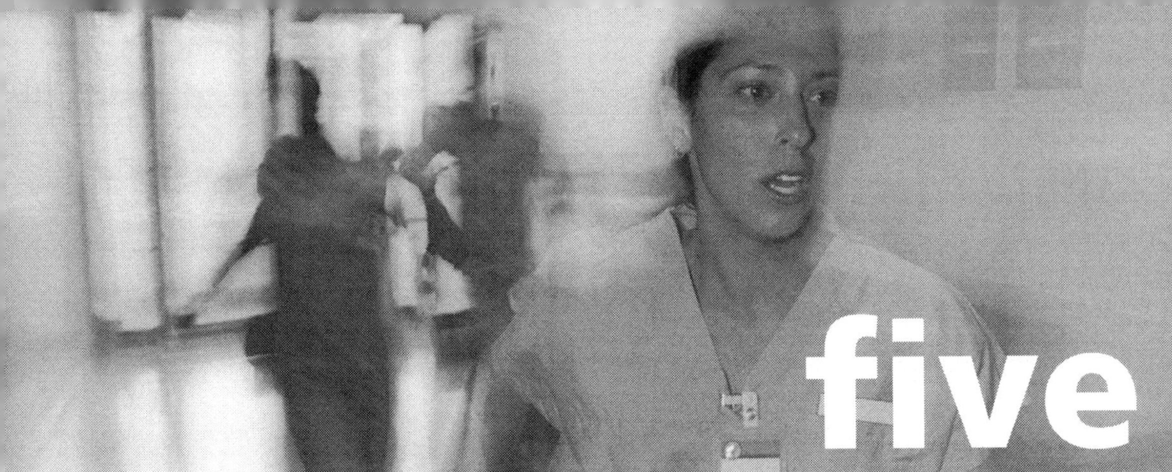

The media and health policy

Overview

This chapter examines the role of the media in the health policy arena. The analysis is divided into three parts. First, media coverage of health and illness is explored. Second, the media's role in the health policy process and its impact on policy is examined. Third, the relationship between the media and other policy actors is analysed.

The media has an important role in the policy process (see Chapter One). It shapes the perception of problems and policies. The media can be manipulated by other policy actors, such as government and pressure groups. But it is also a policy actor in its own right and may influence policy outcomes as well as perceptions.

Media coverage of health and illness

The coverage of health and illness in the media has increased over the last 20 years (Entwhistle and Beaulieu-Hancock, 1992; Ali et al, 2001). Health topics are regarded as particularly newsworthy (see ***Box 5.1***), and are seen by journalists as typical of quality of life issues that will attract the public's interest. The increased coverage of health and illness is also linked to the rise of specialist correspondents in this field, which has extended the media's capacity to report on such activities.

Bias in media attention

Although the media's coverage of health and illness is extensive, some issues receive more attention than others. In the past, several biases have been identified (see Karpf, 1988; Seale, 2002), including:

- an overwhelming concern with hospital-based medicine and technology at the expense of primary and community-based services;
- a preoccupation with 'health scares' at the expense of long-term chronic illness and more serious underlying threats to health; and
- a focus on 'newsworthy' diseases, which do not reflect the actual burden of mortality and morbidity in society.

Stories about health care services are the largest single category in both TV and newspaper health news (Harrabin et al, 2003; Millward Brown, 2004). Hospital news predominates, although increasing coverage is now given to GP and community-based services, public health and alternative therapies (Seale, 2002).

The media tends to concentrate on dramatic health threats, irrespective of the level of risk they pose. To demonstrate this, Harrabin et al (2003) compared the number of deaths in the UK from a particular 'health threat' with the number of news stories on the topic. They found that for every story on smoking reported on BBC News there were 8,571 deaths from smoking-related illness. But for every news item on HIV/AIDS, there were only 19.56 deaths.

Some health issues receive more media attention than others (Henderson and Kitzinger, 1999). One study found that breast cancer received a third of all cancer coverage and was headlined four times as often as other cancers (Saywell et al, 2000). The predominance of breast cancer coverage has been found in other countries (see Clarke and Everest, 2006). The plight of sick children also engages the media (Seale, 2002; Baggott et al, 2005). 'Health scares' such as new infectious diseases are also attractive to journalists (such as SARS (Washer, 2004) and the flesh-eating bug (Gwyn, 1999)).

Interestingly, breast cancer was once a taboo subject that attracted little media attention. Public health issues such as smoking, alcohol abuse and obesity now receive much more coverage than before (Gard and Wright, 2005). Meanwhile, some former 'low-profile' illnesses, such as prostate cancer, bowel disease, stroke and arthritis have received more media attention in recent years, as have traditionally unfashionable topics such as mental health and the care of elderly people. Indeed, recent research (Millward Brown, 2004) found that mental health received the most media attention, followed by cancer, elderly services, heart disease treatment and children's health. This suggests that 'media bias' is not static. The media's desire for new angles and stories may lead to 'neglected' topics being covered. Increased media coverage may also indicate the success of those campaigning for attention for certain conditions and illnesses. It may also reflect new and more favourable circumstances that generate media interest (for example, greater openness about 'taboo' illnesses, or acknowledgement of the consequences of a 'greying population').

Bias in media reporting

The reporting of health issues can reinforce stereotypes and existing assumptions about illness, inhibiting public understanding and the development of appropriate policies. For example, breast cancer, although predominantly a disease affecting older women, is usually portrayed as a threat to much younger women. Charities and consumer groups in this field are concerned about the media's obsession with breast cancer and young women (Baggott et al, 2005; Saywell et al, 2000). More generally, it appears that the media are preoccupied with breast, ovarian and cervical cancer in women, and prostate/testicular cancer in men. This could distort the public perceptions of health risks. Indeed, a study of Canadian/US English-language magazines undertaken in the late 1980s (Clarke, 2004) found that breast cancer and prostate/testicular cancers were closely associated with the respective stereotypes of femininity and masculinity, exacerbating fear of these diseases and diminishing awareness of other, more prevalent causes of death.

According to some, cancer has been portrayed in a way that does not meet with patients' actual experiences. Sontag (1991) argued that the dominant 'military' metaphors of cancer (for example, the battle or fight against cancer) were unhelpful and demoralised patients, justified brutal interventions and stigmatised those diagnosed with the disease. While such metaphors are indeed still evident (Lupton, 1994; Clarke, 1999; Clarke and Everest, 2006), more positive metaphors and coverage by the media have been acknowledged. Seale (2002) found evidence of more positive 'sporting' metaphors and argued that cancer stories (often based on individual experiences) in the media had become more positive.

Media reporting of mental health has been criticised for reinforcing stereotypes. Negative images of mental illness predominate (Lawrie, 2000; Millward Brown, 2004). In particular, the portrayal of mental illness highlights dangerous and psychotic behaviour far more often than chronic mental health problems, even though the former is far less common (Philo, 1996, 1999). This reinforces the stigma of mental illness and possibly discourages people from seeking help. Such coverage may also impact on mental health policy, in ways discussed later.

Another example is childhood illness, which not only attracts media attention, but is covered in a particular way. The vulnerability and helplessness of the child, the heroism of parents and medical staff, the disruption of 'normal' childhood, are all emphasised, and perhaps most seriously, the chances of successful intervention are exaggerated (Seale, 2005). This can produce an unhelpful distortion of reality for sick children and their families, raising expectations, preventing children from participating in their own care and also possibly restricting their activities more than clinically necessary. Some of these features were evident in the Child B case, where a father took a health authority to court for refusing to fund further cancer treatment for his daughter. A study of the media coverage of this case (Entwhistle et al, 1996), found that some (although not all) newspapers focused strongly on the benefits of treatment and ignored the costs – including the possible side-effects of treatment on the child's quality of life. The 'red-top' tabloids in particular, and some broadsheet newspapers, emphasised the importance of giving priority to life-saving treatments for children and constructed the issue largely in terms of a flawed rationing decision based on lack of funds or inappropriate priorities. Some failed to mention that a team of clinicians recommended that further intensive treatment was not in the child's best interests.

Stereotyping also happens to health professionals and producers of health care products and services. There are 'villains' (Seale, 2002), such as the drugs industry and the tobacco companies, and, more recently, the food and alcoholic drinks industries. NHS health authorities, managers and administrators are often depicted as heartless bureaucrats denying services to those in need (see Seale, 2005). They are portrayed as an unnecessary drain on the NHS that prevents resources reaching the 'front line'. Doctors and nurses, meanwhile, tend to get treated as 'heroes' by the media (Karpf, 1988; Seale, 2005) although individual practitioners face vilification when exposed as a danger to the public. In the past, cases of clinical incompetence have been regarded as isolated, and the reputation of medical and nursing professionals as a whole has not been tarnished. However, some perceive a more critical approach by the media in recent years (Ali et al, 2001), which has opened up 'chinks in the medical hero's armour' (Seale, 2002, p 146), leaving practitioners more exposed to media criticism than before. Arguably, the coverage of cases where practitioners have deliberately harmed patients (such as the Shipman and Allitt cases) has also created an atmosphere more conducive to media criticism of health professionals.

What influences media coverage?

Many factors affect the attention given to a topic by the media and shape the way it is reported. To understand this, one has to explore the motivations, values and practices of media organisations and journalists as well as the constraints within which they operate. Media organisations contain many different interests and operate in a complex business environment (Keane, 1991; Newton, 2001). But none can ignore 'newsworthiness'. The bottom-line, even for public service broadcasters such as the BBC, is that they must select and cover news items in such a way that attracts and holds audiences. Although newsworthiness is highly subjective, there is broad agreement on what attracts media interest. These features are listed in ***Box 5.1***.

Box 5.1: Newsworthiness

- The availability of 'visuals' or 'images' that clearly illustrate or attract attention.
- A human interest aspect, if possible portraying actual individuals or families.
- Affects children.
- Potentially wide implications, could affect a large proportion of the population.
- Newness of the story, or at least a new angle on something familiar.
- Unusual, rare occurrence, out of the ordinary event.
- Likely to provoke a strong emotional reaction from most people.
- Raises ethical or moral issues.
- Can be related to current news agenda, perhaps continuing a current story but in a different way.
- Fits in with underlying public preconceptions.
- Involves sex/sexuality.
- Involves a celebrity.
- Could involve a significant future threat to the public.
- Relates to an unpredictable pattern of events that lie ahead.
- Involves an invisible or powerful threat.
- Involves dramatic consequences, in particular, death.
- Involves conflict, crisis or scandal.
- Involves fault or blame.
- Involves new technology or a scientific breakthrough.

Sources: see Karpf, 1988; Bell, 1991; Negrine, 1994; Entwhistle, 1995; Entwhistle and Sheldon, 1999; Franklin, 1999; Gwyn, 1999; Jennings, 1999; Doyle, 2000; Harrabin et al, 2003

Of course, stories do not require all these ingredients in order to be newsworthy. Some media will emphasise some factors over others. The tabloids are more likely to respond to 'sex', 'celebrity' and sensationalist aspects. Nonetheless, this list suggests why certain issues get more media attention than others: breast cancer, new infectious diseases, food safety scares and health care rationing decisions, all score highly against these criteria. The list also indicates why certain issues are treated in a particular way. For example, the relatively few people with violent psychotic disorders who kill are far more newsworthy than the much larger number of people whose lives are seriously disrupted by anxiety and depression.

Journalists and their editors are driven by an urge to entertain as well as inform (Miller and Reilly, 1994). As Seale (2003, p 519) has noted, 'people do not make TV programmes or publish newspapers solely in order to provide the public with accurate health information'. Journalists reject the idea that health reporting must be purely factual and that coverage must be commensurate with actual health risks (Harrabin et al, 2003). As one health correspondent has stated 'we're a business; we are there to make money. To be cynical we are almost a branch of showbiz, we have to entertain, have at least to interest people so they keep shelling out their xp each day' (quoted in Doyle, 2000, p 154). To focus wholly on informing the public might actually be counterproductive and may reduce sales and audience ratings. Ultimately, media organisations (including public service broadcasters) must sell their product and therefore the audience's desire to be entertained cannot be ignored.

There are additional technical pressures and constraints that lead to stories being 'packaged' in a way that oversimplifies them. Cottle (2001) has described how the packaging of news in particular formats, often with a strong influence on visuals, can simplify messages and prevent certain critical and non-mainstream views from being heard. Similarly, Kitzinger (2000) discusses how media templates are used to portray issues in particular, stylised ways to reinforce interpretations, meanings and values. Although these can be reversed for dramatic effect (the classic 'Man bites Dog' story) which may in turn prompt a reinterpretation of an issue, the story is still subject to a process of simplification. The result of packaging and stylisation may be that, as Franklin (1999) has argued, complex issues – and more complicated *treatment* of issues – are pushed off the media agenda. There is much evidence of this in the health field, where stories on mental health (Philo, 1996, 1999), new infectious disease and food safety threats (Miller and Reilly, 1994; Gwyn, 1999; Doyle, 2000; Washer, 2004; King and Street, 2005), sick children (Seale, 2005), and rationing (Entwhistle et al, 1996) have tended to follow a particular style of presentation.

The competitive pressure to entertain, along with technical constraints, impels the media towards simplification, exaggeration, stereotyping and the selection of particular issues over others. However, as Harrabin and colleagues (2003) observed, journalists maintain that they act in the overall public interest when reporting health. Journalists point to examples of where they have acted in the public interest by highlighting NHS scandals and risks to health, and by campaigning on 'neglected' issues – some examples of which are discussed later. It may be that the need to simplify and entertain is counterbalanced by specialist correspondents (Harrabin et al, 2003). These are better informed about health issues and more likely to avoid sensationalism than other journalists (see also ***Box 5.2***).

Interviews with health policy actors identified a decline of investigative reporting and highlighted the distorting effect of the media. Comments included: 'the media lens magnifies issues' (think tank spokesperson); 'the media are mainly interested in scare stories' (peer); 'often the media have their own agenda and only want bad news' (trade unionist); 'it blows some things up while not covering other issues that merit attention' (former senior NHS manager), and 'the media simplifies the health debate. Most journalists don't understand the issues' (NHS management organisation spokesperson). On the other hand, there was some acknowledgement of the quality of specialist health reporting, with several informants praising health correspondents for their efforts to inform the public and to promote rational debate about policy issues and dilemmas.

Box 5.2: AIDS and the media

The level of media interest in HIV/AIDS during the 1980s was high, despite the fact that the disease affected relatively few people at this time (Street, 1988; Day and Klein, 1989; Berridge, 1996; Miller et al, 1998; Seale, 2002). When the disease emerged into the public domain it had several key characteristics that triggered media attention (see ***Box 5.1***). It raised issues of sex and death, both of which are newsworthy in their own right. The manifestation of 'full-blown AIDS' was graphic and highly visible. It afflicted celebrities (the prominent US actor Rock Hudson was an early victim of the disease). It was also a mysterious illness and although numbers currently affected were small, it was seen as posing a potentially catastrophic threat to society.

The media described the disease as a plague, invoking 'gothic horror' symbolism while emphasising military metaphors (Wellings, 1988; Day and Klein, 1989; Sontag, 1991). The disease was initially depicted as a problem affecting homosexual men, a 'gay plague' (see Berridge, 1991). Some argue that this symbolism represented an attempt to moralise about the culture and practices of these and other 'high-risk' groups (including prostitutes, intravenous drug users and some ethnic groups) and demonise them as the cause of the problem (Watney, 1997; Seale, 2002). It was argued that the media tended to attribute blame to these people, while other 'innocent victims' (such as those infected by blood products, babies born to HIV positive mothers, and the families of people with the disease) received compassionate coverage.

Although the initial coverage of AIDS certainly emphasised these aspects, as Berridge (1991, 1996) observed, there were differences between broadcast and non-broadcast media, with the former placing emphasis on the need for a consensual and liberal approach to the issue (the line subsequently taken by the UK government). Berridge points out that the AIDS issue underwent several phases, with the early sensationalist press coverage yielding to a more responsible and informed approach dominated by the broadcast media. Most observers agree that the tabloids were the most 'anti-gay' and discriminatory in their tone, though some (such as the *Daily Mirror*, whose proprietor headed an AIDS charity) were less sensationalist and more sympathetic to gay people. Not all broadsheets took a liberal or enlightened approach, for that matter. Some right-wing broadsheets tailored their message to their conservative readership. Williams (1999) observed conflicts and tensions within media organisations on how to approach the issue, particularly between specialist health and science reporters on the one hand and non-specialist journalists, editors and sub-editors, on the other, with the latter group being more prone to exaggeration and sensationalism. It appears that the issue generated a range of views and accounts in the media and that not all were negative, enabling dissenting voices (notably organisations representing gay men and HIV/AIDS patients) to challenge the way in which the issue was being presented (see Berridge, 1996; Miller et al, 1998; Williams, 1999). Although coverage was initially negative, the media facilitated greater openness in public debates surrounding taboo subjects such as sexuality and sexual practices, not only improving public understanding of such matters but perhaps also producing greater tolerance of minorities (Seale, 2002).

The media impact on AIDS policy is very difficult to assess (see Day and Klein, 1989; Garfield, 1994; Berridge, 1996; Seale, 2002). Public opinion surveys supported discriminatory and punitive action endorsed by most tabloids (Berridge, 1996, p 135). Paradoxically, the government took an enlightened liberal stance, remarkable given the predominance of the new right philosophy in British government during this period, and its emphasis on family values and its links to right-wing Conservative moral pressure groups (Durham, 1991). However, the policy was adjusted to avoid offending these interests – the language of health education campaigns was deliberately toned down and the Prime Minister Margaret Thatcher refused to allow public funding for a survey of sexual lifestyles (Rhodes and Shaughnessy, 1990; Garfield, 1994).

The media successfully raised AIDS to the top of the political agenda by adding to a sense of public panic (Day and Klein, 1989; Williams, 1999). But the more sensationalist tabloids, despite playing a key part in this, were unable to get the government to adopt their discriminatory and authoritarian policy recommendations. Meanwhile, the more measured tone of the liberal press and the broadcast media helped to create an environment whereby the government's actions were less likely to provoke a public backlash. This was facilitated by the use of scientific and medical experts in policy formation and implementation, who also acted as media figures to endorse and justify the measures taken (Garfield, 1994; Berridge, 1996). To some extent this insulated government from pressure from the tabloid press and conservative moral groups (Day and Klein, 1989).

The journalist David Brindle (1999) has argued that the production of news is more chaotic than is realised and journalists have considerable freedom to select issues and report on them. To see them as mere puppets of media organisations is too simplistic (although it is true that proprietors seek to influence content and some are more intrusive than others in this respect).

Over the years, campaigning journalism in the health field has challenged dominant and mainstream views, and has highlighted neglected groups, sometimes in the face of strong commercial opposition. Examples include the Thalidomide case of the 1960s, where *The Sunday Times* exposed the scandal of children severely disabled by a drug taken by their mothers during pregnancy. There was also the series of articles written in the mid-1980s by *The Times* journalist Marjorie Wallace on problems facing people with schizophrenia and their families, which put this particular issue on the political agenda. She later went on to form the pressure group, SANE (Schizophrenia a National Emergency) and remains an active campaigner in this field. Another example, was the major campaign in the late 1990s led by the *Observer* ('The Dignity on the Ward Campaign') highlighting the plight of elderly people in hospital.

Drama

Drama and fictional accounts also shape how issues are perceived by the public, and can have implications for policy (Philo, 1999; Davis, 2005). They can also affect health behaviour. When a character in the popular television drama *Coronation Street* was diagnosed with cervical cancer, the charity CancerBACUP experienced a large increase in calls to its helpline and the number of smear tests rose by a fifth in Manchester alone (Wright, 2003).

The principal function of drama is to entertain. Representations of health issues are therefore tailored to fit the requirements of entertaining storylines and characters in a way which tends to simplify, exaggerate and reinforce stereotypes (Henderson, 1999). Particular attention has been paid to television soaps, regular mass-audience dramas based on the lives of a fictional community. As Seale (2002) has observed, soaps focus on acute illness and on young or middle-aged people with health problems. Deaths among soap characters are higher than in the population at large and tend to be disproportionately violent (Crayford et al, 1997). There is stereotyping of certain types of illness (mental illness), population groups (elderly people) and gender roles (doctors/nurses), reinforcing biases in news media described earlier (Seale, 2002). Even soaps that make strong claims for social realism contain inaccuracies that can distort public perceptions of illness (Henderson, 1999; Philo, 1999). However, dramas can challenge existing stereotypes – as in the *EastEnders* storyline on schizophrenia in the late 1990s (Baggott et al, 2005) – or cover issues that previously have attracted little media attention – such as depression (covered by both *Coronation Street* and *EastEnders* in the past).

While health issues often appear in drama programmes they are obviously central to medical dramas, such as BBC TV's *Casualty*. Such programmes are popular and there is evidence that the public both trust and use information received from these sources (Kingsley, 1993; Davis, 2005). The need to be credible, and to avoid providing misleading information, is particularly important to these programme-makers. Indeed, medical dramas retain clinical advisers, to ensure a level of accuracy. Other programme-makers also consult outside experts when portraying health issues, particularly those of a sensitive or controversial nature. In some cases, notably with regard to HIV/AIDS and mental illness, health consumer and patients' groups have been consulted on scripts (Baggott et al, 2005).

Celebrities and illness

The modern celebrity culture has transformed the media (Sampson, 2004). Although celebrities are not political figures like ministers or MPs, their actions can have a political impact (see ***Box 5.3***). In the health field, celebrities can highlight specific conditions by lending explicit support to a particular health cause or charity. Perhaps the most prominent example was the public support given by the late Princess Diana to the work of HIV/AIDS charities. Celebrity support can, however, be a double-edged weapon. Charities are often worried about celebrities portraying an inappropriate image (Batty, 2001). Also, celebrity support is often unequal, being less evident for stigmatised conditions such as mental illness (Cope, 2002).

Celebrity illness is doubly compelling as both 'celebrity' and 'illness' are newsworthy in their own right (see ***Box 5.1***). When a famous person suffers from a condition, especially a high-profile condition such as breast cancer, media interest is intense, particularly when this person is youthful and vibrant. Hence the media frenzy that followed news of singer Kylie Minogue's breast cancer diagnosis in 2005.

The impact of media coverage of celebrity illness can be enormous. Following the death of Linda McCartney from breast cancer in April 1998, there was a 64% increase in telephone calls to CancerBACUP (Boudioni et al, 1998). Sometimes celebrities galvanise public perceptions of a disease or condition and may campaign to improve research and treatment, as in the cases of the actors Christopher Reeve (paralysed due to a broken neck, now deceased – see Reeve, 2004) and Michael J. Fox (young onset Parkinson's Disease – see Fox, 2002). An American study found that celebrities who talked about their experience of cancer screening helped persuade individuals to attend for tests (Larson et al, 2005). Another found that although celebrity illness could improve public awareness of a condition, it could mislead the public about what should be done to prevent it (Hopkins, 2000). It has been suggested that by focusing on the experience of young female celebrities with breast cancer, the media has misled women about the age-related risks of the disease (Cancer Research UK, 2006). Choice of treatment also may be affected. When Nancy Reagan, the wife of the then US President, had a mastectomy in 1987, the number of women choosing breast-conserving surgery fell by a quarter, although it later returned to baseline levels (Nattinger et al, 1998).

The media and the policy process

Public opinion

One can find other examples where people have responded to media coverage by changing their behaviour in a significant way. For example, extensive media coverage given to research in the late 1990s that suggested a link between the MMR vaccine, autism and chronic inflammatory bowel disease may have misled the public about the balance of scientific evidence. The media focused on the emotive accounts of parents who blamed MMR for their children's illnesses. This fuelled fears about the safety of the vaccine and prompted a fall in MMR immunisations (see Begg et al, 1998; Horton, 2004; Speers and Lewis, 2004). Similarly, periodic health scares about risks associated with the contraceptive pill have prompted women to stop taking the drug, even though the risks associated with consequential pregnancy and abortion are higher (Wellings, 1986; Allison et al, 1997).

The media can foster a climate that encourages policy initiatives, as the following examples indicate. The media coverage of breast cancer has encouraged policy developments (screening, waiting-time targets, funding for new treatments) by helping to install the disease as a top priority for the NHS. ***Box 5.2*** illustrates how sections of the media played a part in creating an atmosphere of consensus for policies on HIV/AIDS. Furthermore, the media portrayal of the NHS as permanently in crisis created a climate for reforms introduced by the Conservative government of the 1980s, and more recently by the Labour government (Harrabin et al, 2003).

The media can also promote public resistance to policies. This 'blocking' or 'veto' aspect to media influence has been identified as an important element in mental health, for example (Rose, 1998; Philo, 1999). It is argued that the media has reinforced an extremely negative view of mental illness among the public, which harbours an exaggerated fear of dangerously mentally ill people. This, coupled with criticism of community-based care, makes it difficult for politicians to pursue a balanced policy in this field, and they are impelled by public safety rather than therapeutic concerns.

Although the media can shape public attitudes, it cannot determine them. As Seale has put it 'audiences may be treated like dupes, but they do not necessarily behave like them' (2002, p 43). Resistance may result from direct personal experience, the identification of contradictions in media accounts, or certain cultural attributes or value systems (Philo, 1999). However, media influence is often subtle and operates not by telling people what to think, but by shaping fundamental assumptions and the way in which issues are comprehended (Eldridge et al, 1999). These assumptions and interpretative frameworks may outweigh personal experience and other factors that promote resistance to media messages.

The media's role in the policy process is strengthened further by the response of policy makers, particularly politicians, to its activities (Harrabin et al, 2003). They regard the media as an important barometer of public opinion, as well as an important influence upon it. Policy makers know that the media can generate debate on issues, which can lead to public pressure. They also acknowledge that media shape public judgements about the effectiveness of government policy and the competence of individual politicians.

The media can exert a subtle effect on policy makers. It can shape policy debates by using particular language and symbolism. For example, an American study of abortion politics illustrated how the media was able to structure the debate in such a way that policy actors had to operate within these constraints in order to be successful (Terkildsen et al, 1998). There are other examples of where the media has developed a policy discourse that defines problems and possible solutions (Miller et al, 1998; King and Street, 2005). With regard to obesity, some have argued that it has deployed 'epidemic/universal threat/crisis/timebomb' terminology to exaggerate the threat (Gard and Wright, 2005). At the same time powerful imagery (in particular the 'fat child/couch potato') is used in such a way that stigmatises people and prioritises certain problems (obese and overweight children) and solutions (ban junk food, increase consumption of fresh fruit, increase exercise and sport), while ignoring other key issues, such as under-nutrition and deprivation among the poor.

Interview data from those involved in the policy process supports the view that the media can influence both public opinion and government agendas. Only a minority of respondents thought that the media could drive the policy agenda, but most believed it strongly influenced the way in which the public thought about health issues and had the ability to push issues up the agenda (see also Doyle, 2000). In the words of one interviewee (an MP), for example, 'they can identify issues which need attention'. Most saw the media as a negative rather than a positive force. Media power was described by some as a 'negative force' and as 'blocking policies'. Others commented that 'it exerts a veto' and that 'it makes it difficult to pursue policies in a particular way'. An ex-civil servant at the DoH commented that 'the media portrays a particular *idée fixe* which prevents policies from being developed', and gave mental health policy as an example. Several interviewees identified the tabloids as a particularly negative force, inhibiting policy options, especially in areas such as public health where government policy had been dominated by a fear of being labelled 'nanny state' by the tabloid press.

Some interviewees noted that the media could have a significant effect on the timing of proposals. A respondent from a health professional organisation commented that the media could slow down the process of reform by highlighting problems with a proposed policy. In other situations, as a policy adviser noted, the efforts of the media could lead to policies being brought forward, in order to reassure the public that something was being done. The result was often an ill-thought-out policy, as one interviewee, from a think tank, commented: 'the media can be pretty destructive forcing government to act in a knee-jerk way'.

Box 5.3: The 'Feed Me Better' campaign

School meals raise important public health issues (see Gustaffson, 2002). Amid public concern about rising obesity levels in children, the Labour government reintroduced minimum standards for school meals in 2001, to encourage the provision of fruit and vegetables. However, problems remained, largely due to the lack of investment in the school meal service, low level of funding for ingredients (an average of 37p for primary schoolchildren), a system of competitive contracting that emphasised low-cost provision and the fact that children – influenced by large-scale advertising and peer pressure – tended to choose junk food.

Little more was done to address the problem until a media campaign in 2005, headed by the celebrity chef, Jamie Oliver, forced the government to improve school meals in England (other parts of the UK having already adopted new policies following devolution). The trigger was Oliver's series 'Jamie's School Dinners', shown on Channel 4 in February 2005. In the show, Oliver set himself the challenge of providing low-cost but nutritious school meals. The series was compelling viewing, illustrating the appalling state of school meals and the magnitude of the task of improving the diets of schoolchildren.

The public reaction to the series sustained the 'Feed Me Better' campaign, which called for higher nutritional standards and more investment in school meals. A website generated 5 million hits and over 270,000 people signed a petition in support of the campaign. The campaign was picked up by TV news and the national press. Other celebrities endorsed the campaign (including sporting figures such as the footballer Frank Lampard and the yachtswoman Ellen MacArthur). The issue was raised in Parliament and an EDM (see Chapter Four) attracted 159 supporters.

The government, which faced a General Election later in the year, was caught off-guard. The Secretary of State for Education, Ruth Kelly, claimed that she was already looking at ways of improving school meals. Prime Minister Tony Blair publicly acknowledged the strength of the campaign and paid tribute to Oliver's efforts. Despite the political clout of private sector contractors, and the junk food industry, the campaign was difficult to oppose. The government responded with a three-year funding package for school meals (£280m – partly subsidised by National Lottery funds) and new mandatory nutritional standards aimed at cutting salt, sugar and fats and increasing fruit and vegetables. It extended school inspections to cover food standards and established an independent school food trust to encourage higher standards in school meals. Subsequently, in response to a follow-up programme on the campaign in 2006, the Prime Minister pledged that he would consider further recommendations from Oliver on how to improve school meals.

Although the new funding could have been more generous (it raised ingredient cost to only 50p per meal in primary schools and 60p in secondary schools), the campaign influenced public opinion and secured a positive response from government. The main factors behind this success were as follows:

- the campaign was led by a well-known celebrity, genuinely committed to doing something about a problem. The involvement of other celebrities added further strength to the campaign;
- the scale of the problem and the response required was clearly demonstrated;
- the issue related to one already on the political agenda – child obesity;
- the campaign used electronic media to engage the public and enlist support;
- the campaign was effectively cascaded to other media outlets, both broadcast and non-broadcast;
- government faced a General Election, and, as the issue concerned many voters, it had to be seen to be doing something about the problem;
- the issue was taken up in Parliament; and
- the campaign was widely supported by pressure groups and public health organisations.

Not all media outlets have the same influence. Interviews with policy actors revealed different judgements about which were the most important. The *Daily Mail* and the 'red-top' tabloids were credited with having the most influence. Of the daily broadsheet papers, only *The Times* was mentioned as having significant influence on health policy, although Sunday papers (tabloids and broadsheets) were seen by some as important in setting the media agenda for the following week. With regard to broadcast media, the agenda-setting role of BBC Radio 4's *Today* programme was mentioned. The BBC was seen as a key 'shaper' of the news agenda. As one policy actor (from a leading research charity) noted, for example, 'the BBC is good at cascading stories'.

Government health policies do not automatically change according to the whim of the BBC, *The Sun* or the *Daily Mail*. Rather it is the way in which one media outlet triggers others, and how this is interpreted by policy makers. As Harrabin et al (2003) commented, 'opinions really start to shift when a story breaks in the newspapers, is taken up by television and radio programmes and carried over to the next day's papers' (p 25). However, these dynamics are not well understood. Rather than being informed by one newspaper or programme, people's experience of the media is fragmentary (Seale, 2003) and they pick up information and meanings in different ways and in various settings (see also Eldridge et al, 1999). On some issues, but perhaps not on others, current media coverage may be able to stimulate public interest on the basis of accumulated understandings and information built up over time. Hence media coverage of the same breadth and intensity may well impact differently on public opinion and policy because of different contexts and circumstances.

Influencing the media

Government influence over the media

The Blair government was not the first to adopt techniques of 'news management' or, as it is more commonly known, 'spin'. Previous governments from the 1960s onwards became increasingly concerned about presentation, and attempted to portray themselves and their policies in a more positive light. However, it is widely acknowledged that the Blair government pursued a particularly robust and systematic approach to media management (see Brindle, 1999; Newton, 2001; Jones, 2002; Harrabin et al, 2003; Oborne and Walters, 2004).

Within government, public relations has become centralised with Number Ten exerting greater control over the government's communications. There has also been an increasing politicisation of government communications, with press and information officers being subjected to stronger pressure from their political masters, who include special advisers as well as ministers. A strong emphasis on 'rapid rebuttal' has been evident, whereby criticisms of government policies or actions in the media are closely monitored and immediately countered, often in an aggressive manner. A closer integration of policy and presentation has been observed, and the need to 'sell' the policy is now recognised as a key factor in its development (Fairclough, 2000; Newton, 2001). Finally, and related to this, it is argued that government seeks to describe policies in increasingly imprecise and simple terms (Fairclough, 2000; Newton, 2001).

These features are particularly evident within health policy, which is not surprising given its attractiveness to the media and its role as a basis for judging the competence of governments. As Entwhistle and Sheldon (1999, p 125) have commented, 'media reports of events in the health service are of key importance to politicians as one of the main currencies of success or failure'. Such concern among politicians is not new. In 1994 the Major government was so concerned about media coverage of the NHS that a senior figure warned (in a leaked memorandum) that 'the best result for the next 12 months would be zero media coverage of the National Health Service' (Beckett and Brown, 1994). It also established a 'good news' health unit to warn ministers of potentially damaging incidents and counter adverse publicity about the NHS.

Since 1997, the management of health issues in the media has been strengthened. A new rapid rebuttal system was introduced into the DoH and attacks on the government's handling of the NHS were monitored and vigorously challenged (Jones, 2002). This led to a direct attack on media coverage, as in November 2000 when Downing Street criticised the BBC for exaggerating claims about a forthcoming crisis of capacity in the NHS (Laurance and Grice, 2000). However, government 'spin' in relation to health policy has been criticised (see, for example, BBC TV, 2000). The DoH spends over £50m a year on publicity and advertising (although this includes spending on health promotion campaigns). It employs former journalists and PR experts to get its message across. The DoH has explored how coverage of health policy issues can be more favourable and less adverse. It has commissioned research to identify which media correspondents had the most impact and whether they were positive or negative in their coverage (see Millward Brown, 2004). There has also been an attempt to bring policy and presentation closer together. Policy documents – notably Green and White Papers – are now more like brochures. They are glossy in appearance, use attractive images and pictures but place less emphasis on explaining policy options and decisions and are thin on background evidence. Furthermore, there is careful management of information from the DoH, from health agencies and the NHS in order to minimise criticism of policy.

Individual complaints about alleged neglect, maltreatment or service failure taken up by the media are now firmly rebutted by government. The Rose Addis case (Jones, 2002) was an example of how issues are now managed. The family of this elderly lady complained that she had been left unwashed and neglected in the Accident and Emergency unit at the Whittington Hospital in London. Her case was taken up by opposition politicians and by the media. However, the DoH and the NHS trust concerned challenged the details of the case – implying that the patient and her family were not telling the truth and that the patient had been unwilling to accept treatment from ethnic minority staff. The trust subsequently denied any allegations of racism against Mrs Addis. Even so, its rebuttal strategy successfully countered the initial adverse publicity by undermining the credibility of the allegations.

More generally, the government has used performance targets and data to counter allegations of service failures and shortcomings. The achievement of targets, although crude and sometimes counterproductive, has been cited as evidence that the government's reforms are working and that cases suggesting the opposite are merely anecdotal. Government has also moved quickly to counter criticism in relation to its 'flagship' policies, such as PFI, foundation trusts and patient choice, including that from within the Labour Party itself

Pressure groups

Professions, health consumer and patients' groups, voluntary organisations, single issue groups and corporate interests are all keen to shape the way in which issues are portrayed. According to Karpf (1988), media discourse of health matters is dominated by medical definitions and perceptions. She argued that this was still the case, despite the greater diversity of media reporting, associated with the rise of lay perspectives, for example. Since she wrote, these trends have become stronger. Media coverage of medicine today is more critical (Gabe et al, 1991; Bury and Gabe, 1994; Seale, 2002). There is greater scope for expressing alternative views in the media, including lay perspectives (Entwhistle and Sheldon, 1999).

Although medical concepts and perspectives are more open to challenge today, professional organisations – such as the BMA and the Royal Colleges – remain active in seeking to influence the media. These organisations are well-resourced and skilled in media relations. They are also proactive, and do not simply respond to stories already in the media. For example, the BMA is regarded as 'an active source for stories' (health correspondent, quoted in Doyle, 2000). According to several policy participants, journalists often turn to the BMA for potential stories and for scientific advice on medical issues. Other NHS 'producer' groups also place great importance on influencing the media, including trade unions (such as UNISON) and groups representing NHS organisations (such as the NHS Confederation).

Interviewees from such groups indicated the importance of good relations with the media. The media was perceived as an important forum for advancing policy ideas, opposing policies, for portraying their members in a positive light and countering negative stereotypes. When seeking to influence the media, there are apparently no simple rules. As noted earlier, some programmes and newspapers are seen as particularly important in cascading stories. However, most organisations prefer a 'blunderbuss' approach, rather than targeting only a few media outlets. To concentrate on too few is risky as it could mean the story is not reported at all.

Others argue that patients have a stronger presence in the media nowadays and can exert greater influence than previously. Seale (2002), for example, has observed that the media identifies lay heroes and sponsors consumer power, including 'victims' of medical mistakes and 'survivors' of serious illnesses. The consumer/patient voice is heard more strongly and this is to some extent down to greater openness in the media to alternative and lay perspectives on health (Entwhistle and Sheldon, 1999) and its more critical approach to medicine and producer groups. It is also partly due to the 'halo effect' of the voluntary sector (Lloyd, 2001) and charities (Deacon, 1999), which increasingly claim to represent patient and carer interests.

Stronger advocacy by organisations representing patients and consumers, including charities and voluntary organisations, has had an impact. These groups have correctly perceived the importance of the media in raising awareness about medical conditions, their role in portraying health and illness, and as a means of influencing government policy (Baggott et al, 2005). Groups representing patients, users and carers have extensive contact with the media – in 1999 just under half reported being in contact at least once a month.

Groups representing patients, users and carers try to change media images of illness. For example, MIND and other mental health groups and professional organisations have been extremely critical of media coverage (Philo, 1996). An organisation – Mental Health Media – was established to challenge media stereotypes in this field. Similarly, the Stroke Association has tried to correct negative stereotypes about the condition, in particular the negative images associated with decline and old age. As noted in ***Box 5.2***, HIV/AIDS campaigners influenced the media coverage of this issue. But, as Baggott et al (2005) found in their study, many groups find it difficult to counteract media stereotypes. Often the media have a particular agenda or angle on a story that is not negotiable. As noted earlier, health consumer and patients' groups complain about the media's reinforcement of the inaccurate image that young women are disproportionately at risk from breast cancer. But if groups do not comply with media demands and requirements, they may forfeit opportunities to raise awareness about the condition. As one mental health group (quoted in Baggott et al, 2005, p 280) stated 'because you're so desperate to get the coverage, you'll just do whatever they say'.

Commercial interests also strive to influence the media. The pharmaceutical and medical technology industries have a profit motive to shape the perception of health issues and policies (Collier, 1989; Moynihan, 1998; Moran, 1999; Ferner, 2005). Their profitability depends heavily on funding for research and development and ultimately on the funding of health care services. It is in their interests for the media to adopt an uncritical approach to medical technologies and drugs.

The Health Committee (2005) concluded that a climate has been fostered where drug therapies are the intervention of choice. Medicines take up a large and increasing slice of the NHS budget (11% in 2004). In the management of depression, for example, drug therapies have been adopted in preference to other interventions (such as counselling) despite concerns about their relative efficacy, efficiency and safety. Drugs companies have been able to control the flow of information about their products, and have even suppressed adverse research findings (Health Committee, 2005). In addition, they have massive promotional budgets to shape the preferences of clinicians and the public (approximately £1.65 billion in the UK in 2004 (Health Committee, 2005, p 58)). Although direct to consumer advertising of drugs is not currently permitted in the European Union, the industry can still impact on the public through influence over professionals and by promoting public awareness of diseases and drug treatments (Moynihan et al, 2002; O'Donovan and Glavanis-Grantham, 2003). Moreover, as the Health Committee (2005) noted, a major part of promotional activities involves working with journalists and patients' groups.

A similar situation is found in relation to medical technology, where equipment such as scanners and screening techniques are promoted without much consideration for alternative approaches that might be more cost-effective. In many cases, the adoption of new techniques is not simply due to lobbying by manufacturers, but an alliance with professionals who want to get their hands on the latest equipment. In addition, health consumer and patients' groups, charities and journalists can be useful allies in the fight for approval of techniques and resources to fund them.

The media tends to portray medical technology in an positive light and to emphasise the benefits rather than the costs of these technologies (Karpf, 1988; Moynihan, 1998; Entwhistle and Sheldon, 1999). Nonetheless, the media is unable to resist negative stories about drugs and other technologies, even when faced with the possibility of legal action and other threats from large corporations. It is doubtful that any of the major drug scandals would have seen the light of day had it not been for the efforts of journalists and the courage of their editors (notably, in the Thalidomide affair mentioned earlier). Despite their huge economic and political power, the drugs industry has a persistent bad image, uncorrected by the large amount of money spent on promotion, marketing and public relations.

Other industries have an interest in health policy. The food, alcoholic drink and tobacco companies have been identified as major culprits in some of today's main public health problems, including obesity, food poisoning, chronic alcohol-related disease, alcohol-related accidents and injuries, lung cancer and heart disease. These are profitable industries, and have an incentive to oppose policies that reduce their commercial freedoms (for example, bans on promoting their products).

These industries are highly politicised. They fund organisations that undertake 'socially responsible' activities (such as the Portman Group, financed by the drinks industry). They fund massive PR operations to combat adverse media coverage and promote a more positive image. In addition, the promotion of their products builds customer loyalty and shapes wider public perceptions about the legitimacy of products and, in particular, their benefits and harms. Furthermore, as large advertisers, they are able to put pressure on commercial media outlets covering health issues related to their products.

Although the various interests that shape media portrayal of health are distinct, they rarely operate in isolation. Health issues are usually propelled into the media by combined activity of professional, consumer and business interests (Moynihan, 1998; Baggott et al, 2005; Health Committee, 2005). For example, demands for action on prostate cancer have been articulated by a coalition of charities, patients' groups and clinicians' organisations including the British Association of Urological Surgeons, CancerBACUP, Cancer Research UK, the Prostate Cancer Charity, the Men's Health Forum and the Prostate Research Campaign. At the same time the medical technology companies and drugs companies in this field have lobbied for more resources to be allocated to the prevention and treatment of the disease. In another case, Attention Deficit Hyperactivity Disorder was propelled onto the agenda by parents' organisations, experts and drugs companies all of which had an interest in pushing for medical diagnoses and treatment (Lloyd and Norris, 1999). Coalitions also seek to influence the portrayal of issues already on the agenda. Hence, as noted earlier, mental health user groups and clinicians have united to campaign against the negative images prevalent in this area.

There is nothing intrinsically wrong with such coalitions of interest. But there may be situations where 'resource poor' groups are exploited by those with plenty of resources. It has been claimed that some health consumer and patients' organisations, for example, are too reliant on drugs companies and/or professional interests (see Moynihan, 1998; Hogg, 1999; Baggott et al, 2005) and that this could affect their independence. Similarly, there are dangers in assuming that 'front' organisations funded by the food, alcohol and tobacco industries are actually independent. Clearly, links between organisations need to be transparent – and well publicised in the media – in order to ensure that the public is not misled.

Conclusion

It is clear from this analysis that in health policy, as in other areas of public policy that attract media and public attention, the media cannot be ignored. However, its role in health policy is complex. As Eldridge and colleagues (1999) have noted, the media is not a single ideological conspiracy, nor does its power exist in a social vacuum. The media is both a means of describing and making sense of policy issues and a force for shaping policy (Terkildsen et al, 1998; King and Street, 2005). It has its own interests, but it also used by other interests, including government, to portray issues in particular ways and to support or oppose policies. The influence of the media tends to be indirect and involves other policy actors such as pressure groups, government agencies and Parliament.

In health policy, there is much evidence that the media is more effective as a negative force or veto power. This reflects the situation in other areas of public policy (Newton, 2001). Although instances can be found where the media has been used to exert direct and positive influence on decision making, as in the case of the 'Jamie Oliver' school meals campaign, such examples are fairly rare. Usually, the media operates at a more subtle level, helping to define and reinforce particular meanings and values, constructing issues and shaping agendas.

Summary

- Media coverage of health issues is extensive, and health issues are particularly newsworthy.
- The coverage of health issues in the media contains significant biases. Some diseases and conditions receive more (and more positive) coverage than others.
- Drama, not just news, can shape public perceptions of health and illness. Celebrities can also have an impact on public perceptions.
- The media can influence public opinion, which can affect both health behaviour and policy.
- The media is regarded mainly as a negative force, blocking policies, rather than a driver of the policy agenda. However, it can prompt government intervention by highlighting problems.
- Government seeks to influence media coverage of health policy issues and these efforts have increased in recent years.
- Pressure groups also seek to influence the media, including professional and producer groups, commercial organisations, charities and health consumer and patients' groups.

Key questions

1. What factors make a health issue 'newsworthy'?
2. Why do some health issues get more favourable coverage in the media than others?
3. How does the media influence the public perception of health issues?
4. How does the media influence health policy?
5. Why do (a) the government, and (b) pressure groups seek to influence the media?

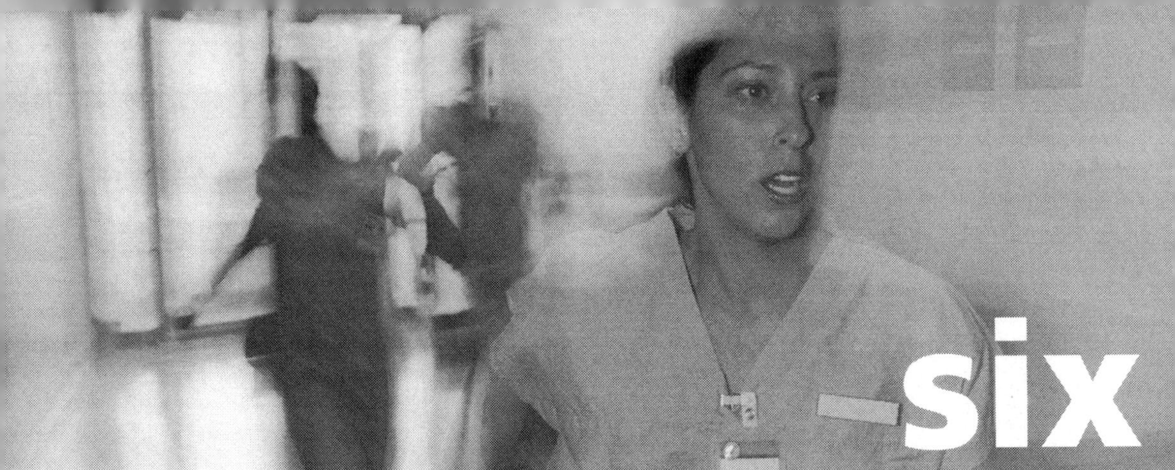

Pressure groups and health policy

Overview

The health policy area is host to a range of pressure groups, including professional and labour organisations, think tanks and research bodies, commercial organisations, voluntary groups and charities. This chapter examines their interaction with governing processes and institutions, their strategies and tactics, and discusses those factors which enable them to exert influence over health policy.

As noted in Chapter One, policy can be seen as a process of interaction between various pressure groups, interests and government. From this perspective, groups and government form networks, which shape policy in specific fields such as health. Many different groups are engaged in seeking to influence health policy (see, for example, Wall and Owen, 2002). These are now examined, along with the various lobbying tactics they use, and the resources that help them to exert influence.

Pressure groups in health

Professional and labour groups

The medical profession

Over the past century, the medical profession has exerted strong influence over health policy. Its influence increased further during the second half of the twentieth century, due in part to the 'concordat' between the profession and the state on the NHS (Klein, 1995; Salter, 1998). This allowed the state to nationalise health care to bring it to a wider population, while the medical profession secured both autonomy and influence within the decision-making process. In addition, the medical profession possessed considerable political resources, including specialist expertise and knowledge, high social status, excellent political contacts and strong representative institutions. Indeed, the doctors' 'trade union', the BMA, gained a reputation as one of the most effective pressure groups in the country, while the prestigious Royal Colleges of Medicine, which accredit specialists and represent their interests, could rely on the 'old boy network' to gain access to the highest levels of government. Meanwhile, the General Medical Council (GMC), with its responsibilities for medical regulation, standards of practice and the quality of medical education, continued to guard the privileges of professional autonomy.

Medical influence took a number of forms. The representative bodies of the profession – in particular the BMA – were enmeshed in the policy process and consulted extensively (see Eckstein, 1960). Indeed, the relationship between the DoH and the BMA was described by Klein (1990) as 'the politics of the double bed'. Until the 1970s, the relationship was close and consensual. Occasionally, open conflict occurred. For example, there was a major dispute over GP pay and conditions in the mid-1960s, where doctors threatened mass resignations from the NHS. However, despite a 'repetitive cycle of confrontation' conflict was constrained and managed through an 'engineered consensus' (Klein, 1990). The medical profession also exerted influence through advisory mechanisms established by the DoH, in which doctors participated. Medical civil servants working for the DoH, including the CMO, were an important channel of influence (see Chapter Three).

During the 1970s, the consensual approach began to unravel, evident in the dispute with the medical profession over pay beds, discussed in Chapter Two. Conflicts intensified under the Thatcher premiership. Her hostility to the public sector brought confrontation with doctors on issues such as NHS spending, GP contracts, restrictions on prescribed medicines and health service reorganisation. The government's relationship with the BMA deteriorated and, at times, degenerated into open hostility.

Routine contact between the DoH and the medical profession's representatives continued during this period. As one civil servant remarked, 'the relationship never foundered, there was never a situation in which we weren't talking to one another … conversations still took place but on a rather more distant basis than has been the case previously' (McGregor-Riley, 1997a). Even so, the BMA was frustrated, believing that its advice was being ignored (see Lee-Potter, 1997). Relationships between the professional organisations and the DoH varied according to the approach of each Secretary of State. Kenneth Clarke's style as Conservative Secretary of State in the late 1980s was particularly confrontational and his leadership at the department marked a low point in relationships between the profession and the government (Ham, 2000).

During the 1990s, the Major government adopted a more conciliatory approach towards the BMA and the profession at large, and the traditional approach of 'mutual accommodation' was to some extent restored (Day and Klein, 1992). Following the departure of Clarke, subsequent Secretaries of State pursued a more consensual approach. Even so, relationships with the BMA never returned to their former intimacy. Indeed, DoH-initiated contacts with the BMA declined in the early 1990s along with the number of formal meetings between the two organisations (Baggott and McGregor-Riley, 1999).

The election of the Blair government was heralded as a fresh start (Webster, 1998). Initial signs were good, with new reforms introduced in an atmosphere of consensus. Dialogue between the government and both the BMA and the Royal Colleges became more cordial. Relationships with the GMC were more fraught, however, as the government made clear its intentions to strengthen medical regulation in the light of several scandals including the Bristol case (see Irvine, 2003). The BMA gradually became disillusioned with the Blair government. Although delighted with increases in NHS funding, it complained about doctors' workloads and the pace of the government's modernisation agenda. It was angry with Blair for identifying the organisation as one of the 'forces of conservatism' blocking public services reform. As the government's reforms evolved, drawing on some of the market-oriented proposals adopted by the Conservatives in the 1980s and 1990s, the BMA became even more hostile.

Some of the policy participants interviewed saw this as an indicator that the BMA had become weaker and lost influence in recent years. For example, a policy adviser stated that 'the BMA has for the most part been marginalised ... it has been powerless for most of this period'. However, others believed it remained a big player and retained influence over government. In the words of a former DoH civil servant, for example, it 'remains a potent force'. The Royal Colleges appear to have consolidated their position, with the Royal College of Physicians regarded as particularly influential by some interviewees (see also Sheard and Donaldson, 2006). Other Royal Colleges, including the Surgeons and the Paediatricians, are also believed to have increased their influence. This is attributed to the effective leadership of these organisations and their willingness to work constructively with the government. As one informant stated, 'the Royal Colleges tend to play along with government'. Unlike the BMA, they are reluctant to challenge the government in public.

Meanwhile, other opportunities for medical influence have arisen. The Blair government identified key priority areas, subject to explicit service standards in the form of national service frameworks (NSFs) and clinical leadership in the form of national service directors (or czars, see Chapter Three). NSF processes are dominated by doctors, although other policy actors are represented, such as health consumer bodies and patients' groups (Hogg, 1999; Baggott et al, 2005). Meanwhile the czars (mostly drawn from the medical profession) have been a key channel for medical influence (Edwards and Fall, 2005). One interviewee noted that 'they have enormous influence … and provide a further route through which professional groups and other pressure groups can influence policy'. These channels have to some extent compensated for the reduced influence of medical civil servants over policy in recent years (see Chapter Three).

The supremacy of the medical profession as a political force has been challenged, both in the UK and elsewhere (Wilsford, 1991; Moran, 1999; Harrison and Ahmad, 2000; Hartley, 2002). The policy arena has become more crowded and doctors' organisations have not found it easy to dominate the health policy process, although they still retain considerable influence over policy (Haywood and Hunter, 1982; Moran, 1999). Increasingly, they share access with representatives of other professional groups such as nurses, managers and other health workers, as well as organisations representing patients and users, the voluntary sector, commercial interests and single issue campaigners.

Some interviewees felt that the medical profession as a whole had experienced a serious loss of influence in recent years. One, from a think tank, stated that the profession had taken 'a real battering'. However, most believed that the medical profession had retained considerable influence over policy, despite having lost ground. Some pointed out that medical influence was evident from the outcomes of recent negotiations over doctors' contracts, widely perceived as favourable to their financial interests. It was felt that government was still concerned about the 'public voice' of the doctors. According to a former civil servant, for example, 'doctors are still seen as powerful by ministers and civil servants'.

The medical profession continues to exert much influence over the public. Despite recent scandals and an increase in patient assertiveness, trust in the medical profession remains high. The media still adopts a broadly favourable view of the medical profession and the BMA is regarded as very effective in dealing with the media (see Chapter Five). The profession influences how we think about health care and its power remains entrenched in health care institutions, and in the values of the health care system. According to Alford's model, mentioned in Chapter One, the dominant professional monopoly interest can maintain its supremacy by way of its ability to define the values of the health care system, its professional status and knowledge, and its control over the supply of professional services. This has been challenged in recent years by the corporate rationalisers – the bureaucratic, corporate and managerial interests that seek greater accountability and efficiency in health services – and to an extent by community interests, but nonetheless medicine retains its overall pre-eminence as a structural interest (see Harrison, 2001).

Nurses

When the NHS was created, nurses were excluded from policy formation and decision-making machinery (Hart, 2004). In the intervening years, nursing has become a more vociferous lobby. Nurses have campaigned on pay and conditions and have sought to improve their professional status through improvements to education and training and by seeking to extend their role in health care (Sibbald et al, 2004; McKee et al, 2006). There have been significant achievements – the creation of a pay review body in the 1980s and the Project 2000 reforms, which raised the status of nurse education and training. Moreover, recent reforms have emphasised nursing skills and knowledge (for example, NHS Direct, Walk-in Centres, nurse prescribing) and have created new posts for higher qualified nurses (nurse consultants, nurse practitioners, clinical nurse specialists and modern matrons). Some, however, believe that these changes have actually undermined nurses' political influence by further fragmenting the profession, creating an elite of qualified and advanced level nurses and removing the protection previously afforded to nursing by the medical profession (Salter, 1998). It has also been argued that other government policies have posed a direct threat to nurses' interests, such as the introduction of internal markets in health care, privatisation and the growth of managerialism in the NHS (Salter, 1998; Hart, 2004)

Nurses do possess a number of resources within the policy process. They are the largest section of the workforce, and have much public support. Acknowledgement of the extended role of nurses has placed a premium on their knowledge and expertise and they are now consulted more extensively on policy issues. Government has realised that many reform initiatives depend on political and practical cooperation from nurses' organisations. Although nurses' representatives are now more involved in policy discussions, their influence remains weak relative to the medical profession (Hart, 2004).

Several interviewees commented on nurses and the policy process. It was noted that the Royal College of Nurses (RCN) had a succession of high-profile leaders regarded by other policy actors as 'good operators' in relation to government and the media. UNISON, which represents a broader range of public service workers, was also credited with raising the profile of issues relevant to nurses. However, leadership of the nursing profession as a whole was regarded as problematic. Nursing remains a fragmented profession and therein lies its weakness. As Hart (2004, p 201) has written 'the division and lasting enmity between nursing's trade unions and professional associations is almost unique in British labour history'. More recently, the RCN and UNISON have begun to move closer together, but still have different perspectives on key issues (Hart, 2004).

In summary, nursing organisations participate in the networks that shape policy, but do not have the same quality of access as doctors on the most important issues. They represent a large and important professional group but lack real 'clout'. Nurses are popular with the public, so government does not welcome an open fight with them. But they have gained comparatively little and what has been achieved is somewhat 'double-edged' in that it may undermine unity, and ultimately the strength of the profession within the policy process.

Managers

The growth in managerialism within the NHS during the 1980s and 1990s strengthened managers' status in the eyes of government. However, they lacked public support partly because of their poor media image, which persists today (see Chapter Five). While senior NHS managers have exerted influence over policy as individuals (see Edwards and Fall, 2005), they have lacked a powerful collective voice. The Institute of Health Service Management (IHSM), which had quite a high profile on policy matters some years ago, is not as prominent now (and has been rebadged as the Institute of Healthcare Management, focusing more on professional standards). In contrast, the NHS Confederation, which represents statutory NHS authorities such as strategic health authorities, PCTs and trusts (that is, management bodies rather than managers), is perceived as more active than its predecessors (the National Association for Health Authorities, and the National Association for Health Authorities and Trusts) on policy matters.

According to interviewees from within the policy process, after an initial period of distrust, the Blair government began to involve the NHS Confederation more closely in policy development. It is seen as in tune with the government's reform agenda and is credited with 'having the ear of ministers', according to one insider. Another respondent commented that it had 'grown enormously in stature' in recent years. A former NHS manager stated that its success was partly due to a favourable political context, which facilitated the influence of managerial interests. It was to some extent pushing at an open door. However, others attributed the rise of the organisation to good leadership, clever tactics and effective political contacts. Some informants, in contrast, argued that the NHS Confederation was too pliant. In the words of one former DoH civil servant it is regarded as being 'in bed with government'. Another, from a health think tank, stated that it was 'now almost an arm of government'. Even those that disagreed with this view acknowledged that the

NHS Confederation's broad support for government policies could sometimes put it in a difficult position. But as one respondent, from the organisation itself, stated, this did not prevent it from being critical when necessary. As this respondent went on to observe, 'the trick is to walk the line between being critical enough but not so as to be cast into the outer darkness'.

Other professions and health workers

It is impossible to examine in detail all the different professional and labour groups that have an interest in health policy. Other professional organisations engaged in the policy process include the dentists' and pharmacists' associations, and organisations representing midwives and therapists. Other staff members are represented by trade unions such as UNISON, which speaks for a range of NHS employees including nurses, midwives, health visitors and health care assistants. These and many other organisations are actively involved in seeking to influence policy and engage with government, Parliament and the media.

Commercial interests

The drugs industry

The drugs industry has a major interest in health policy. The NHS is an important 'customer' for the drugs industry and health policy decisions can affect both sales and profits. Moreover, many aspects of the industry are regulated by government, including safety and marketing. The industry is also affected by government policy in areas such as science and technology, research and development and trade/industry matters. This brings an added incentive to engage in the policy process. Furthermore, as multinational corporations, drugs companies are active in the European and international policy processes (see Chapter Ten).

The drugs industry is economically and politically powerful. It is one of the most successful manufacturing sectors (Pharmaceutical Industry Competitiveness Task Force, 2001). It is a major exporter (with a positive trade balance of £2 billion per annum), a significant employer (60,000 direct employees), a major contributor to research and development spending (£2.85 billion in 1999), and makes a significant contribution to tax revenues. These factors give it economic leverage, which, coupled with excellent political contacts, makes it an extremely powerful political force. The industry is well-connected in government and it is sponsored and regulated by the same department (the DoH), with which has had a good relationship. It has good parliamentary links and employs former civil servants who are knowledgeable about the corridors of power. It has strong links with researchers and other professionals who advise government on policy and regulatory matters. Furthermore, it has built relationships with charities, health consumer bodies and patients' groups representing the interests of patients, users and carers (Baggott et al, 2005).

The drugs industry has a rather sinister public image (Collier, 1989; Moynihan, 1998; Abraham, 2002). Its primary motive is to make profits, and although it is not necessarily against the public interest, there are instances where the industry has clearly acted against this (Health Committee, 2005). Such activities include: targeting of health professionals with marketing, sponsorship and inducements; selective publication of research findings on the efficacy of drugs and in some cases suppression of evidence on side-effects; use of patients, professionals and the media to 'market' illness and drug treatments, a process labelled as 'disease mongering' (Moynihan, 1998 – see also Chapter Five). It is believed that the industry exerts undue influence over regulators as well as prescribers and patients. Indeed, the regulatory regime has been criticised for being captured by the industry and not acting fully in the public interest (Abraham, 2002; Health Committee, 2005). Individual cases, where drugs have been later found to have been associated with adverse events (including Thalidomide, Opren, Seroxat and Vioxx), have exposed the industry and its practices to wide media coverage and have undermined its public image (Collier, 1989; Health Committee, 2005).

Interviews conducted with policy actors, including from the industry, indicate that it remains a formidable player in the health policy arena. There was disagreement, however, on the extent of its power. Most believed that the industry remained influential. For example, it was described by one senior parliamentarian as having 'a lot of clout' and being 'a strong lobbyist'. Another, from a think tank, believed 'its contribution to economy gives it considerable influence'. Other respondents commented that the industry was 'listened to closely by ministers' and had 'good relationships with government'. However, some interviewees thought that the industry's influence had waned since the late 1990s. A former DoH civil servant commented that 'the industry's influence is exaggerated'. The introduction of NICE – to provide guidance on the cost-effectiveness of treatments including medicines – was believed to have moderated its influence. The Blair government was also seen as adopting a more adversarial approach on several issues – notably on drug pricing – creating tensions in the relationship with the industry (see also Kay, 2001). On the other hand, a number of respondents believed that the relationship between the DoH and the industry was too cosy and were particularly critical of the department's dual role, as both regulator and sponsor of the industry. A similar point was made by the Health Committee (2005), which recommended that the responsibility for promoting the interests of the industry should be moved to a more suitable department, namely the DTI.

The private health industry

The creation of the NHS left a 'rump' of private operators within the British health care system. However, private health care expanded from the 1970s onwards partly due to uncertainties surrounding the future of NHS pay beds. Additional opportunities arose from favourable conditions created by the Thatcher government, which wished to see a flourishing private sector. Subsequently, the Blair government encouraged the private sector by promoting competition and plurality of supply in NHS services (see Chapter Eight).

The private health sector is diverse. Paradoxically, despite having unprecedented market opportunities, domestic private health operators have struggled. The real beneficiaries of recent policy developments have been the large insurance companies (which offer health insurance as part of a wider portfolio of products) and private health care providers from overseas, including companies from Sweden, Germany, South Africa and the US, which now run independent sector treatment centres.

Little is known about how exactly these overseas-based organisations have influenced policy. They appear to have been pushing at an open door. The Blair government was desperate to expand capacity following ambitious targets set out in the NHS Plan and saw overseas operators as part of this solution. Nonetheless, it stretches credibility to believe that these providers did not encourage the adoption of policies that directly benefited them. Moreover, overseas operators now have a platform, as producers of NHS services, which they can use to shape further initiatives. As Pollock (2004, p 80) observed, 'with each new insertion of private provision into the NHS, the political clout of the private sector increases'. In contrast, the domestic private health care sector has lacked influence in recent years. Indeed, several informants from the health arena confirmed that the UK-based operators have been fairly uninfluential compared with the overseas operators.

There is now something of a 'revolving door' between government and the private health sector. Executives from the private sector have been seconded to the DoH to work on issues such as PFI and IT. Meanwhile, the private sector employs former government personnel. For example, Simon Stevens after leaving his post as Prime Minister's adviser on health in 2004, joined United Health Europe, a subsidiary of a US health corporation (Lister, 2006). The private health sector has good links with Parliament and works closely with several MPs (including former ministers), some of whom are retained as advisers.

Other private contractors and suppliers

The NHS has always depended on commercial suppliers. Medical equipment, instruments and devices are manufactured by private companies. This includes products ranging from expensive scanners through to small disposable items, such as syringes. The medical equipment industry is large, consisting of 1,800 companies and is worth £4.5 billion per annum (DoH, 2004b). The government acknowledged its importance by establishing a joint industry–government task force to explore issues of mutual interest, including market access, international trade, research and development and regulatory matters.

Other private contractors have also benefited from policies that have given them additional business. These include management consultancies, marketing agencies and providers of 'outsourced' services (which began with the Conservative government's contracting-out policy in the 1980s – see Chapter Two). The Blair government encouraged private sector involvement in the building and maintenance of health care facilities, again building on the policies of its Conservative predecessor. Public–private partnerships (PPPs), and in particular the private finance initiative (PFI), have created huge opportunities for the private sector (see Chapter Eight). Moreover, PPP/PFI consortia, given the profitability of these schemes, have an incentive to lobby for more contracts in the hospital sector and other parts of the health service. The influence of PFI firms and other contractors over health policy was noted by some interviewees. One, for example, commented that 'PFI players have been very influential' (think tank spokesperson). Another, a trade unionist, stated that 'PFI-related commercial interests are influential, as are management consultants and private supply agencies'.

Commercial interests and public health

Many industries have an interest in minimising the impact of health policies on their businesses. One of the classic examples is the tobacco industry, which has tried to resist measures to curb smoking. The impact of other industries on health is more complex. The food industry plays an essential part in maintaining a healthy population, but certain practices, such as the marketing of high fat/salt/sugar products (particularly to children), mass production techniques and the use of harmful additives pose a threat to health (see Baggott, 2000; Nestle, 2003; Health Committee, 2004). The industry has defended its practices and sought to minimise public fears (see Chapter Five). More recently, it is currently working with government on initiatives to improve the nation's diet, although the outcome of this is as yet unclear. The alcoholic drinks industry (see ***Box 6.1***) is in a similar position. Its products are not necessarily harmful, although their misuse seriously undermines public health.

Box 6.1: The political influence of the drinks industry

Historically, the alcoholic drinks industry has been regarded as a potent political force. When, in Victorian and Edwardian times, the drink question became a major issue of national politics, the industry successfully defended its interests (see Greenaway, 2003). Although facing a mass campaign by the Temperance movement and a succession of hostile Liberal governments, the industry had friends in Parliament and was particularly influential within the Conservative Party. It was the imposition of wartime controls in World War One (under a Liberal Party leadership) that eventually forced the industry to concede on many crucial matters of policy (such as the reduction of licensing hours).

In recent times, alcohol problems are once again on the political agenda. In the 1970s, concerns about the rising levels of alcohol consumption, voiced by professional groups, voluntary organisations and statutory authorities in policing, criminal justice, health and social welfare – coupled with wider public disquiet articulated in the media – led the then Labour government to formulate an alcohol strategy. But the industry successfully lobbied against this, and the policy was significantly weakened (Baggott, 1990).

In the past decade, these concerns resurfaced around 'binge drinking' and associated late-night public disorder in cities and towns. Pressure on government to tackle this problem led to an alcohol strategy for England (Prime Minister's Strategy Unit, 2004). This was criticised for ignoring evidence on interventions that could reduce overall consumption (such as taxation and controls on availability – see Babor et al, 2003) and for giving a drinks industry organisation, the Portman Group, a key role in implementing the strategy (Drummond, 2004; Room, 2004).

The industry has considerable economic leverage, is extremely profitable, generating large tax revenues and is a major employer. The Portman Group, the major drinks companies and trade associations are close to government. They are effective in mobilising Parliament (for example, the All Party Parliamentary Beer Group has strong support among MPs).

The industry ensured that the government's policy did not harm its commercial interests. However, continuing public concern about alcohol misuse, and counter-lobbying by health, welfare and public order pressure groups, have kept the issue on the agenda. More recently, this has produced a tougher approach from government, with new legislation to compel the industry to pay for the local costs of alcohol-related public disorder and measures to increase funding of alcohol harm prevention projects (see Baggott, 2006).

Commercial interests support public health interventions where they increase consumer confidence in their products, open up new market opportunities or bring good publicity. Although there is much cynicism about the credibility of commercial organisations to act as 'responsible citizens', they may be persuaded to do so if this yields profits.

Either way, the corporate interests in public health are powerful. They have excellent political contacts, possess great economic leverage and can persuade government not to adopt health policies inimical to their interests.

Voluntary organisations, charities and single issue groups

Health consumer and patients' groups

These organisations seek to promote and represent the interests of patients, users and carers. Studies of groups in specific areas, such as mental health and maternity services (Durward and Evans, 1990; Pilgrim, 1991; Rogers and Tew, 1998; Barnes et al, 1999), and more widely (Wood, 2000; Baggott et al, 2005) have provided key insights into their activities within the policy process.

There are often different reasons behind their formation. Older groups are associated with a more philanthropic tradition while others have their origins in feminism or self-help. Despite their diverse origins, the political environment has created strong pressures for conformity. Most groups are now active in seeking to involve patients, users and carers more closely in their decision-making processes and are more strongly focused on influencing the policy process. Most health consumer and patients' groups are relatively small in terms of income and membership. Others have large incomes and thousands of members (such as the Multiple Sclerosis Society and Diabetes UK).

Research by Baggott et al (2005) found that health consumer and patients' groups had extensive contact with decision makers. Groups had regular contact with ministers, civil servants, Parliament and the media. There was evidence that these organisations were taken seriously by other policy actors, such as the health professions and the drugs industry, which increasingly sought alliances with them. Even so, groups varied considerably in their policy activities and their influence over policy. The larger and wealthier organisations, those forming alliances, those that could bring the experience of patients, users and carers to the policy process in a coherent way, and those with research and lobbying skills, tended to be among the most effective within the policy process.

Baggott and colleagues found that although these groups were influential, the power of professional and commercial interests remained strong. This supports the conclusions of previous writers such as Alford (1975) and Hogg (1999) about the underlying weakness of consumer, patient and public interests in health care systems, reflected in everyday decisions, in the structures and institutions of decision making and the language and discourse of policy. One of the key weaknesses of health consumer and patients' groups is that they lack economic leverage (unlike commercial interests) and their claims to knowledge have been less highly valued than the scientific and technical expertise of other policy actors, such as the professions. There have been cases where professional groups and commercial interests have 'colonised' health consumer and patients' groups or even created new groups to campaign on their behalf (to support the licensing of a new drug, for example – see Baggott et al, 2005; Health Committee, 2005; O'Donovan, 2005). Indeed, as Salter (2003) has observed, despite the rise of health consumer groups, traditional interests continue to dominate health policy networks.

Interviews with policy actors confirmed that health consumer and patients' groups have further to travel before they become equal partners in the policy process. Efforts by government to incorporate groups and involve them in policy consultations were acknowledged. One respondent, an MP, noted that 'the expertise of patient's groups is highly regarded'. But there were mixed views on their actual influence over policy. Some believed that health consumer and patients' groups could exert influence in particular sectors, notably mental health, and that they were broadly more influential than in the past. A former civil servant at the DoH remarked that patient and voluntary organisations had 'quite a lot of influence'. It was accepted that some of the larger and the more specialised groups could be influential (examples given included the Alzheimer's Disease Society, Rethink and Diabetes UK), although smaller organisations and those lacking knowledge and skills in the political process were regarded as less so. One interviewee, from a think tank, stated that 'patient and consumer groups don't really have much influence', but acknowledged that much depended on the nature of the issue. Another, from a medical organisation, observed that although 'a huge amount of lip service is paid to them', government used them for its own purposes, to develop policies in priority areas, for example, or to counter professional power. Indeed, a health consumer group spokesperson expressed concern about voluntary organisations 'getting too close to government' and compromising their independence and autonomy.

Other voluntary organisations, charities and public interest groups

There is a significant body of organisations that are not health consumer or patients' groups, but form part of the voluntary sector and make an important contribution not only to service provision (see Chapter Eight) but also to the health policy process. This is a diverse group of research and service provider charities (such as the British Heart Foundation, Cancer Research UK, Macmillan Cancer Relief, MENCAP and Scope) about which it is very difficult to generalise. Many have considerable resources and have excellent political contacts. They are also experienced in the policy process and have expertise that is highly valued by government. But this sector also includes small, charitable organisations that are not politically active and which concentrate on raising money for good causes and providing help for those in need.

There are also statutory bodies representing patient and public interests, which have on occasion acted as pressure groups within the political process. The former CHCs often provided a focus for local protest on issues such as budget cuts and the reconfiguration of services. They also acted as a focal point for complaints about substandard services or poor practice at a local level. At a national level, the ACHCEW, also a statutory body, was able to bring together these various local concerns. By highlighting shortcomings in services, the ACHCEW proved an irritant to successive governments. It was abolished along with CHCs and replaced by a new system of patient and public involvement (see ***Box 4.4***).

Single issue groups

Single issue 'cause' groups have a broader public policy focus. They seek to move public policy in their chosen direction by demonstrating broad public support for action on a particular issue. Examples include Action on Smoking and Health (ASH) and its adversary FOREST (Freedom Organisation for the Right to Enjoy Smoking Tobacco) and the pro-choice and anti-abortion lobbies. Other interests also endorse and support causes. Professional organisations, such as the BMA and the Royal Colleges, have supported anti-smoking campaigns. Similarly, commercial interests, on the receiving end of protests and cause group lobbying, have funded or created 'front' organisations to promote their view on a particular issue, in areas such as food, tobacco and alcohol policy.

It is difficult to generalise about the influence of single issue groups. Some have been very successful, particularly over the longer term. For example, ASH, formed in the 1970s (by the Royal College of Physicians), has campaigned successfully for advertising restrictions (including a ban on tobacco advertisements) as well as a ban on smoking in most enclosed public spaces. The Bristol Heart Children's Action Group campaigned successfully for an inquiry into the standards of paediatric heart surgery at Bristol Royal Infirmary (Bristol Royal Infirmary Inquiry, 2001), which later had wide ramifications for policies on clinical governance, medical regulation and patient and public involvement. But much depends on the existence and strength of opposing groups. For example, the anti-abortion lobby has been relatively unsuccessful in reversing the abortion rights embodied in the Termination of Pregnancy Act 1967, a measure promoted and defended by pro-choice groups.

Other organisations

A range of other organisations seek to influence health policy. These include 'think tanks' such as the King's Fund, Institute for Public Policy Research (IPPR), the Adam Smith Institute, Civitas, Demos, Catalyst and Social Market Foundation (see Dorey, 2005; Ruane, 2005). It is difficult to generalise about the influence of these diverse organisations. They can be highly influential, but much depends on how their ideas, findings and recommendations are taken up by others, including politicians, pressure groups and the media. The timing of reports is obviously important. If a policy is in the process of development, new ideas or findings can have a significant influence. Much also depends on the links between these organisations and policy makers. Notably, several prime ministerial advisers have previously worked for think tanks, including Matthew Taylor (IPPR) and Geoff Mulgan (Demos). Highly respected health research bodies (such as the King's Fund) and general think tanks with close links to those in government (such as IPPR and Demos) tend to be the most influential (see Ham, 2000). It should be noted that important polices have been generated from ideas provided by think tanks including foundation trusts and the use of market incentives in the NHS (Ruane, 2005). In contrast, academic researchers are seen as less influential in recent years, although some individual researchers are highly regarded by both government and other policy actors.

Lobbying, 'pressure points' and resources

Groups have a variety of options when seeking to influence policy. Although their strategies and tactics vary according to particular circumstances, they have a broad view on which approaches are most effective. Interviews with key policy actors identified the following points.

Central government

The importance of participating in the institutions, networks and policy processes of central government – discussed in Chapter Three – is acknowledged by groups. Not surprisingly, the DoH is seen as the main point of contact, except where other departments have specific health-related responsibilities (for example, housing, road safety, health and safety at work). Even so, groups are aware of the increased role of Number Ten and the Treasury (see Chapter Three) with regard to health policy and their need to influence these core institutions.

The maintenance of stable relationships with civil servants remains a key aim for most groups despite an acknowledged decline in their influence over policy. Groups tended to target ministers on politically controversial and high-profile issues. Wherever possible, groups seek to build a constructive relationship with the Secretary of State. Relationships with junior ministers are also important because they operate on the Secretary of State's behalf and liaise with groups on matters within their area of responsibility.

Meanwhile, the growing importance of ministerial advisers (at both departmental and prime ministerial level) had not escaped the attention of groups. Interviews with group representatives confirmed that ministerial advisers are an important target for lobbying (see also Baggott et al, 2005). Advisers often play an 'intermediary role' on behalf of ministers, which involves listening to the views of groups and negotiating possible solutions on behalf of ministers when necessary (see Chapter Three). In addition the clinical leaders, or czars, were seen as important figures with influence over policy in their specific field.

Parliament and parties

Parliament remains a key target for lobbying, despite its marginal impact on policy (see Chapter Four). Groups are aware that parliamentary support is sometimes needed to draw the government's attention to a problem. Parliamentary activities (such as debates, amendments to Bills and questions) can be an important adjunct to a media campaign to propel issues on the agenda. Parliamentary activity is also regarded as important when government is neutral or not committed. This applies particularly to cross-party issues (such as abortion, genetic technologies, ethics and so on) where tacit government support is needed. Parliamentary support is also required to gain concessions from government, for example on legislation, although this is acknowledged as difficult when faced with a highly committed and disciplined government with a large majority.

Parliament is highly accessible to groups. As noted in Chapter Four, the level of interest in health matters is high among parliamentarians, and groups are generally pushing at an open door when making contact with them. Groups usually try to identify individual members likely to be helpful to them. Such 'sympathisers' are usually the first port of call when parliamentary briefings are being undertaken. They are also most likely to be approached about tabling debates, motions, questions and other parliamentary activities. To underpin this process, some groups have databases, based on registers of members' interests and previous contributions to health debates, which can enable the identification of 'friendly' MPs and peers and also those who are hostile or opposed to their aims and campaigns.

In some cases, a group will establish a panel of MPs and/or peers with which it will liaise on policy matters, as in the case of the RCN, for example. Other useful fora include APGs, some of which receive administrative and financial support from outside organisations (see Chapter Four). Other parliamentary committees are also targeted by groups. Standing committees, which consider legislation in detail, are lobbied by pressure groups. Similarly, select committees – particularly the Health Committee – are an important target. During the course of their inquiries, select committees receive oral and written evidence from groups (see Chapter Four). Interviewees believe these committees have the potential to create a more favourable climate for their policies and argue that select committee 'endorsement' of policy recommendations can affect the direction of policy, particularly in the longer term (see also Baggott et al, 2005).

When lobbying Parliament or government most groups maintain a neutral stance with regard to party politics. With the exception of most trade unions and some business interests, groups do not wish to be seen as partisan. If the party they support is out of power, the possibilities for influence tends to shrink (although, as the trade unions have learned, a Labour government does not guarantee influence). Nonetheless, it would be wrong to assume that groups have nothing to do with political parties. On the contrary, many seek endorsement for their policies from across all parties, in an effort to improve the chances of implementation by future governments.

Media, public opinion and support

As shown in Chapter Five, the media contributes to the construction of health issues chiefly through definition and reinforcement of particular meanings and values. It can shape the political agenda by highlighting key issues. The media is especially potent as a negative force, discouraging specific policy options, although it can exert a direct and positive impact on policy.

It is a testimony to the importance of the media in the health policy arena that pressure groups put so much time and resources into influencing it (see Chapter Five). Some find it easier to secure favourable coverage than others. Professional groups, particularly the medical profession, still command sympathetic media attention. Although medical concepts and perspectives are more open to challenge than once was the case, they still carry considerable weight. In addition, groups campaigning in condition areas such as breast cancer and children's health tend to get more favourable coverage than those in mental health and the care of the elderly, although in recent years the latter have challenged negative stereotypes with some success.

Although groups use the media to build public support for their aims and campaigns, some try alternative ways of generating grassroots support. Direct action, such as protests, boycotts and 'sit ins' are increasingly used by groups (Ridley and Jordan, 1998; Grant, 2005), especially in the environmental sector. However, the media remains important, as it is the publicity given to direct action methods that mobilises members and the wider public. The internet is increasingly used, with direct action activities organised through e-mails and websites (and the use of mobile phone technology). The health sector has had less experience of direct action, but the growing protests against hospital closures and some campaigns to make new drugs more widely available are perhaps an indicator that this is changing (Mandelstam, 2006).

Access and influence

Good political contacts with decision makers and opinion formers are regarded as essential. As noted in Chapter One, it has been suggested that groups with good access to government that are regularly consulted on policy matters tend to be more influential than those lacking access and not regularly consulted (Grant, 2000). The former are regarded as 'insiders' and the latter, 'outsiders'. More recently, doubt has been cast on this dichotomy. It has been argued that strategies that rely on good contacts with government may not be as effective as those deploying a wider range of tactics, including contacts with the media and the mobilisation of public opinion (Whiteley and Winyard, 1987). In the health field, research by Baggott et al (2005) found that health consumer groups that adopted an open strategy tended to be more successful than those that relied on good contacts with government. Further interviews with health policy actors confirmed that although contact with government is important, other pressure points, such as the media and Parliament, should not be neglected. Moreover, policy actors overwhelmingly emphasise that access to government does not equate with influence. For example, a charity spokesperson stated that: 'access does not equal influence – arguments have to be sold', while a former senior NHS manager commented that 'there is a difference between putting your point across and getting it accepted'.

Furthermore, it would be wrong to assume that 'outsider' groups, which focus on the media and mobilising public opinion, are without influence. Such groups may lack good contacts with decision makers, but they can shape the political agenda and have an enormous impact on decision making. For example, 'outsider' groups allied with social movements have been very effective in getting issues on the health agenda, changing the nature of public debate about these issues and ultimately influencing decisions (see ***Box 6.2***).

Box 6.2: Social movements and health

One must not ignore wider social movements in health, which can have an impact on the underlying assumptions and values in health policy and practice. Although they are undoubtedly important, there is much disagreement over what actually constitutes a social movement (see, for example, Byrne, 1997; Jordan and Maloney, 1997; Martin, 2001). Perhaps the best approach is to see social movements not as a distinct category of collective action but as a more complex activity that consists of certain traits:

- Challenging existing assumptions or ways of doing things from the outside rather than from the inside. One of the key attributes of a social movement is that it poses a challenge by those excluded from current arrangements (Scott, 1990; Tarrow, 1998). These may be socially excluded groups or those facing some form of discrimination (for example, ethnic minorities, women, homosexual people). However, many activists are in fact from higher socio-economic backgrounds and are well educated, while members of the lower classes tend to be poorly represented, particularly in the more recent social movements.
- Promoting societal change rather than localised campaigns or policy-specific changes. Social movements may be active on local and national issues and may impact on policies. However, their focus is usually much wider, promoting values and principles (such as gender or racial equality, for example). Social movements tend to be ongoing (although particular movements may wax and wane over time).
- Social movements are not simply organisations. They encompass a range of activities, including the activities of informal groups and individuals, and are held together by common values rather than organisational structures. However, most social movements contain organisations that raise resources for campaigns and mobilise wider public support (such as Greenpeace and Friends of the Earth within the environmental movement).
- Social movements tend to adopt 'unconventional' tactics, such as protest and direct action rather than meetings with policy makers. However, they and their constituent organisations also use conventional means (encouraging members and supporters to write to MPs, for example – see Ridley and Jordan, 1998). Furthermore, social movements do not have a monopoly on protest and direct action. Other, more conventional pressure groups (such as trade unions and professional bodies) have also engaged in boycotts, strikes and protests from time to time.
- Social movements are concerned with politics and policies, but they are also concerned with the practices of everyday life. Indeed, theorists such as Habermas (1987) have pointed out that they can counter the 'colonisation of

the lifeworld' by the state and other powerful groups such as the professions. Social movements therefore operate at the symbolic level and in cultural networks as much as in the political sphere (Melucci, 1989).

- Social movements are usually international in scope, not confined by the borders of nation states. They are related to broader global cultural and social debates.
- Social movements are primarily concerned with lifestyle and consumption issues rather than economic or material issues. People are part of a movement because they wish to express their values and identity rather than for any pecuniary motive. However, it is recognised that material concerns represent an important focus for many movements including those that seek to redress inequalities in society (such as the women's, disability and racial equality movements).

One can identify various social movements in the health field. Indeed, Brown and Zavestoski (2004, p 679) have defined health social movements (HSMs) as 'collective challenges to medical policy, public health policy and politics, belief systems, research and practice which include an array of formal and informal organisations, supporters, networks of cooperation and media'. These authors see HSMs as posing a challenge on several fronts including political power, professional authority and personal and collective identity. They also identify three types of HSM: health access movements which address issues of access and provision of health care services; embodied health movements that focus on the personal understanding and experience of illness; and constituency-based health movements that address health inequality based on race, ethnicity, gender, sexuality and class.

Perhaps the most prominent examples are the childbirth movement and the mental health movement. In the field of maternity and childbirth, a social movement consisting of informal and formal organisations and individuals campaigned to de-medicalise childbirth and restructure services to provide for a more women-centred approach (Declerq, 1998; Tew, 1998). This has been fairly successful, leading to changes in government policy. However, in practice, implementation has been less dramatic, with women-centred services inhibited by resource constraints and professional and managerial conservatism (Garcia et al, 1998). Also, somewhat paradoxically, patient choice (and other factors such as fears of litigation) has driven an increase in medicalisation of childbirth as reflected in the increase in Caesarean sections to a level that has caused concern, even among obstetricians. With regard to mental health, the mobilisation of a users' movement drove efforts to create more humane mental health services and challenged attitudes to mental illness within government, the health professions and in wider society (see Rogers and Pilgrim, 1991; Crossley, 2006). This also had paradoxical consequences. The flawed implementation of community care created a public backlash paving the way for policies that reflected public safety rather than the needs of users (Rogers and Pilgrim, 2001). However, there are signs of improved cooperation between professionals and user groups in this field, which are increasingly working together on common issues.

These cases illustrate the difficulties of evaluating the impact of health social movements (see also Keefe et al, 2006). These problems are compounded by the kind of definitional issues raised earlier, by the multi-level impact of movements (on ideas, values, agendas, policies and practice) and the long-term nature of their struggle, which can mean that their impact should not be prematurely judged.

Resources

Aside from political contacts, other factors affect the likelihood that a group will exert influence over policy. The resources allocated to lobbying and campaigning is an important factor. The wealthier groups can afford to rent expensive offices close to Westminster and Whitehall (or in Brussels – see Chapter Ten). They can also employ specialist lobbying staff (see below). They are able to commission research and publicity for their cause. The playing field is not level. Large professional membership organisations, trade unions, trade associations and companies have plenty of resources. Larger charities may also have big budgets, although their ability to lobby is sometimes constrained by their charitable status. Others, such as smaller single issue groups, minority professional groups and most health consumer and patients' groups are relatively resource-poor. They rely heavily on voluntary effort and in some cases a small number of administrators. Sometimes the smaller organisations will be able to punch above their weight, particularly if they produce a well-argued case backed with sound research (Baggott et al, 2005).

Skills

Some groups are able to employ specialist staff, who have a thorough understanding of the political process and are experienced in dealing with government, Parliament and the media. In some cases these people have previously worked in government and have an inside knowledge of how the political process operates. The larger and wealthier organisations can afford specialist staff and in some cases these form a self-contained policy unit (for example, the BMA and the RCN). The smaller groups tend to rely more heavily on volunteers to undertake policy roles. Where they can afford to employ officers, these are often less specialised, undertaking general administrative and tasks alongside policy-related functions.

Expertise and knowledge

A key 'resource' possessed by groups is expertise and knowledge relevant to policy issues. Groups hold various types of knowledge. Some hold scientific and technical knowledge (about the cost-effectiveness of a particular intervention, for example). They may hold practical or experiential knowledge (relating to the actual experiences of treatment or the workings of the health system). The distribution of knowledge and expertise varies across groups. Some have high levels of both types. The BMA, for example, possesses medical expertise and knowledge as well as the 'grassroots' experience of individual practitioners.

The government's demand for knowledge and expertise can change over time and this can affect its relationship with particular groups. In recent years, for example, the government's preoccupation with health care costs, privatisation and marketisation has led it to become more dependent on those groups with financial and economic expertise related to health care, or which can help implement new modes of service delivery. Similarly, the government's aim to create a more 'patient-centred' health care system has enhanced the role of health consumer and patients' groups which can give an authentic account of the experiences of patients, users and carers (Baggott et al, 2005). The knowledge and expertise of those representing clinical and pharmaceutical interests is still regarded as extremely important by government and continues to have a major impact on policy.

Economic leverage and sanctions

Groups that possess economic leverage or other sanctions are among the most influential. In the health care system the government is dependent on a range of organisations, notably those representing doctors and other professional groups, commercial organisations and, increasingly, private contractors. Ultimately, if these groups are unhappy with government policy, they can deploy sanctions. Examples include: industrial action by staff, and drug companies moving their manufacturing operations overseas. Even the threat of such action can yield influence, though much depends on the government's resolve. Other groups have few sanctions. Managers have little leverage and lack public support. Moreover, as part of the management structure of the NHS they are in a vulnerable position if they withdraw labour. Groups representing patients, users and carers also have few options to really damage government. Their main weapon is publicity – about issues such as inadequate standards, difficulties in access to services and the effect of budgetary decisions.

Alliances

Finally, an ability to work with other groups on issues of common concern is a major factor in determining policy influence. Alliances of groups tend to be much more powerful than the sum of their parts. Groups of professionals or workers can come together to fight on common issues. There now appears to be much more cooperation between professional organisations and trade unions on issues such as NHS reform and reorganisation, for example. In addition, professional and consumer/patient interests (and in some cases commercial groups and single issue groups too) can join forces on a particular issue. For example, the campaign to ban smoking in public places was backed by a wide range of groups including the BMA, the RCN, the British Heart Foundation, Cancer Research UK and ASH. There are many examples of coalitions that are lobbying for resources or treatments in a particular condition area (such as multiple sclerosis, breast cancer and Alzheimer's disease) that include health consumer and patients' groups, professionals and drugs companies. Several interviewees observed the importance of alliances, especially coalitions between service users, professionals and the drugs industry. Some saw health politics increasingly as a zero sum game where advocates for different conditions fought over scarce resources.

Conclusion

It is very difficult to generalise about the influence of groups on policy and their relationship with government. At any point in time, many groups are trying to influence health policy and the various constellations of groups will vary from issue to issue. Moreover, relationships between groups and government, and between groups themselves, change over time. Despite this complexity and dynamism, it is possible to draw some conclusions about the role of groups in the policy process.

First, the medical profession remains a potent force within the policy process. Although challenged by commercial, managerial and consumer/patient interests and other professional groups, the medical profession and its organisations continue to exert more influence over health policy than any other single group. Second, and related to this, the health policy network (see Chapter One) has become more crowded. The simple 'bilateral' relationships between medicine and the state have given way to a more complex set of relationships. Superficially, this is a more open 'issue network', but in reality the traditionally powerful groups (medicine, the drugs industry) are still in a pre-eminent position. Some 'stars' have risen – parts of the private sector, sections of the voluntary sector, while others such as nursing and management interests have had a more mixed experience. Third, considerable inequalities persist between groups. Political resources – public support, economic leverage, status, possession of knowledge and expertise – are not evenly distributed. Furthermore, there is a variation in the quality of political contact with the media, Parliament and government. Fourth, there is no simple prescription regarding strategy and tactics. To be an insider is not sufficient to guarantee influence over policy, while outsiders are not without influence. Groups should not neglect relationships with other arenas such as Parliament and the media that can help shape political agendas and provide rallying points for opposition to government policy.

Finally, while the focus on organised groups and interests is important, and provides much of the empirical data on the influence of interests and their relationships with policy makers, one should not forget the role of diffuse and amorphous social forces – such as structural interests and social movements. These can exert influence over the context of health policy making and the policy agenda in this field.

Summary

- The medical profession does not have a monopoly of influence over health policy. The health policy network is more open and inclusive. However, doctors' interests and their organisations remain highly influential in the policy process.
- Among the various other interests in health policy – other health professions, trade unions, commercial interests, health consumer and patients' groups, the wider voluntary sector and single issue groups – some have grown in influence, others have had a more mixed experience.
- Groups have various resources that they can bring to the policy process. These include status, expertise and economic leverage. These resources are not equally distributed.
- To be an insider group does not guarantee influence. Groups need to maintain contacts with several 'pressure points', including Parliament and the media.
- Changes in policy making within central government (notably in health policy and the rise of special advisers) have been reflected in the strategies and tactics of pressure groups.
- Broader social movements can exert influence over the context of health policy and the health policy agenda.

Key questions

1. What are the main interests in health policy? What influence have these groups had over health policy in recent years?
2. Has medical influence over health policy declined?
3. Does access to government equal influence over policy?
4. How and to what extent have health social movements influenced health policy?
5. What resources are important for groups seeking to influence health policy?

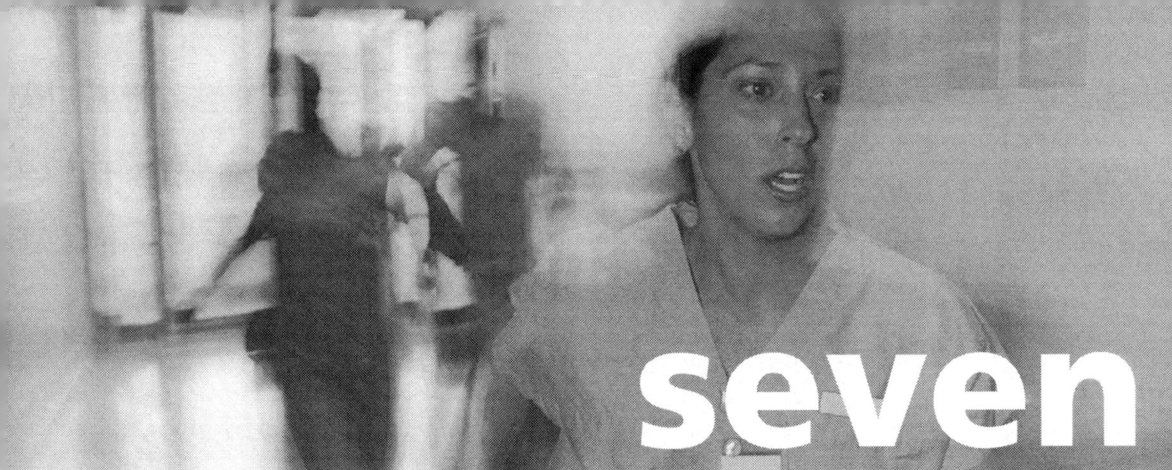

Health policy and the NHS

Overview

This chapter concentrates upon the implementation of health policy within the NHS. It focuses on the relationship between central government and the NHS and to what extent this has changed in recent years. It discusses key concepts such as centralisation and decentralisation and examines the various attempts to reorganise the NHS since its creation.

Implementation is a crucial part of the policy process (see Chapter One). In health policy, much of the task of implementation falls to the NHS, which is a large and complex organisation containing powerful professional interests. There is no guarantee that national health policies will be implemented locally (Ham, 2004). This chapter explores policy implementation in the NHS and the efforts of central government to ensure that its policies are put into practice.

Central–local relations

The legacy of 1948

The NHS was constituted as a tripartite service consisting of: hospitals, owned and funded by the state; state-funded family health services provided by independent contractors (such as GPs and dentists); and community and public health services run by local councils (also responsible for non-NHS social care). The Minister (and later, Secretary of State) for Health was responsible for the NHS and accountable to Parliament for policy, funding and service delivery (see Chapter Three). Centralised responsibility was further reflected in the central funding of health services and appointment by ministers of regional and local boards. However, these factors did not give significant power to the centre in practice. Budgets were based on historical allocations. NHS hospital boards, particularly in the prestigious teaching hospitals, had considerable autonomy. Furthermore, GPs and other independent contractor professions were administered by separate Executive Councils and insulated from central control.

Not only had central government little capacity to intervene, it lacked the inclination to do so. The Ministry of Health was regarded as a relatively weak department with little influence over the field (see Chapter Three). When it decided to intervene, it was mainly through 'exhortation', in the form of guidance or advice to local health bodies (Klein, 1995; Ham, 2004). Even up to the late 1970s and early 1980s, the centre was regarded as weak. Most observers identified a strong medical profession at local level as the key element preserving significant local autonomy (see Haywood and Alaszewski, 1980; Ham, 1981; Harrison et al, 1992; Harrison and Pollitt, 1994).

Nonetheless, central government became increasingly concerned about its lack of influence over service providers (Klein, 1995; Webster, 1996). Initially, the main issues were related to financial control and efficiency, later accompanied by other considerations, such as the quality and effectiveness of health services, and inequities in services between different geographical areas and service users. Fragmentation was also recognised as a problem, particularly on strategic issues such as training and capital investment as well as on specific service issues (such as mental health, disability, maternity, children and the elderly services) where there was a history of poor cooperation between different parts of the NHS (see Allsop, 1984).

From the 1960s onwards, central government tried to exert much stronger influence over the NHS. Efforts were made to reorganise the service, set clear objectives, strengthen management systems and improve local accountability to the centre. Alongside this centralisation process was an element of decentralisation, giving local NHS organisations greater responsibility. Before looking at the various ways in which central government attempted to increase control and strengthen policy implementation, it is important to clarify the concepts of centralisation and decentralisation.

Centralisation and decentralisation

Deeming (2004, p 60) has defined decentralisation as a situation where 'significant decision-making discretion is available at lower hierarchical levels, with the managers and staff who are closer to the people receiving services'. In contrast, he defines centralisation as where 'significant decisions are taken upstream at the centre of government within a tighter system of control and accountability.' Similarly, Saltman and colleagues (2007) define decentralisation as 'the transfer of authority and power from higher to lower levels of government or from national to subnational levels'. The potential benefits of decentralisation (see Milburn, 2001; Peckham et al, 2005) include greater responsiveness to local service users' needs; enabling local managers to manage services without interference; efficiencies arising from the shedding of bureaucratic tiers and processes; empowerment of staff leading to greater motivation and service innovation. But even 'genuine' decentralisation has disadvantages in terms of inequalities, fragmentation and confusion over accountability (Walker, 2002; Mosca, 2006).

Several writers have identified different types of centralisation and decentralisation (see Pollitt et al, 1998; Peckham et al, 2005; Saltman et al, 2007). Rondinelli (1981) specified three major types of government decentralisation (in addition to privatisation): deconcentration – shifting of administrative workload, but not authority, to regional and/or local offices of an organisation; delegation – to semi-autonomous agencies with given powers; and devolution – where decision making and management authority is shifted on to provincial and local governments. An alternative typology, applied specifically to UK health policy, is the 'arrows framework', devised by Peckham and colleagues (2005), which identifies key dimensions that may be subject to centralisation/decentralisation (see ***Box 7.1*** below).

Box 7.1: The arrows framework

Peckham and colleagues identified three main dimensions subject to degrees of centralisation and decentralisation: *inputs, process and outcomes*. These dimensions were mapped against various tiers ranging from the global level and Europe through national, regional and local organisation down to sub-units and, ultimately, the individual user. *Inputs* included budgets, organisational change, pay, education and training, as well as political devolution with regard to Scotland and Wales (see Chapter Nine). *Process* included policies such as earned autonomy/star ratings, patient choice, commissioning, clinical governance and foundation trusts. *Outcomes* included payment by results, performance management targets, evidence-based policy, inspection and regulation. The mapping of policy impacts on the direction of centralisation/decentralisation in each of these areas (with the use of arrows, which gives the framework its name) gives an overall picture of centralisation/decentralisation trends over time. Using this method, Peckham and colleagues found that the impact of policies with regard to inputs was mixed, policies affecting process were decentralist, while those impacting on outcomes were centralist.

Source: Peckham et al (2005)

According to the arrows model, centralisation and decentralisation may occur during the same time period. Peckham and colleagues (see ***Box 7.1***) found that centralisation and decentralisation varied across different dimensions of policy. This explains the paradox that decentralisation can be accompanied by centralisation (Pollitt et al, 1998; Dopson et al, 1999; Peckham et al, 2005). Central government may delegate some functions and even allow local managers greater autonomy on some issues, but retains overall control over strategy and, when necessary, intervenes in implementation.

That decentralisation often involves a strong dose of central intervention is acknowledged (Pollitt et al, 1998; Taylor, 2000). Indeed, decentralisation is often seen as a symbolic policy, masking tighter control of local organisations (Mohan, 1995; Ross and Tomaney, 2001; Smith et al, 2001; Tallis, 2004). More recently, 'centralised decentralisation' (Hoggett, 1996) has evolved into 'earned autonomy', where local NHS organisations are promised greater freedoms within a performance framework set by the centre.

Structural reorganisation

The NHS in England has been reorganised many times (health service reorganisations in other parts of the UK are discussed in Chapter Nine). The original 'tripartite' structure described earlier lasted until 1974. Following several years of debate (see Chapter Two), a new structure was introduced, which incorporated the community health services run by local authorities within the main NHS structure (see Klein, 1995; Webster, 1996). The hospital boards were abolished. Three tiers of health service management were created, at regional, area and district level, overseen by new regional and area health authorities. For the independent contractor professions, such as the GPs, family practitioner committees (FPCs) replaced the Executive Councils. However, the new structure attracted criticism, chiefly for being 'top-down' and bureaucratic (Edwards, 1993). Subsequently, the Royal Commission on the NHS recommended the abolition of one of the tiers below the regional level (Cmnd 7615, 1979). The Thatcher government responded by abolishing area health authorities and creating health authorities at the district level.

Further structural reorganisation took place following the 1989 White Paper, *Working for Patients* (Cm 555, 1989). Its aim, discussed in more detail in a later section of this chapter, was to create a quasi-market in health care. As Harrison and Wood (1998) observed, this represented a different approach to reform. Rather than having an organisational blueprint, as with the 1974 and 1982 reorganisations, the government opted for 'manipulated emergence' of a new system. This reform also marked a deeper shift in philosophy from the conventional 'welfare-state' approach to a neo-liberal perspective (see Greener, 2004d). The government introduced some organisational reform combined with new incentives. NHS bodies became 'purchasers' or 'providers' of health care. Purchasers included district health authorities (DHAs) and fund-holding GPs (who, along with the other independent contractor professions, were managed by new Family Health Services Authorities (FHSAs), which by now had replaced FPCs as the bodies overseeing primary care). The providers were established as new self-governing NHS trusts, removed from health authority control and promised greater freedom to manage their affairs. The providers would earn their income through service contracts negotiated with the purchasers.

The creation of GP fund-holders and trusts occurred in several 'waves' and so did not transform the NHS structure overnight. However, their emergence created pressures for further structural changes. In the mid-1990s, DHAs – whose purchasing role was increasingly transferred to GPs – were reduced in number and eventually merged with FHSAs to form unitary health authorities. Trusts also merged, as some were simply too small to survive in the new health service market. Meanwhile, the regional health authorities (RHAs), which had divested most of their service-provider functions, were abolished and replaced with regional offices of the NHS Executive (see Chapter Three), staffed by civil servants.

The election of the Labour government in 1997 brought further organisational changes. The division between purchasers of health care (by now known as commissioners) and providers of health care was retained, but the GP fund-holding scheme was abolished. New bodies, known as primary care groups (PCGs), were created in each local area to commission services. It was envisaged that PCGs would eventually become primary care trusts (PCTs), free-standing bodies that could take on service provision as well as commissioning roles.

The move from PCG to PCT was expected to be voluntary and dependent on the local context. However, in 2002, all PCGs were converted into PCTs as part of a programme of 'shifting the balance of power' in the NHS to the local level. The unitary health authorities were abolished and 28 Strategic Health Authorities (SHAs) created. This was accompanied by a reduction in the number of regional offices, which were later abolished. In 2006 there was yet another restructuring involving mergers of both SHAs and PCTs. The number of SHAs fell to 10 and PCTs to 152, moving to some extent back to structure of the mid-1990s. The current NHS structure is shown in ***Figure 7.1***.

A further organisational change introduced by the Blair government was foundation trusts (see also Chapter Four). Initially, foundation status was only available to those trusts that had received the highest performance ratings (discussed further later in this chapter). Foundation trusts were promised certain freedoms to manage their affairs (including ability to retain surpluses, borrow, sell assets, enter into private partnerships and to reward staff). In

Figure 7.1: Current structure of the NHS in England

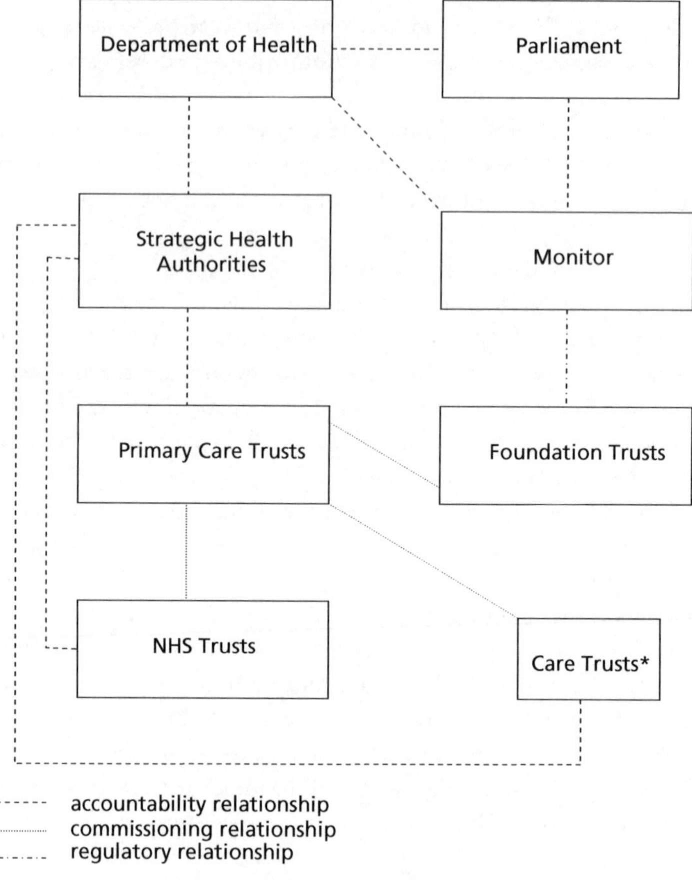

*Note:** Care trusts are discussed further in Chapter Eight.

reality, constraints were imposed on these activities. Moreover, foundation trusts are subject to an independent national regulator (called Monitor) that can intervene in certain circumstances. Foundation trusts are also accountable to the local community through governing boards that contain a majority of representatives elected by local people and patients.

Why reorganisation?

Many observe that governments find it difficult to resist reorganising the NHS. Klein (1995) refers to the search for an 'organisational fix' while McLachlan (1990, pp 117-18) writes of an 'almost irrelevant obsession with structure' in central government. Ministers find it difficult to resist playing 'organisational lego' with the NHS (Edwards, 1993) – even when they previously criticised reorganisation in opposition (Edwards and Fall, 2005, p 187). One reason for this is that reorganisation is a useful tool for politicians. It is highly symbolic, and gives the impression that something is being done about the problems of the NHS. Reorganisation shifts attention to the administration and management of the service and therefore can be used to deflect criticism of central government policies. But there may be a less cynical explanation: that the impact of reorganisation is simply ill-thought out. Brown's (1979, p 200) observation, that 'reorganisation is normally undertaken in a spirit of over-optimism about the net advantages', remains true today.

The pace of reorganisation increased from the early 1980s, and even more dramatically from 1997 onwards (Webster, 2002; Tallis, 2004). Various commentators described this in terms of a 'permanent revolution'. Interviewees from the health policy process complained of 'constant reorganisations' (according to one peer) and believed that 'government should stop changing things around and give things a chance to work' (spokesperson, health professional organisation). Another, an MP, said that the message from staff was 'for God's sake, leave us alone, let us get on with what we are doing and stop messing around with us'.

In this context Tallis (2004) and Smith et al (2001) use the term 'redisorganisation' to describe the perpetual restructuring that undermines the ability of the NHS to improve. Meanwhile the Health Committee (2006, p 5), commenting on the latest round of NHS restructuring noted that 'the cycle of perpetual change is ill-judged and not conducive to the successful provision and improvement of health services'. More specifically, reorganisation can lead to loss of skills and knowledge that it is difficult, if not impossible, to replace. It can disrupt relationships with other agencies (see Chapter Eight) and damage staff morale. There are also a host of additional financial costs (including, redundancies, changes to logos, movement of staff to new offices), although most reorganisation costs are hidden (Brown, 1979).

Reorganisation has become so discredited in recent years that critics have called for a moratorium (Smith et al, 2001). However, even they accept that where there is good evidence that reorganisation will be cost-effective and is likely to produce improvements, it should be undertaken. Others argue that if reorganisation is necessary it should be smaller scale, evidence-based and piloted (Tallis, 2004). Indeed, it is the 'big bang' approach to reorganisation that attracts the most criticism, with considerable support remaining for organic change that builds on the strengths of existing organisations (Health Committee, 2006, p 6).

Planning and priorities

In the early years of the NHS, little consideration was given to how services might be planned in order to meet existing and future needs. Webster (1996, p 27) observed that 'given the precipitous and haphazard manner in which the NHS was put together, there was no opportunity to incorporate arrangements for comprehensive and integrated planning, or even to guarantee the efficient use of resources'. As planning developed, the focus was initially upon manpower and resources. The high point of this approach, as noted by Mohan (2002), was the Hospital Plan of 1962. This was essentially a plan of capital expenditure, although it did set norms for bed provision in each locality. Although acknowledged as a long-term, national plan, and therefore an advance on the haphazard, short-term approach that preceded it, it was not really a strategic plan at all. Moreover, it did not deliver the level of capital expenditure envisaged (Klein, 1995; Webster, 1996; Mohan, 2002). The Hospital Plan was not comprehensive; it did not cover community health services or social care (which were the responsibility of local councils). A community care plan did follow, but failed to indicate common standards or costs. This represented a form of planning, according to Webster (1996, p 126) 'only in the most rudimentary sense'.

Subsequently, planning was extended to other areas. Concerns in the late 1960s and early 1970s about poor standards in the so-called 'Cinderella services' (particularly the long-stay facilities for people with mental illness, severe physical and mental disabilities and elderly people) prompted greater regulation and brought efforts to reorient priorities. In 1976 a new planning system was introduced. Each health authority produced plans that were then passed up to the central department, the DHSS, which produced a priorities document setting out a framework (DHSS, 1976a). The idea was to shift resources into services that had been neglected, and was accompanied by changes to the resource allocation mechanism within the NHS. Even so, the planning process remained persuasive rather than directive and the government's priorities encountered considerable resistance at local level.

The Thatcher government attempted to simplify the planning process (Hambleton, 1983). Local health authorities were given a general statement of priorities rather than detailed guidance (DHSS, 1981). However, as the decade unfolded, central guidance became more prescriptive. An annual priorities document was produced and various goals and targets were set for specific services. In addition, plans were subject to much closer scrutiny by higher tier authorities. The increase in central planning stemmed from changes in NHS management processes, discussed later, which reflected a desire to strengthen line management in the NHS. New policy initiatives also played a significant part, particularly in the 1990s, by which time Thatcher had been replaced by John Major. Perhaps the most important was *The Patient's Charter* (DoH, 1991), which set out a range of standards and rights (such as maximum waiting times, for example). Health authorities were expected to achieve targets set by government in relation to these commitments. Much less influential was the Major government's *Health of the Nation* strategy (Cm 1986, 1992), which set targets for improving public health, discussed further in Chapter Eight.

The Blair government's approach to planning indicated some similarities with its Conservative predecessor (Cm 3807, 1997). Plans were introduced, targets set and performance was monitored. There were also new features. An attempt was made to integrate health and social care by combining planning guidance for the NHS and local authorities. In addition, NHS organisations and local government had a duty of cooperation imposed upon them (see Chapter Eight). Local health plans became 'health improvement programmes', which focused on health as well as health care, and health authorities were expected to include local stakeholders such as local government and the voluntary sector in their formulation (see Chapter Eight).

Other changes introduced by Labour included three-year plans (to replace annual plans) and a promised reduction in planning requirements. At national level, however, there was actually a proliferation of plans. The NHS Plan (Cm 4818, 2000) was based on a wide-ranging review of the service (see ***Box 3.3***). It set a range of policy objectives and targets. These included new waiting-time targets (including maximum waiting times of 48 hours to see a GP, three months for an outpatient appointment and six months for an inpatient appointment). This was followed by the NHS Improvement Plan (Cm 6268, 2004), which set further goals, including an 18-week maximum waiting time from GP referral to receiving treatment. In the meantime, further White Papers outlined policies on choice (see Cm 6079, 2003), public health (Cm 6374, 2004) and health care outside hospitals (Cm 6737, 2006), set out a range of new policy aims and objectives, while priorities were reiterated through successive planning and priorities documents (DoH, 2001a, 2005).

On top of this, the Blair government formulated specific service plans and frameworks. The previous government's Cancer Plan was revised, and other condition areas and services were given NSFs, including mental health, coronary heart disease, diabetes, older people and children's services. These plans, which set out service standards and models of care and covered prevention as well as care and treatment, were expected to be implemented at the local level. However, the proliferation of plans was confusing. It was clear that plans, including the NSFs, could only come to life by making resources available (Tallis, 2004). For example, one interviewee, from a health charity, observed that the early NSFs did receive additional resources and were perceived as more successful than later ones, which stalled due to a lack of resources. Prioritisation also caused problems for services not earmarked for improvement. As Tallis (2004, p 68) put it 'where there is overall scarcity, the prioritisation of one problem leads to the posteriorisation of another'.

One of the central features of the Blair government's approach has been the setting of targets for NHS organisations. The number of targets was once estimated at over four hundred (Stephenson, 2003). Efforts have since been made to streamline the targets and highlight those of greatest importance. However, following fresh policy initiatives, additional targets have been introduced. There is a great ambivalence towards targets. On the one hand, they are credited with successfully highlighting key priorities. Some interviewees agreed that policy implementation had improved in recent years to a large extent because of them. A professional organisation spokesperson stated that: 'targets have no doubt helped … they helped to change the culture ... they have given a new sense of priority for outcomes'; an informant from a think tank commented that 'the government have focused on a narrow set of key priorities and have been relatively successful in achieving their aims'. Another, a former civil servant at the DoH, observed that 'the target culture has been beneficial in the main – by strengthening accountability'.

Targets also clearly have disadvantages. As one interviewee, a trade unionist, commented, 'too many targets have impeded implementation'. Another respondent, from an NHS management organisation, observed that 'target culture has improved implementation but this has disadvantaged areas that are not priorities, that are not amenable to measurement', while another, a former civil servant with a health professional background, noted that 'areas not covered by performance targets and plans tend to get ignored'. Further criticisms of targets related to their unintended consequences. Several interviewees were concerned about the 'unforeseen effect' of targets and the scope for dysfunctional or fraudulent behaviour. A spokesperson from a medical organisation commented that they 'are subject to gaming, and clinical need suffers'. Inquiries into the use of targets in the public sector have echoed such worries (see Audit Commission, 2003; Select Committee on Public Administration, 2003). Negative consequences of targets have been found in the NHS, including the manipulation of data and the distortion of clinical priorities (Goddard et al, 2000; Public Accounts Committee, 2002; Mannion et al, 2005a; Smith, 2005; Bevan and Hood, 2006). Patients are often inconvenienced by targets. For example, Accident and Emergency admission targets were found to have resulted in patients being kept waiting in ambulances outside hospital (CHI, 2003). There have also been complaints about the impact of waiting-time targets in primary care, which make it difficult for patients to book advance appointments (Healthcare Commission, 2004).

Targets can be useful in focusing on key priorities, but crude targets, designed without thinking about the consequences, can be damaging. Suggestions for improvement include fewer and better-designed targets, more involvement in their formulation by service users and providers, the use of more sophisticated measures of progress and improvement, more sensitivity to local settings and conditions, better policing of 'gaming' and fraudulent activities, more 'joint targets' (to improve joint working between different agencies) and independent assessment of performance (see Select Committee on Public Administration, 2003; Bevan and Hood, 2006).

Management

Issuing plans and targets is irrelevant in the absence of mechanisms to manage performance. Up until the 1980s NHS managers played an important though low-key role (Harrison, 1988; Harrison et al, 1992). Lay administrators acted as 'diplomats', sorting out 'turf wars' between professional groups and specialties. They tended to react to problems rather than initiate changes, accepted the status quo and were deferential to the medical profession. Senior doctors effectively controlled their own territory. Although they engaged in forms of clinical leadership (through educational and research activity, for example) they were reluctant to engage in a management role. Moreover, the medical profession was regarded as very powerful at the local level and able to block implementation of central policies and plans.

Other professional groups, although weaker than doctors, also demanded a role in decision making. This led to the development of 'consensus management' introduced formally by the 1974 reorganisation. This involved management teams drawn from a variety of backgrounds (administration, finance, nursing and medicine). In theory, no member of the team had superior status and each had a veto over decisions (although the doctors remained the most powerful group). The advantages of this system lay in the emphasis on agreement and consensual decision making. Less positively, it was held responsible for delays in making decisions, blurred accountability and a failure to take tough decisions (Harrison, 1988).

The Thatcher government believed that management reform was essential to bring the NHS into line with its priorities. Although it initially encouraged local diversity within a national statement of priorities, pressures for stronger parliamentary accountability, coupled with large-scale industrial action in the NHS, led the government to pursue a more directive approach. The Griffiths Inquiry was appointed to explore NHS management, which found an absence of clear responsibility in the NHS. It reported that 'if Florence Nightingale were carrying her lamp through the corridors of the NHS today, she would almost certainly be searching for the people in charge' (DHSS, 1983, p 12). The Griffiths Inquiry criticised the confusion of responsibilities between the DHSS and the NHS, echoing an earlier investigation that found excessive central intervention in the affairs of health authorities (DHSS, 1976b). It was also critical of the failure of the NHS to meet national policy objectives and to address the needs of consumers.

The Griffiths Inquiry recommended separate supervisory and management boards to clarify the roles of policy makers and managers. Its report argued that 'the requirement for central isolated initiatives should disappear once a coherent management process is established' (DHSS, 1983, p 16). In practice this did not happen, and the chairman of the NHS management board resigned amid allegations that ministers took all the key decisions. He was eventually replaced by a minister. A further attempt was made to separate policy from implementation in the form of the NHS Management Executive, which replaced the management board. This body, later renamed the NHS Executive (NHSE), survived until 2000 (see Chapter Three). Notably, these bodies remained part of the DoH and had no separate accountability for the NHS (see Edwards and Fall, 2005).

Griffiths recommended that general management should replace consensus management. Henceforth, a general manager would be held to account for the management performance of each health authority or service provider. The idea of chief executives for NHS bodies had been raised previously, but was rejected. Now, the idea had come of age. Although strongly opposed by professional groups and by the Labour Party at the time, it became an entrenched feature of NHS management. Contrary to initial predictions, general managers did not (apart from a few spectacularly unsuccessful examples) openly take on the medical profession (see Strong and Robinson, 1990; Harrison et al, 1992).

In addition, the Griffiths Inquiry recommended stronger 'line management' of the NHS by extending the annual accountability reviews (currently used to monitor the performance of health authorities) to health service providers. Throughout the 1980s and 1990s, the DHSS/DoH subjected the performance of the NHS to closer scrutiny. Performance indicators were developed and league tables introduced. In addition, as noted in the previous section, targets were set, to provide a basis for reviews at each level of the NHS. Other Griffiths recommendations included a stronger leadership role for health authority chairs, greater involvement of clinicians in management at the local level, and better quality information about effectiveness and efficiency of the NHS.

The implementation of Griffiths' recommendations heralded a more business-oriented approach to running the NHS and emphasised corporate responsibility (of staff to their host organisation) and upward accountability (of NHS organisations to higher level authorities and ultimately the DoH). Other important changes that followed included the reshaping of health authorities as 'corporate bodies' (including senior managers on their boards, abolishing the requirement to have local authority nominees and strengthening the role of chairs – see Mohan, 1995). Moreover, central government took a closer interest in the appointment of health authorities and this led to allegations

– with some foundation (see Baggott, 1994a, pp 129-31) – that these bodies were dominated by Conservative Party supporters and people from a business background. Furthermore, the replacement of regional health authorities in the mid-1990s by regional offices of the NHSE staffed by civil servants enhanced the performance management role of this tier and strengthened the position of the centre against the local NHS (Dopson et al, 1999; Ham, 2004, p 164).

Ironically, the introduction of the internal market in the 1990s also strengthened line management. As Pollitt and colleagues (1998, p 180) observed, the freedoms of self-governing trusts were limited by a 'nervous central government' and they were subjected to a tight regime of monitoring, regulation and direction (Paton, 1993; Mohan, 1995; Hughes and Griffiths, 1999; Arrowsmith and Sisson, 2002). The tone was set early, when the market was introduced during a pre-election period. Ministers were keen to avoid controversy and dictated that a 'steady state' be preserved. Given the potentially dysfunctional nature of the health market, central government subsequently regulated behaviour that could lead to higher costs, increased surpluses and reductions in access and quality of services.

The Blair government reinforced this trend. The early years of this government were characterised by 'command and control' in health policy (see Klein, 1999; Carvel, 2000; Hunter, 2000; Taylor, 2000; Dixon, 2001; Ross and Tomaney, 2001; Edwards and Fall, 2005). Most policy participants interviewed supported this interpretation, although they disagreed over whether it was good or bad. According a former DoH civil servant, 'England has the most centralised and effective management the NHS has ever had'. From his perspective, a measure of centralised management was necessary to give a strong national lead to the NHS. However, most believed that management had been over-centralised to the detriment of the NHS. One interviewee, a former senior NHS manager, observed that the system was producing 'Stalinism of the worst kind' and claimed that managers were afraid to speak out. Another, from a think tank, pointed out that the performance regime was 'brutal' with ministers 'not afraid to give chief executives a bollocking'.

The Blair government introduced a host of national inspectorates and standard-setting bodies, discussed later in this chapter. The government took on new powers (under the 2001 Health and Social Care Act) to intervene in health authorities, PCTs and trusts in cases where they had been shown to be performing inadequately, including the removal of a body's powers and/or board members. There was greater intervention in the appointment of NHS managers and new arrangements were introduced to 'franchise' out the management of NHS bodies to other management teams, including the private sector. Meanwhile, ministers continued to intervene in health authority and trust appointments to ensure their initiatives would not be resisted at local level. Amid concern about political appointments (Select Committee on Public

Administration, 2000), ministers handed over the process to a special health authority, the NHS Appointments Commission, in 2001.

Central interventions were bolstered by the plethora of plans and targets discussed earlier. Managers knew what would happen if they failed to meet the key targets, such as those on waiting times (which became known as 'P45 targets'). Moreover, entire health authorities were threatened with removal if they did not comply with central directives. Nonetheless, disquiet about the centralisation of management began to grow. From 2000 onwards, a new approach was enunciated. Alan Milburn, as Secretary of State for Health (described by some as an 'arch centraliser' – Edwards and Fall, 2005, p 174 – see also Chapter Three) called for a new 'localism' (Milburn, 2001; see also Stoker, 2004). This was a major theme of the NHS Plan, which identified a new system of performance assessment – 'earned autonomy' – that proclaimed a 'lighter touch' for those who complied with central objectives. This regime promised greater autonomy, additional resources and less intrusive inspection of NHS bodies that performed well. Initially, a traffic-light system was suggested (green – greater autonomy; amber – limited autonomy; red – tighter controls from the centre). This was later dropped in favour of a star rating system. The 'localist' approach also fed into other policies, such as the creation of foundation hospitals and the expansion of the private sector's role as a supplier of services on behalf of the NHS. The government's policy was outlined further in subsequent policy documents, which set out the aim of shifting 'the balance of power ... towards front line staff who understand patients' needs and concerns' (DoH, 2001a, p 5; Cm 5503, 2002). Further policy documents emphasised these themes while developing further initiatives on patient choice and privatisation of NHS services (see Cm 6079, 2003; Cm 6268, 2005; DoH, 2005).

Those interviewed about recent developments in health policy broadly welcomed any efforts to decentralise and devolve NHS management, but were cynical about central government's actual intentions. Most maintained that despite the commitment to 'Shifting the Balance of Power', central government maintained a tight grip on the NHS. One, a trade unionist, observed that 'the government has not learned from its mistakes. It still seeks to impose from above.' Another, from a health charity, stated that 'central government still exerts strong influence ... local services often don't have the freedom to respond ... most decisions are taken in a centralised way'. Doubts were expressed that ministers would ever be able to leave the NHS alone (see ***Box 7.2***). According to a think tank spokesperson, the real test would be whether 'ministers can walk away or will they get frustrated and intervene'. Some believed that the excessive centralism of the 1990s had damaged local decision-making, a former senior NHS manager pointing out that 'capacity and capability on the ground has been eroded'. Others agreed that more could be done to promote 'real' or 'proper' devolution, with a bigger role for independent inspectorates and, possibly, the creation of autonomous regional health bodies.

Other studies support the view that earned autonomy has not yielded the benefits promised. Autonomy is restricted by central targets, and incentives associated with autonomy are not sufficiently powerful to promote improved performance (Hoque et al, 2004; Mannion et al, 2005b). There are also doubts about the capacity for greater local autonomy. Anecdotal evidence indicates that central government will continue to intervene where the political stakes are high. For example, ministers intervened in decisions by PCTs about independent treatment centres. In the case of South West Oxfordshire PCT, for example, pressure was exerted by the DoH and the SHA when it refused to sanction a new independent treatment centre for cataract surgery, leading to resignations of some of the PCT's non-executive directors, including the chairman (Carvel, 2004).

Box 7.2: Taking the NHS out of politics?

Throughout its history, and particularly in recent decades, there have been calls to take the NHS out of politics. It is argued that the high political profile of the NHS, coupled with its centralisation under successive governments, have combined to undermine the service. On the one hand, it is claimed that the priorities of the NHS are too heavily influenced by the government's desire to get re-elected, reflected in politically driven targets on waiting times. On another, the NHS's ability to provide services on a day-to-day basis is inhibited by efforts to micromanage the service in order to minimise media and public criticism.

Concern about political interference has inspired a range of proposals to give the NHS greater independence from central government (see, for example, Hutton, 2000; King's Fund, 2002; NHS Alliance, 2002). Although varying in detail, these recommend that the NHS be given some kind of formal status to protect its independence. Suggestions include establishing it as a non-departmental public body or as a public corporation. Ministers would retain a role in setting the overall objectives of the NHS, but would not be allowed to interfere in day-to-day management. More recently, senior politicians in both Labour and Conservative Parties have suggested greater independence for the NHS (BBC, 2006).

One problem is that such a move could insulate the NHS from democratic pressures and reduce public accountability. A possible compromise is to simultaneously strengthen accountability by introducing more effective structures of patient and public involvement in the NHS, especially at the local level. Another idea is to give local authorities greater powers of oversight and scrutiny than they currently enjoy, or perhaps even a commissioning role in relation to NHS services (Glasby et al, 2006). A further alternative is to 'regionalise' the NHS, possibly with some oversight from Regional Assemblies (which at present are not directly elected, see Chapter Nine). Indeed, over 25 years ago, the Royal Commission on the NHS recommended that regional health authorities be given direct accountability to Parliament for the operation of NHS services (Cmnd 7615, 1979).

A second problem is that, as the NHS is funded mainly out of national taxation, the government is compelled to intervene. Indeed, many of the pressures behind central government intervention have come from Parliament, with MPs urging the government to strengthen NHS accountability to the centre to ensure that funds are spent effectively. The NHS is unavoidably politicised. It is a large employer, its services affect many people in a significant way and it is a major institution in the country. As Douglas Black (1987, p 38) wrote back in 1987, 'it is not possible, as some wish, to take the health service out of politics – both the amount of money involved and the sensitivity of anything to do with health will keep the health service a major political preoccupation'. His comments were echoed by Christopher France, former Permanent Secretary at the DoH (quoted in Edwards and Fall, 2005, p 197), '... the NHS was never an industry to be managed by an independent board. It is a branch of the body politic and will be for as long as it is publicly funded.'

Regulation and inspection

According to Walshe (2003, p 14), 'since 1997, there has been a rapid and continuing growth in healthcare regulation in the UK, especially in England'. This has taken the form of centralised regulation, embodied in new national regulatory agencies. Previously only finance (discussed in a later section of this chapter) was subject to such a degree of central regulation (by the Treasury and DoH) and scrutiny by independent bodies, such as the NAO and, since 1990, the Audit Commission (see Chapter Four). There was little central regulation of standards of health care and treatment. Regulation mainly took the form of professional self-regulation, underpinned by the state. The exposure of poor standards produced changes in self-regulation rather than the creation of government regulatory bodies. An exception was the Hospital Advisory Service (HAS – later the Health Advisory Service), created in the 1960s to monitor and inspect services in long-stay hospitals, following several scandals (Robb, 1967; Butler and Drakeford, 2005). Any suggestion that the remit of the HAS be extended to all NHS hospitals in the future was blocked (Webster, 1996).

Not until the 1990s were plans for an NHS-wide inspectorate revived. As already mentioned, attempts to set and monitor service standards began under the Conservatives, with the setting of targets and *The Patient's Charter* standards.

The DoH highlighted the cost-effectiveness of clinical procedures, while stressing the importance of evidence-based practice and the use of national clinical guidelines within the NHS (Klein et al, 1996). Medical (and later clinical) audit was promoted in an effort to monitor the quality of care and to encourage improvements in practice. The Conservatives' internal market led to further regulation. Market rules were established and a Clinical Standards Advisory Group created to assess the impact of the market on access, standards and quality of NHS services.

The Blair government subsequently created a new statutory body, the Commission for Health Improvement (CHI) to monitor NHS performance against service standards (Day and Klein, 2004). These standards were set out by national bodies such as NICE (whose role is discussed later) and in NSFs. CHI was responsible for ensuring that NHS provider organisations introduced 'clinical governance', a system of internal quality assurance that reflected responsibility for the quality of care newly imposed on NHS chief executives. CHI also investigated serious service failures and had a general duty to promote health care improvement in the NHS. Subsequently, CHI was given additional powers to inspect NHS bodies and recommend closure or suspension of services. It was charged with producing information on performance, which included a system of star ratings. NHS organisations were given 3, 2, 1, or no stars, depending on an assessment of their performance. Those with higher ratings were promised greater autonomy, those with the lowest would face detailed scrutiny and intervention. The star rating system has since been replaced by an 'annual health check'. This employs a scoring system reflecting the organisation's effectiveness in using financial resources and the quality of care provided. Health care organisations are monitored against core standards covering patient safety, clinical effectiveness and public health and their performance against government targets.

CHI was later reconstituted as the Commission for Healthcare Audit and Inspection (CHAI), and is now known as the Healthcare Commission. It absorbed some functions from other bodies (including the Audit Commission's responsibility for value for money in the NHS) and has overall responsibility for assessing the performance of NHS organisations, reporting on the state of health care, regulating the private health care sector and promoting improvements in health care provision. It is expected that the Healthcare Commission will be merged with a further body, the Commission for Social Care Inspection (CSCI), to create a single quality assurance body for health and social care. The Healthcare Commission is a statutory non-departmental public body accountable to Parliament as well as health ministers. To safeguard its independence, its board is appointed by the NHS Appointments Commission. However, it must have regard to government policy and some aspects of its work are subject to direction from ministers, discussed further later.

Another new body, the National Patient Safety Agency (NPSA), was created following concerns about the level of adverse incidents in health care. Its task is to ensure the introduction of a new system of incident reporting and that appropriate guidance is given to health care organisations to avoid such events. Another new body, the National Clinical Assessment Authority (NCAA), was given the task of assessing the needs of doctors and dentists who fell short of the required standards and advising their employers on how to deal with poor clinical performance. The NCAA has since been taken over by the NPSA.

The creation of these bodies was partly inspired by a series of medical scandals, including the poor standards of paediatric surgery at Bristol Royal Infirmary (Bristol Royal Infirmary Inquiry, 2001), illegal and unethical organ retention at Bristol and at Alder Hey Hospital, Liverpool (Royal Liverpool Children's Inquiry, 2001), the case of Harold Shipman, the GP found guilty of murdering his elderly patients (Shipman Inquiry, 2001), and other individual cases of negligence and malpractice, such as the notorious gynaecologist Rodney Ledward (Ritchie, 2000). As with the HAS (whose work has since been taken over by other agencies) three decades earlier, public and media concern strengthened ministers' commitment to stronger regulation.

Professional self-regulation has also been reformed in recent years (Allsop and Saks, 2002; Irvine, 2003). The Blair government introduced changes to make it easier to alter legislation relating to professional self-regulation. It introduced a UK council for the regulation of health care professionals (the Council for Healthcare Regulatory Excellence – CHRE) to oversee health professional self-regulatory bodies, promote cooperation between them, and in exceptional cases require them to make new rules. CHRE has powers to over-rule the decision of these bodies in certain circumstances. The existing self-regulatory bodies were expected to review and strengthen their procedures for dealing with complaints and maintaining high standards of practice. The GMC, for example, acquired new powers to suspend doctors or impose restrictions on them with immediate effect. It also pledged to introduce a new system of revalidation for doctors – under which they would have to prove their fitness to practice. Following further criticism (Shipman Inquiry, 2001, 2004) and a review (DoH, 2006a), further changes in the system of medical regulation are expected.

An important part of the government's regulatory approach was the setting of clinical standards through NSFs and the activities of NICE (the National Institute for Health and Clinical Excellence, originally known as the National Institute for Clinical Excellence). NICE was established in 1999 as a special health authority to provide evidence on the cost-effectiveness of new and existing health care interventions, develop clinical guidelines for various conditions, and assist the NHS with clinical audit. It also has responsibility for checking the safety and efficacy of new clinical procedures and has acquired the responsibilities of the former Health Development Agency for the evidence base in public health.

NICE guidance to the NHS has been mandatory since 2002, although implementation varies by trust and by topic (Sheldon et al, 2004; Raftery, 2006). In the absence of guidance, PCTs and trusts may decide not to fund a particular course of treatment. This leads to particular problems for patients seeking access to new treatments, as indicated by the case of the breast cancer drug, Herceptin. This drug was not approved for women with early-stage breast cancer, despite claims that they could benefit from it. A number of women took their PCTs to court, with some success. In 2005, the Secretary of State for Health stated that PCTs must not refuse to fund the drug purely on grounds of cost. As a result, NICE's judgement was effectively bypassed, at least in the short term. In some other cases NICE has been accused of changing guidance in response to political pressure from government, the drugs industry and patients' organisations (see Ferner and McDowell, 2006). More generally, NICE has been criticised for lacking in transparency, for basing judgements on a limited range of evidence, for taking too much time to evaluate new treatments and for limiting clinical freedom by effectively preventing certain treatments that might in particular individual circumstances be justified (see Consumers' Association, 2001; Health Committee, 2001). Given the controversial territory it inhabits, perhaps one should not be surprised by such criticism.

With the creation of foundation trusts in 2003 another regulatory body was born. To meet criticisms that foundation trusts might undermine the principles of the NHS, the government created a national regulator, accountable to Parliament and to health ministers. This organisation, known as Monitor, was constituted as a non-departmental public body. Monitor is responsible for authorising the framework for each foundation trust, including conditions on the range of services it provides, the level of private practice, restrictions on borrowing and asset sales. It authorises initial financial plans and governance structures. Monitor may intervene where a foundation trust has breached its 'authorisation', for example if it incurs high financial deficits or severe problems with services. In such circumstances Monitor may replace senior managers and members of the governing board. It should be noted that the quality of health services provided by foundation trusts remains subject to regulation by the Healthcare Commission.

There has been a huge amount of new regulation in the NHS, much of it arising from these new regulatory bodies. The regulatory regime has been overwhelmingly centralist, with strong emphasis on national standards, frameworks and processes (Davies, 2000; Walshe, 2003). Moreover, the independence of the new regulatory regime is not guaranteed. Some regulatory agencies are constituted as special health authorities and as such are potentially subject to a degree of ministerial intervention. In contrast, Monitor has greater constitutional independence as a non-departmental public body reporting directly to Parliament. However, it is also required to report to the Secretary of State for Health, who appoints its members. Furthermore, it is required to act in a way consistent with ministers' general duties in relation to the NHS. The Healthcare Commission has some independence, being constituted as a non-departmental public body and accountable to Parliament as well as ministers. It is appointed by the NHS Appointments Commission, rather than by ministers directly. The Healthcare Commission is subject to ministerial involvement in some aspects of its work, notably with regard to setting standards of health care, the criteria for performance ratings, and the initiation of reviews and investigations. It must also have regard to such aspects of government policy as the Secretary of State for Health may direct in relation to annual reviews of performance and reviews, and investigations of NHS bodies. The Secretary of State may ultimately issue directions if he/she believes the Healthcare Commission is not fulfilling its functions properly and has powers to remove its chair and individual members on grounds of incapacity or failing to discharge their duties. Some experts argue that the creation of the Healthcare Commission represents a significant step away from a centrally directed bureaucratic structure (Walshe, 2003). Although, so far, this body appears to have maintained its independence, it remains to be seen whether strong ministerial pressure can be withstood.

A major criticism is that health care regulation is fragmented. An opportunity to create a single, overarching framework was missed when the government rejected two key recommendations from the Bristol Royal Infirmary Inquiry (2001): that NICE be given responsibility for all action relating to the setting and issuing of clinical standards and keeping them under review; and that there should be a single regulatory body to bring together all the agencies involved in health care regulation. There have been further calls for NICE's work to be more closely integrated with NSFs (see Health Committee, 2001; Wanless, 2002).

Finally, the new regulatory regimes have imposed substantial costs on the NHS (National Audit Office, 2003; Walshe, 2003). Most costs are hidden because they involve institutional compliance with regulation rather than the actual financial costs of operating regulatory bodies. Moreover, doubts have been expressed about the quality of the system of quality assurance introduced in recent years (Walshe, 2003; Benson et al, 2004; Day and Klein, 2004; Gray and Harrison, 2004). Particular concerns include the capacity of regulators to engage with practitioners at the front line and most important of all, their ability to actually improve service standards, an issue taken up in the next section.

Culture and networks

Despite efforts to control and regulate the NHS, considerable power remains at local level in the hands of the medical profession. Many writers have observed that doctors are able to resist initiatives, not just by direct opposition but by lack of cooperation with local managers (see Harrison et al, 1992; Harrison and Pollitt, 1994; Ferlie et al, 1996; McNulty and Ferlie, 2002). Doctors are notoriously difficult to manage and have a high degree of autonomy especially in technical matters (Fitzgerald and Dufour, 1997; Dopson and Fitzgerald, 2006). Indeed, managing doctors has been likened to 'herding cats' (Mui, 1997, p 67). Doctors are generally opposed to being line-managed and dislike taking on management responsibilities.

Since the Griffiths reforms, discussed earlier, there have been several attempts to bring doctors into management. Some have taken on management roles, such as general manager, medical director or director of clinical speciality. But within the profession, these jobs are not seen as prestigious. Doctors undertaking management roles complain about heavy workloads – partly due to a desire to continue some level of medical practice, and offer limited opportunities for career development (see Simpson and Scott, 1997; Millar, 2000). Clinical directors can be treated with suspicion by colleagues and are regarded as having little influence over medical practice (Fitzgerald and Reeves, 1999).

Since the 1980s, governments have tried to bring about changes in medical practice by promoting audits of medical and clinical work. New schemes were introduced with limited success. They did not challenge professional autonomy, were poorly implemented and did not provide any clear benefits (Public Accounts Committee, 1996; van Herk et al, 2001). The Blair government introduced clinical governance as a means of encouraging audit and service improvements (Gray and Harrison, 2004). This involved establishing clearer lines of responsibility for care; a comprehensive programme of quality improvement; procedures for identifying and remedying poor performance; clear policies for identifying and minimising risk; and appropriate institutional arrangements within each trust.

Early evidence suggests that although institutional arrangements have been put in place, clinical governance has not had a major impact (see CHI, 2002, 2003; Leatherman and Sutherland, 2003; National Audit Office, 2003). On a more positive note, there are signs that clinical quality issues have become more mainstream, and that accountability for performance may be becoming more explicit. There are indications of more open, collaborative and transparent ways of working in professional cultures. However, there is also evidence of poor implementation of policies and variations between trusts and departments within the same trust. Failure in communication and learning both between and across organisations has been found.

Others have pointed out that the limited impact of clinical governance so far has been largely due to the 'top-down' and bureaucratic approach adopted by government (see contributions in Gray and Harrison, 2004). They argue that the model of clinical governance pursued by government has emphasised formal requirements, surveillance and compliance. From this perspective, more could be achieved by building high-trust relationships with the professions and involving them more closely in improving quality and standards (see also Leatherman and Sutherland, 2003). This approach emphasises the importance of informal and cultural aspects of professional work and the need to create conditions to encourage self-improvement within the professions.

These views were reflected among policy actors interviewed. Several interviewees emphasised that, despite its rhetoric, the government had failed to engage with clinicians at the local level. One (a trade unionist) commented, 'if you are trying to implement change, you have to take people with you', while another (a peer) observed that 'only cultural change will work'. Another (a former senior NHS manager) pointed out that 'it was essential to engage with clinicians, but they had become disillusioned with the government'.

The Blair government may claim that it had responded to such criticism by highlighting the need to shift the balance of power to the 'front line' and by emphasising the 'new localism' in the NHS (see discussion earlier). However, as noted earlier, these initiatives were strong on rhetoric and there is little evidence to suggest that change is actually happening in practice. However, other initiatives have placed greater emphasis on cultural change and collaboration, particularly those established under the auspices of the DoH and the Modernisation Agency (the latter now superseded by a new body, the NHS Institute for Innovation and Improvement). For example, 'beacons' were introduced in the NHS to spread good practice. These were examples of innovative practice identified by a competitive selection process. Those deemed exemplary were then disseminated around the NHS and others were encouraged to learn from their experience (see SHM, 2002). Other initiatives included collaborative networks (Bate, 2000), which seek to challenge existing ways of delivering services. These are part of national programmes connected to service plans and frameworks (such as the Cancer Plan, for example). However, these initiatives also emphasise the importance of involving local clinicians and other stakeholders. In principle, they should be driven by cultural change and knowledge management rather than by structural reconfiguration and managerial reform.

Beacons and collaborative networks have the potential to change the culture of the NHS and improve services from the bottom up. However, they have been introduced within a framework of central control and targets and emphasise structural change rather than knowledge sharing and cultural change (CHI/Audit Commission, 2001; Kewell et al, 2002; Mohan, 2002, p 217; All Party Group on Cancer, 2004; Entwhistle and Downe, 2005; Addicott et al, 2006). It is important that they are not seen as a top-down exercise but must genuinely empower local managers and clinicians to pursue improvements to services. As the link between organisational culture and performance has been acknowledged (see Mannion et al, 2005a), 'command and control' models of decision making have been increasingly discredited (Degeling et al, 1998). Critics such as Chapman (2002), for example, argue for new systems of policy-making and governance that empower professionals, service users and other stakeholders, and that encourage innovation, learning and experimentation.

Financial incentives

One feature of the NHS has always been centralised: its funding. Because the NHS is funded overwhelmingly out of general taxation, national insurance contributions and centrally fixed charges, there is little scope for NHS organisations to develop independent sources of finance. Aside from relatively small-scale income-generating activities (car parking charges, asset sales) and endowments and charitable donations (which can be substantial for some prestigious hospitals), the NHS is dependent on income from central government.

Although this gives central government considerable power, it was not until the 1960s that funding was really used to stimulate centrally led service developments. The Hospital Plan, referred to earlier, was probably the first major exercise in stimulating service changes through the funding regime, but it fell short of expectations. This was followed in the 1970s by the 'RAWP' (Resource Allocation Working Party) formula, introduced by the Labour government to shift resources from over-funded areas relative to needs to those that were under-resourced. During this period resources were also earmarked for the development of particular services, particularly the 'Cinderella services', mentioned earlier. Efforts to allocate resources based on measures of need continued throughout the 1980s and 1990s, although Conservative ministers intervened to protect services in the generously funded Tory-voting heartlands of London and the South East. Meanwhile, 'earmarked funding' continued as a means of promoting particular service developments and to reduce the size of waiting-lists.

A significant change occurred with the creation of the internal market during the 1990s. As already noted, this divided the NHS into purchasers and providers of services. The former, which included health authorities and fund-holding GPs, were given a budget, which they could use to secure services for their populations. Hospitals and other providers were expected to compete for this 'business'. Although heralded as creating powerful incentives for change, the reforms were managed and regulated. Competition was limited and the incentives to change were not dramatic (Le Grand et al, 1998; Mays et al, 2000). However, the internal market did have an impact in some respects. First, there was evidence of entrepreneurialism among fund-holding GPs (Ennew et al, 1998) – although due in part to the early entrants to the scheme being more entrepreneurial in their outlook than the average GP. Second, trusts became more efficient. Productivity, measured by changes in activity relative to resources, increased around by 7 per cent between 1991 and 1996 (Maniadakis et al, 1999). Third, there was evidence of inequities arising from the reforms, particularly differential access to hospital services between the patients of fund-holders and non-fund-holding GPs (Kammerling and Kinnear, 1996; Dowling, 1997), although the impact of the market on overall quality of care was different to ascertain.

As discussed earlier, the Blair government replaced the Conservatives' internal market. GPs, both fund-holder and non-fund-holder alike, were corralled into PCGs and then into PCTs. Under the 'Shifting the Balance of Power' initiative, PCTs acquired responsibility for over three quarters of the NHS budget. However, they did not have the autonomy that the government proclaimed. PCTs' discretion was limited by a range of factors including the requirement to attain government targets, limited management capacity and scarce resources. Politically, it proved extremely difficult for PCTs to dramatically alter funding flows to the acute and specialist providers. Studies of PCTs confirm that they have had limited discretion (see Greener and Powell, 2003; Deeming, 2004; Roche, 2004).

The Blair government embarked on a journey that would take it some way back to the system inherited from the Conservatives (Allsop and Baggott, 2004). It began to introduce supply-side reforms, such as the introduction of independent treatment centres, franchising of NHS management and foundation trusts. Together, these reforms represented a significant change; in the view of some observers nothing less than a redefinition of the NHS (see, for example, Pollock, 2004; Edwards and Fall, 2005, p 179).

Market forces were reintroduced. A new system, called 'payment by results', was launched to reimburse providers for individual treatments supplied, based on the standard cost of a group of procedures (known as a 'tariff'). Trusts could no longer rely on large-scale 'block' agreements to generate income, but would have to 'sell' their services to PCTs, GPs and their patients. Although reform was introduced gradually, the government maintained that failure by providers to generate sufficient income would ultimately lead to the closure of services. Meanwhile, on the demand side, the Blair government sought to reintroduce elements of GP fund-holding by committing to devolve budgets to the practice level. In addition, it went further than the Conservatives by allowing NHS patients to choose from a menu of potential service providers, including the private sector.

These changes, if fully implemented, herald the breakdown of old NHS hierarchies and could lead to a more decentralised health care system. There may also be a significant shift in the balance of power between professionals and service managers. If attracting patients in order to generate revenue becomes paramount, significant power may accrue to managers, which they may use to drive changes in professional practice and service provision. Nonetheless, there are reasons for scepticism. It should be remembered that the Conservatives' internal market was introduced with a similar fanfare, but became a tightly managed market. Moreover, as the experience of the 1990s showed, it is possible that some professional groups (for example, GPs, and specialists whose skills are in short supply) may increase their leverage as a result of the changes.

Conclusion

According to Edwards and Fall (2005, p 187), 'ever since the NHS was created, governments have struggled to manage it'. This continues today, despite the political pressures on central government that have led it to take a closer interest in the NHS. Although an oscillation between centralisation and decentralisation has been perceived by some commentators (for example, Klein, 1995), the longer-term trend has been the centralisation of key elements of policy and the increasing use of 'command and control' in implementation. Other ways of improving policy implementation have been recognised, notably organisational learning, trust building and cultural approaches. However, these have been secondary to the top-down bureaucratic model. There also has been a clear attempt to pass responsibility down the structure of the NHS. While there may be good reasons for devolving responsibility – especially where power is also devolved – the persistence of command and control means that this has largely been interpreted as an exercise in shifting blame away from central government to the local NHS. A further feature of this has been the increasing pace of change. 'Redisorganisation', discussed earlier, is only part of this. There is a broader problem of 'initiativitis', which means that reform has been 'relentless, almost hyperactive' (Appleby and Coote, 2002, p 5). This seems to have had a negative effect on the NHS and its staff (*Health Service Journal*, 2005). Such disillusionment among those who, ultimately, implement government policy is likely to lead to further gaps between policy and practice in the future.

Summary

- In general, central government has centralised many aspects of health policy. This process has increased markedly in the past 20 years. Centralisation has been accompanied by a process of decentralising responsibility to the local level of the NHS.
- The NHS has undergone many reorganisations. Constant reorganisation can be counterproductive and costly.
- The centre has taken a more active role in setting plans and targets for the NHS in recent decades. Although planning is regarded as important, crude targets are seen as counterproductive.
- Management reform has been an important feature of the NHS since the 1970s. Managers are regarded as key players in implementing government policies.
- There has been a large increase in regulation and inspection in the NHS, reflected in the creation of new regulatory bodies. There have also been efforts to strengthen self-regulation by the professional bodies.
- The medical profession remains powerful within the NHS.
- Improvements in the NHS depend to a large extent on cultural changes within the professions and in health care institutions.
- There have been calls to take the NHS out of politics. But these ignore the fact that the NHS is highly politicised due to its funding and organisation and the prominence of health on the political agenda.

Key questions

1. Why has the NHS been reorganised so often?
2. Can the NHS be taken out of politics?
3. How important is cultural change to the implementation of policies? How can cultural change be promoted within the NHS?
4. Has the NHS become more centralised? If so, in what sense?
5. Name the key regulatory bodies in health services and specify their particular functions.

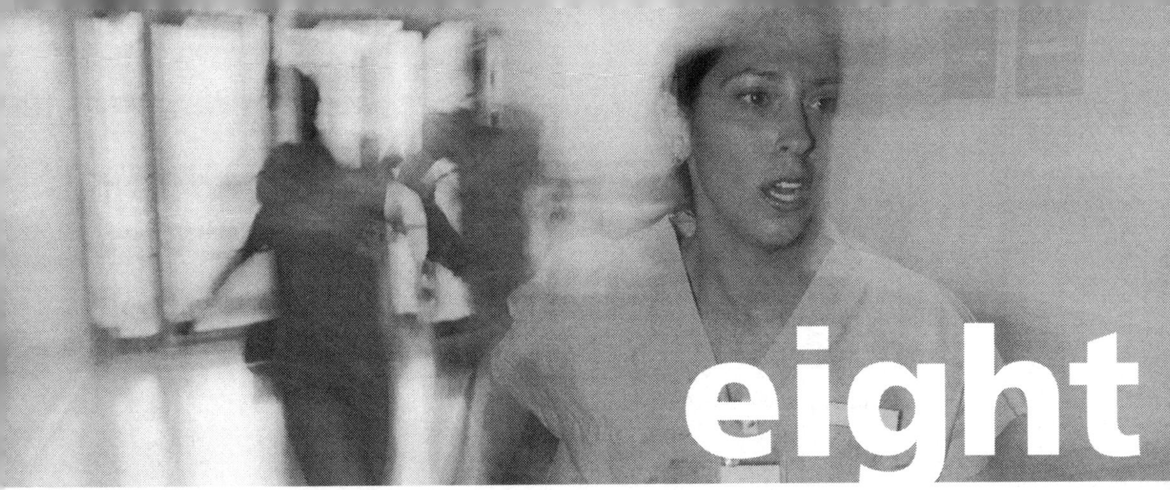

Partnerships and health policy

Overview

This chapter explores the role of other organisations involved in the implementation of health policy. After discussing the concept of partnership, it explores partnership working, first in the field of social care and then in relation to public health. The chapter also examines public–private partnerships and relationships between the NHS and the voluntary sector.

Health policy is not a matter for the NHS alone. The implementation of health policies depends heavily on other organisations that provide health and social care services, support people with health problems, and promote health and well-being. This includes local authorities, the private sector and voluntary organisations. This chapter examines the need to form effective partnerships between these organisations, the difficulties involved in working collaboratively, and the impact of policies to improve partnership working,

Partnerships

Ling (2000, p 82) observed that the literature on partnerships is characterised by 'methodological anarchy and definitional chaos'. This is exacerbated by assumptions that partnerships are necessarily a good thing (Powell and Glendinning, 2002), which means they are often invoked as a vague ideal. The Audit Commission (1998) sought to pin down the concept by describing partnerships as a joint working arrangement where partners are otherwise independent, agree to cooperate to achieve a common goal, establish new organisational structures or processes to achieve this goal, plan and implement a joint programme, and share relevant information, risks and rewards. Although this is a useful starting point for analysis, the reality is more complex. Partnerships vary according to the formality of arrangements, inclusiveness, styles of interaction, the means of governing partnership-working, and the degree of voluntarism and autonomy involved. The characteristics of a partnership – and in particular its dominant mode of governance – can change as it develops (see Lowndes and Skelcher, 1998).

This complexity makes it difficult to compare and evaluate partnerships (Dowling et al, 2004). However, principles of successful partnerships have been identified, based on empirical studies (Hudson and Hardy, 2002). These are as follows:

- acknowledgement of the need for partnership
- clarity and realism of purpose
- commitment and ownership
- development and maintenance of trust
- clear and robust partnership arrangements
- monitoring, review and organisational learning.

Similarly Frye and Webb (2002) specified a range of 'essential features' that partnerships must possess: the inclusion of all relevant bodies, a high level of trust, motivation by a common vision, clear objectives, collaboration based on collective responsibility and continued support from key sponsors. They also believed it important that partnerships should have flexibility, sufficient, long-term funding and conflict resolution mechanisms.

There are several reasons for forming a partnership (see Audit Commission, 1998; Lowndes and Skelcher, 1998; Balloch and Taylor, 2001;Newman, 2001; Perri 6 et al, 2002; Sullivan and Skelcher, 2002), which can be listed as follows:

- To create an integrated, holistic approach to policy and service delivery.
- To overcome narrow organisational or departmental perspectives (ie, the 'silo' mentality).
- To reduce transaction costs.
- To reduce overlap and duplication.
- To improve coordination.
- To develop innovative approaches.
- To pool resources and expertise.
- To share knowledge.
- To tackle complex issues that are beyond the capacity of one agency.

Although partnerships are not new, there is now a much stronger impetus to work together. The Blair government has promoted partnership working to tackle social problems and improve public services delivery. As Newman (2001) and others (see Clarke and Glendinning, 2002; Perri 6 et al, 2002) have observed, added impetus arose from the government's attachment to the 'Third Way' (see Chapters One and Two), which emphasised 'holistic and joined-up' government and pragmatic solutions based on new modes of governance. New partnership arrangements were established in a number of policy areas, including health. Even so, the 'silo-mentality' continued (Performance and Innovation Unit, 2000), reinforced by hierarchical performance management systems (ironically introduced by the Blair government's own public services modernisation programme). However, government continued to place faith in partnerships to integrate multiple central initiatives and to address fragmentation arising from other key components of its modernisation agenda – privatisation, pluralism and competition in public service provision.

Partnerships, local government and social care

Much of the debate about partnerships has centred on the 'troubled relationship' (Glendinning et al, 2005) between the NHS and local authority social services. When the NHS was created, local councils ceded hospital services but retained other health service responsibilities including ambulance services, school health services, home nursing and other community health services. These were transferred to the NHS in 1974, leaving local authorities with responsibility for social services. Although reorganisation was meant to address problems of collaboration, particularly between the hospital services, primary care and the community health services, it actually reinforced the existing division between social services and health services (see Brown, 1979; Allsop, 1984; Webster, 1996).

Over the years there have been many calls for an integrated health and social care service (Health Committee, 1999). Sir John Maude, a member of 1956 Guillebaud Inquiry into the NHS and former Permanent Secretary at the Health Ministry, argued that health services should be returned to local government (Webster, 1996). Others have since articulated the case for an extended local government role in health services (see Regan and Stewart, 1982; Hudson, 1998; Morley and Campbell, 2003; Glasby et al, 2006). Other proposals centred on unifying services under the NHS rather than local government (as in Northern Ireland, which established joint health and social service boards in the 1970s). The Major government explored the idea of bringing all mental health services under NHS bodies. More recently, the Blair government introduced care trusts, NHS organisations running both health care and social services for specific client groups (such as elderly people or people with mental illness).

Box 8.1: Local authorities and health scrutiny

The 2001 Health and Social Care Act required local authorities with social service responsibilities to establish Overview and Scrutiny Committees (OSCs) on health. NHS organisations must provide information to OSCs, and their senior managers are required to attend OSC meetings to answer questions. NHS bodies must also consult OSCs when substantial changes in services are proposed. Local authorities have adopted a variety of approaches when implementing health scrutiny (Campbell, 2002; Coleman, 2004). Although health OSCs are relatively new, there is some evidence of their early impact (Edwards, 2006; NPCRDC, 2006). They appear to have improved communication between councils and the NHS. OSCs have also enabled local authorities to raise issues, such as transport for elderly and disabled people, which are important to health and well-being but which have tended to be of marginal interest to the NHS. Councils seem to be taking a greater interest in health and well-being. However, conflicting perspectives between OSCs and the NHS have also been found. OSCs have been particularly frustrated by poor consultation by the NHS, a reluctance to share information, and a lack of engagement with local communities. There has also been a lack of clarity in both local authorities and the NHS about how health scrutiny fits with the wider patient/public involvement agenda.

Government has tried to improve collaboration between the NHS and local authorities (and other relevant partners, such as voluntary organisations – discussed later) in various ways (Sullivan and Skelcher, 2002). The first phase, during the 1960s and 1970s, involved policy coordination at both national and local levels. In central government a new joint approach to social policy was introduced (Challis et al, 1988). Meanwhile at local level, new planning arrangements were established involving the creation of joint consultative committees, planning teams and finance for collaborative ventures. This approach was regarded as unsuccessful. The second phase involved the use of market forces. Following the Griffiths Report on Community Care (DHSS, 1988), government gave social service departments the lead role in commissioning community care, while encouraging private and voluntary sector service provision. Although commissioning of health and social care remained separate, the government expected the NHS and social service departments to collaborate with each other. Although some did engage in joint commissioning to create seamless packages of care for individuals, fragmentation of services and a lack of coordination persisted (Audit Commission, 1997;

Clinical Standards Advisory Group, 1998). Incentives for NHS agencies and local authorities to collaborate were minimal, while the temptation to engage in activities that undermined collaboration – shifting costs on to each other, for example – remained strong (Salter, 1994). The third phase was marked by the programme of reform introduced by the Blair government. Both NHS and local government policies placed emphasis on partnership and collaboration (see Cm 3807, 1997; Cm 4169, 1998; Cm 4014, 1998; Cm 4818, 2000). In addition, specific partnership guidance was issued (DoH, 1998a) alongside joint national guidance on health and social care priorities (DoH, 1998b). Lead responsibilities were designated for specific priorities. Some resided with the NHS (for example, primary care), others with local authorities (for example, inter-agency working) and others were shared (for example, health inequalities). On top of this, the 1999 Health Act launched a new statutory framework that imposed a duty of cooperation regarding health and welfare on NHS bodies and local government. Furthermore, local authorities were given a role in scrutinising health services (see ***Box 8.1***).

Local authorities were also given a greater role in NHS planning. They were required to participate in Health Improvement Programmes, which focused on promoting health as well as improvements in health care. In addition, joint investment plans (JIPs) were introduced, initially for older people and then for people with mental illness and those with learning disabilities. JIPs involved participating agencies setting out needs, current service provision, future service developments and investment needed. Meanwhile, NSFs were introduced for groups such as the elderly and mentally ill people, whose needs spanned health and social care, emphasising further the importance of joint working across agency boundaries. Furthermore, specific policy initiatives were introduced for particular groups, such as elderly people (see ***Box 8.2***) and children. With regard to children, for example, new Children's Trusts were established in an effort to integrate services. This was accompanied by new duties of cooperation and the establishment of multi-professional teams across various agencies including the NHS, social services, education, the police, voluntary sector and the private sector.

Box 8.2: Partnerships for older people

Over 40 per cent of both NHS and social service budgets is spent on services for people aged over 65 (who represent approximately a sixth of the population). The needs of some elderly people are complex, particularly those of frail and very elderly people, many of whom have multiple illness and disabilities and depend on a range of agencies and professionals.

Health and social care services for elderly people have long been regarded as fragmented and poorly coordinated (Glasby and Littlechild, 2004). There has been a history of poor relationships between health and social care agencies, and other services which can affect an older person's quality of life, such as transport and housing. There are many reasons for this. Older people have often been regarded as no one's priority. This has been exacerbated by differences and tensions between agencies providing services for them, and between professional groups involved in their care. Although problems are long-standing, pressure to do something has increased in recent years. This has been partly influenced by increased media coverage of poor standards of care and weak collaboration between agencies, coupled with rise of the elderly as a political force – in particular the growing importance of the grey vote, and the influence of well-organised pressure groups such as Help the Aged and Age Concern.

Efforts to improve coordination between health and social care – such as joint planning and joint commissioning – did little to improve services for elderly people. Various attempts to integrate services were tried at local level (see, for example, Foote and Stanners, 2003), but projects were often difficult to sustain in the context of organisational and interprofessional rivalries. The Blair government introduced new joint planning arrangements, pooled budgets and health action zones (HAZs) (some of which focused specifically on the needs of elderly people). Further proposals, heralded by the NHS Plan of 2000, prioritised services for the elderly. New initiatives included an expansion of intermediate care, cross-charging for delayed hospital discharges, care trusts and an NSF for older people.

Intermediate care is a generic term for integrated services provided for a particular group (such as elderly people) aimed at preventing unnecessary hospital admission and promoting timely discharge. Elderly people can benefit from intermediate care services by avoiding long hospital stays and enjoying greater independence, by being cared for at home, for example. Schemes vary considerably, although their common features include comprehensive assessment of needs, arrangement of a package of appropriate services; multi-agency partnership and interprofessional working arrangements.

A system of *cross-charging* for delayed hospital discharges was introduced in 2004. Under this scheme local authorities are charged if patients cannot be discharged from hospital because there are no facilities to support or care for them in the community. This was introduced to create incentives for local authorities to cooperate in establishing community-based facilities, although it was criticised for creating new tensions between the NHS and local authorities. Delayed discharges have since fallen and in some local areas the policy seems to have strengthened joint commitments between the NHS and local government to invest in intermediate care services.

Care trusts were proposed as a means of integrating services by enabling health and social care to be delivered by a single NHS organisation (Glasby and Peck, 2003). It was argued that they would encourage a consistent and integrated approach to a particular client group across health and social care services. This proved to be a controversial measure, however. There were fears that it represented a take-over of social services by the NHS. The implementation of care trusts faced a series of practical problems and only a few were actually established. Some of the new care trusts covered older people's services, while others focused on mental health or learning disabilities.

The linchpin of government health and social care policy for the elderly is the *NSF for Older People* (DoH, 2001b). This is a 10-year programme, which includes a commitment to intermediate care and stronger partnership working in assessing and caring for older people and promoting their health and well-being. Undoubtedly, the NSF has raised the profile of services for older people (Glasby and Littlechild, 2004). A national clinical leader (or czar) for older people was appointed by the DoH, complemented by local champions and teams to implement the NSF. Since the introduction of the NSF, some improvements have been witnessed in partnership working, including more intermediate care provision, fewer delayed discharges, evidence of some improvements in integration, and better relationships between different agencies (SSI, 2002; Audit Commission, 2002; DoH, 2004c; CSCI et al, 2006). However, a number of problems remained (CSCI et al, 2006). A single assessment process for old people, promised by the NSF by 2002, was not fully implemented by 2006. Integrated services for dealing with the problem of falls by elderly people, promised by 2005, remained at an early stage of development with a significant minority of trusts not participating in collaborative arrangements (see Royal College of Physicians, 2006). Overall, a lack of shared vision among local agencies was evident, leading to the persistence of fragmented services and variations in the quality and range of services between different areas.

A further White Paper (*Our Health, Our Care, Our Say,* Cm 6737) in 2006 proposed further changes in health and social care that if implemented could improve joint working in elderly services. The commitment to a single assessment of needs and proposed joint health and social care teams was reiterated. More joint appointments between the NHS and local government were proposed. Clearer responsibility for older people's health and social care needs was identified within the roles of both NHS directors of public health and local authority directors of adult social services. Individual joint health and social care plans were proposed for those, such as the elderly, who used both services, along with the introduction of integrated health and social care records. Meanwhile, at the strategic level, new planning and financial arrangements were promised to improve collaboration between PCTs and local authorities on issues such as prevention and health promotion, as well as social care.

The 1999 Health Act enabled the NHS and local government to pool budgets, transfer funds and delegate commissioning and provider functions to each other. These new flexibilities were accompanied by organisational changes aimed at improving the relationship between health and local government. The creation of PCGs (and later PCTs) was expected to produce closer ties with local government, as councils were formally represented on them. Meanwhile, new area-based initiatives, HAZs, were introduced. These were based on principles of partnership and intended to promote health and reduce inequalities, as well as improve services. HAZs are discussed later in the context of local government's status as a partner in public health.

Following the NHS Plan of 2000, further initiatives were introduced, including an expansion of intermediate care (defined as a range of integrated services to provide faster recovery from illness, prevent unnecessary acute hospital admission, support timely discharge and support independent living – see ***Box 8.2***). This required greater cooperation of health and local government bodies (and others such as the private and voluntary sectors). Another initiative was the formation of care trusts as a means of integrating health and social care (Glasby and Peck, 2003). Care trusts were created as NHS bodies with responsibilities for delivering both health and social care services for groups such as older people, people with mental illness or people with learning disabilities. In the event only a small number were established because of hostility towards the idea, especially in local government circles, and the practical problems of integrating services in one organisation. The policy was criticised by some for promoting unnecessary organisational upheaval, further undermining relationships between the NHS and local government (Hudson and Henwood, 2002).

Local authorities were also subjected to 'cross-charging' when patients were unable to be discharged from hospital due to a lack of social care. The government argued that this would incentivise councils to invest in social care services, enabling people to be discharged earlier. There have been some improvements (see ***Box 8.2***) but concerns remain about premature discharge from hospital, and inappropriate placements in social care. Finally, under the 2001 Health and Social Care Act, the Secretary of State for Health acquired powers to compel local organisations to use various options to promote joint working, such as pooled budgets and delegation.

Given the number, diversity and timing of these initiatives, it is extremely difficult to evaluate their impact. However, most observers agree that relationships between the NHS and local government on social care issues showed some improvement by the early years of the new Millennium (Local Government Association, 2000; Regen et al, 2001; Banks, 2002; Glendinning et al, 2003). More specifically, Health Act flexibilities were being used, including pooled budgets (Audit Commission, 2005). PCGs/PCTs were forging links with local authorities and improved communication was evident, notably by the participation of local authority personnel on PCG/PCT boards (Glendinning et al, 2001; Peckham, 2003). New staff had been appointed to manage relationships between PCGs/PCTs and local authorities, on issues such as intermediate care, for example (Wilkin et al, 2002). Moreover, the introduction of health scrutiny (see ***Box 8.1***) appeared to have had a broadly positive impact on communication between local authorities and the NHS.

Despite all this, the NHS and local government continued to occupy separate worlds. Notwithstanding a requirement to engage in joint planning, there was little dovetailing of health and local authority plans (Peckham, 2003). Although there were signs of improved communication between health and local government bodies, liaison was weak or non-existent in many areas (Wilkin et al, 2002). Local government representatives believed they lacked influence over the NHS (Glendinning et al, 2003). Despite the increase in the use of pooled budgets, around 40 per cent of local authorities and PCTs reported problems with these arrangements (Audit Commission, 2005)

Joint working on social care continued to be undermined by several factors. First, the turbulence caused by constant reorganisation of both the NHS and local government disrupted relationships between them (Banks, 2002; Glendinning et al, 2003). Second, the inconsistency between NHS and local authority boundaries, another long-standing problem, added to the complexity of inter-agency relationships. A further reorganisation in 2006 added to the turbulence, although it created a better fit between PCT and local authority boundaries (around 70 per cent of PCTs now have boundaries consistent with local authorities). Third, while a measure of central intervention is needed to provide a framework for local collaboration, centralisation in the NHS (see Chapter Seven) and in local government adversely affects partnerships (Newman, 2001; Banks, 2002; Glendinning et al, 2003; Ranade and Hudson, 2003; Snape, 2003; Glendinning et al, 2005). Centralisation undermines local capacities and initiatives by driving local agencies to respond to their own particular hierarchy rather than local priorities. Central government acknowledged this problem by introducing Local Area Agreements (LAAs), which attempt to join local priorities across different agencies. These are discussed in a later section in the context of public health. A fourth problem has been the confusion caused by multiple partnerships. Partnerships are often established for specific reasons – regeneration, social care, public health and inequalities. However, until recently little thought has been given to how these partnerships should relate to each other. The Blair government has championed local strategic partnerships (LSPs) to manage these local partnership arrangements, also discussed later.

The final problem with partnerships is that too much emphasis has been placed on organisational structures and processes. Yet cultural barriers to partnership working are also significant (see Hudson and Hardy, 2002). Both organisational and professional cultures can be resistant to new ways of working (Hudson et al, 1997; Maddock and Morgan, 2000; Balloch and Taylor, 2001; Banks, 2002; Hudson, 2002; Hultberg et al, 2005). This has been addressed to some extent through efforts to create a common culture around integrated services, reinforced by joint posts, co-location of workers from different agencies, new workforce roles and joint training programmes (Glendinning et al, 2001; Dinsdale, 2004; Little, 2005a). Indeed, this is the lesson from Northern Ireland, where health and social services have been integrated since 1973. Although there is some evidence that a more holistic approach has been adopted in the Province, cultural factors have been at least as important as structural factors. Shared vision and values among professions and service providers has been crucial in promoting integration. This did not happen automatically because of the structure, but through active interventions to support multiprofessional and multidisciplinary working, including education and training (see Heenan and Birrell, 2006).

Public health and local authorities

The wider role of local authorities in the promotion of health and well-being has often been overlooked. Snape (2003) has argued that the attention given to the health and social care interface has marginalised local government's potential contribution to health promotion and geared the NHS–local government relationship to narrow social care priorities. In the 19th and 20th centuries, local councils were in the front line of public health improvement through providing education, housing, sanitation, and health and welfare services (Baggott, 2000). Public health responsibilities were lost in 1974, when the Medical Officer of Health post was abolished. Health service and planning functions were transferred to the NHS, although local government retained environmental health functions.

Some progressive local councils – chiefly in metropolitan areas – retained an interest in public health (Snape, 2003). During the 1980s, a period when British central government chose to ignore the social, economic and environmental causes of ill health (Baggott, 2000), these authorities faced severe health-related problems associated with deprivation and inequality. They were inspired by global public health initiatives (see Chapter Ten), such as the World Health Organisation's *Healthy Cities* and *Health for All* initiatives and *Local Agenda 21* (which followed from the 1992 Rio Summit on sustainable development), based on key principles such as prevention, community action, multi-agency working, multi-sectoral approaches and public health. In contrast, the NHS showed little interest in public health, aside from health education about lifestyle-related illness (for example, smoking), and clinical prevention programmes (such as cancer screening, vaccination programmes and incentives for GPs to engage in preventive medicine).

During the 1980s public health moved up the political agenda, prompted in part by the threats posed outbreaks of infectious disease (HIV/AIDS, BSE/CJD, legionnaires' disease, salmonella and E. coli), partly by shortcomings in the system of health protection, and to some extent by the government's own concern about the future burden of chronic illness arising from unhealthy lifestyles. In the 1990s, the *Health of the Nation* strategy was issued (Cm 1986, 1992) setting out key targets for risk factors (such as smoking and obesity) and for the reduction of mortality and morbidity rates for diseases such as cancer, heart disease and stroke, mental health and sexually transmitted diseases.

The *Health of the Nation* strategy was regarded as a missed opportunity, by failing to bring local authorities, the NHS and other agencies into an effective partnership to tackle public health. Local authorities were, however, identified as players in 'Healthy Alliances', established to promote health in specific settings (such as schools, for example). Some local alliances worked well, notably on issues such as heart disease prevention, smoking, drugs, HIV/AIDS awareness and accident prevention, especially where existing relationships between local authorities and the NHS were good and where additional funding was available. Other than this, local authorities found it difficult to shape policy initiatives in this field. Importantly, key public health-related services over which they had influence (notably housing) were ignored by the government's strategy (DoH, 1998c).

The Blair government proposed a greater role for local authorities in improving public health and reducing health inequalities (Cm 4386, 1999). It explicitly recognised the social, economic and environmental aspects of health. Local authorities were identified as key partners in health promotion and public health. As noted earlier, they were expected to contribute to local health improvement plans and liaise with PCTs on public health matters. The limited evidence available indicates improved liaison between the NHS and local government on public health issues (Gillam et al, 2001; SOLACE, 2001; Peckham, 2003; NPCRDC, 2006) and provides examples of good practice on issues such as smoking cessation, housing improvements, accident prevention and sexual health.

Local authorities now have a duty to produce a community strategy, which outlines how they intend to improve the quality of life of local communities and their actions to improve the social, economic and environmental well-being of their area. Research has shown that over 90 per cent of community strategies refer to health and social care issues (ODPM, 2005a). While public health issues are covered, there is a strong focus on services and, particularly, social care (Hamer and Easton, 2002; Snape, 2003). Local authority capacities for contributing towards health improvement are currently limited. For example, a report on their environmental health functions (Burke et al, 2002) found that environmental health services had become narrowly focused and fragmented. Statutory enforcement duties, performance management regimes and limited resources were among the factors responsible for their limited participation in the public health agenda and their inability to participate fully in the new organisational structures for public health.

Local authorities have also acquired powers to promote or improve economic, social or environmental well-being. There is little evidence about how they are using these, although it is generally perceived that the powers are under-utilised (Snape, 2003; ODPM, 2005b). Even if this is the case, it could be because local authorities have other ways of securing improvements to public health, such as the use of existing powers in areas like housing. In 2006, in its Local Government White Paper, the government proposed changes that would enhance the strategic role of councils (Cm 6939, 2006). It was envisaged that these measures (which included improvements in local authority scrutiny of the NHS and more effective joint strategies between local authorities and the NHS) would enable local authorities to exert more influence over health and health services, and strengthen their role in partnerships to improve health and well-being.

The Blair government earlier introduced new area-based partnership initiatives which had implications for public health. These included HAZs (Powell and Moon, 2001; Matka et al, 2002; Barnes et al, 2005), established to improve inter-agency collaboration in areas of high health needs. HAZs were given a brief to encourage integrated services, promote public health and reduce inequalities. HAZ schemes were diverse, making overall evaluation difficult. However, they varied considerably in their capacity to build partnerships. HAZs have since been incorporated within PCTs. Opportunities to improve partnerships were created through other programmes, notably Sure Start – a programme aimed at improving the health and well-being of pre-school children in deprived areas. Also, various regeneration schemes, notably the Neighbourhood Renewal Fund (NRF) – which had an explicit health dimension – required partnership working between various agencies including the NHS and local government (Snape, 2003; Coaffee, 2005).

In addition, there are LSPs, overarching partnerships that bring together various agencies including the NHS, local authorities and the private and voluntary sectors. They provide an overall framework for partnership and in most cases are responsible for the production of local community strategies, mentioned earlier. LSPs are fairly new entities. Available research suggests that their governing arrangements vary considerably. Some have made little progress in integrating plans and strategies and have been slow to make headway with performance monitoring and management (Local Government Association, 2000; ODPM, 2003, 2006). LSPs have limited resources. They are regarded by some as another layer of bureaucracy (Coaffee, 2005).

The need for better integration between the NHS, local government and other partners is a theme of many recent policy documents. *Choosing Health*, a further White Paper on public health (Cm 6374, 2004), called for closer working relationships between PCTs and local government. The government stated that it would encourage PCTs and local authorities to pool resources on issues such as improving diet and nutrition, anti-smoking programmes, sexual health services and reducing alcohol dependency. In addition, LAAs were proposed as a means of establishing joint aims, targets and resources across different agencies on public health and inequalities. LAAs are based on negotiations between local partners and government regional offices. They specify outcomes and resources as well as the ground rules for the partnership and any flexibilities and freedoms it may have. Early evaluation of LAAs showed that, despite the excitement and energy surrounding their introduction, many participants were confused about their purpose, and that they underestimated the scale of the task faced (ODPM, 2005c). There were problems in engaging partners at an early stage. A tendency to 'muddle through' was found, although the process of establishing LAAs did stimulate partnership working, which could have a longer-term positive impact. LAAs, along with LSPs, have been identified as key instruments for promoting improvements in collaboration between local agencies, particularly on public health and inequality issues (Cm 6939, 2006).

Following its Green Paper on adult social care (Cm 6499, 2005), the government produced a White Paper on care outside hospital: *Our Health, Our Care, Our Say* (Cm 6737, 2006). This document reiterated the importance of improvements in partnership working. Specifically, it proposed:

- A redefinition of the role of the Director of Public Health at local level so that public health resources across the public sector are allocated to health promotion and well-being. More joint appointments, pooled budgets and multi-agency teams in public health were also proposed.

- Closer integration between health and social services, including joint health and social care teams, as well as joint commissioning of health and social care. Directors of Adult Social Services were expected to have clear roles in coordinating agencies.
- Closer working between the NHS and local authorities, with streamlining of budgets and planning cycles, shared outcomes and alignment of performance management through LAAs. More coterminosity was recommended (that is, consistent geographical boundaries) between SHAs and Government Regional Offices, as well as between local authorities and PCTs.

These measures in turn stimulated efforts to integrate health policy with other relevant policies at the regional level, which are discussed further in Chapter Nine.

Partnership with the private sector

The British health care system has always depended to some extent on the private sector. A small private health sector survived the creation of the NHS and has since grown. Meanwhile the NHS retained pay beds and therefore remained a significant supplier of private health care. Hospital doctors retained significant private practice as well as working for the NHS, while GPs, dentists and other family practitioners kept their independent contractor status. On top of this, the NHS has always depended on a range of private companies for medical equipment, drugs and other supplies.

The Conservative governments of the 1980s and 1990s actively promoted the privatisation of health and social care. Social care became increasingly funded and provided by the private (and voluntary) sectors. The NHS was urged to involve the private sector in planning and joint projects, such as the sharing of expensive medical equipment. It was also encouraged to use spare capacity in the private sector to reduce waiting lists for treatment. Market testing of NHS services was undertaken, beginning with ancillary services such as laundry, cleaning and catering. Finally, with the introduction of the PFI in the 1990s, the government gave private consortia an opportunity to design, finance, build and operate new hospitals.

In opposition, the Labour Party expressed strong criticism of what it saw as the privatisation of the NHS and was particularly opposed to PFI. However, in office the Blair government adopted public–private partnerships (PPPs), including PFI, as a key part of its public services modernisation programme (IPPR, 2001). It subsequently embarked on an ambitious hospital capital programme using PFI. This major U-turn shocked many Labour supporters, particularly the trade unions (Ruane, 2000; Pollock, 2004; Shaw, 2004). PPPs were also introduced into primary care in the form of local improvement finance trusts (LIFTs). LIFT schemes involve creating local public–private joint ventures to fund and modernise practice premises.

PPPs were controversial, but ministers banked on the public popularity of new facilities outweighing criticisms of trade unionists. In this regard they were successful, at least initially, although revelations about poor design, cuts in services due to the financial burden of PFI, and the huge profits made by consortia members later stirred public concern. By this time, New Labour had begun to develop a much larger role for the private sector in health care. Again, this demonstrated a remarkable turnaround. The Blair government's initial White Paper on the NHS (Cm 3807, 1997) made no mention of the private sector. But only three years later the NHS Plan (Cm 4818, 2000) set out a clear policy of engagement. Subsequently, a Concordat was agreed between the Independent Healthcare Association and the DoH (2000), setting out rules of engagement. The key principle of this document was that 'there should be no organisational or ideological barriers to the delivery of high quality healthcare free at point of delivery to those who need it, when they need it' (p 1). Among other things, the Concordat called for more explicit collaboration in planning between the NHS and the private sector and identified specific areas where partnership working could be strengthened, including intermediate care, workforce planning, elective care and critical care. PCTs were told by the DoH to make full use of the capacity in the private sector. Use of the private sector was further reinforced by the imperatives to reduce waiting-lists and waiting times in line with government targets.

The Concordat and waiting-list/time initiatives were outflanked by further developments (Pollock, 2004). The Blair government proposed the creation of 'fast-track' NHS diagnostic and treatment centres, some in partnership with the private sector, as well as a network of independent sector treatment centres (ISTCs), franchised to overseas health corporations, which would undertake work on behalf of the NHS. In addition, a new system of franchising for NHS trusts was introduced by which the private sector could bid to take over the management of trusts deemed to have performed badly. The creation of foundation trusts had further implications for PPPs, as it gave NHS service providers more scope for joint working with the private sector. Finally, the government announced that it intended the private sector to expand its share of NHS work even further, stating that the private sector could provide up to 15 per cent of operations by 2008. The right of NHS patients to choose and book hospital treatment was also extended to include at least one private supplier (Cm 6268, 2005).

In addition, central government encouraged partnerships in the realm of public health. LSPs, which have an important remit to coordinate action on matters of health, welfare and inequalities, are meant to engage with the private sector and other stakeholders. Central government has also emphasised the importance of working in partnership with commercial organisations on national public health policies. Its public health strategy (Cm 6374, 2004) made clear an intention to work with industry, even on controversial issues such alcohol misuse (see ***Box 6.1***).

The private sector now has a more significant role in relation to health and health care. Despite the rhetoric, however, the degree of actual engagement between public and private sectors remains low. In health care, although there has been an increase in private sector activity, there is little evidence of long-term partnerships being formed (Sussex and Goddard, 2002). In broader public health matters too, it appears that strong business engagement is not widespread (ODPM, 2006). However, the planned expansion of NHS-funded private health care may provide a stronger impetus for strengthening partnerships.

The key problem in forging such partnerships is that the NHS – and the public sector more generally – operates on different principles (Ruane, 2002; Pollock 2004). Private sector organisations are profit-oriented and have a primary duty to benefit shareholders, whereas the public sector has an ill-defined commitment to the public interest. While in particular circumstances there may be common ground, the philosophical differences are important. The private sector will make money at the public's expense where it can. Indeed, there have been several high-profile cases where PFI schemes have been found to have cost the taxpayer dear. The Public Accounts Committee (2006a) report on Norwich and Norfolk NHS Trust hospital project, for example, found that the consortium made large gains – a 60% rate of return. It described this as an 'inappropriate outcome' and 'the unacceptable face of capitalism'. Moreover, the higher prices charged by the private health sector has also undermined the spirit of partnership. One study found that prices were 40 per cent higher on average in the private sector compared with the NHS (Health Committee, 2003).

The contrasting aims and principles of the public and private sectors also have implications for the quality of care. Partnerships between public and private organisations are often undermined by 'principal–agent' problems (Deakin and Walsh, 1996; Sullivan and Skelcher, 2002). Contractors have incentives to reduce costs and under-perform, particularly when services are difficult to specify or standards difficult to enforce. Both the US experience of health care (see Pollock, 2004) and UK experience of competitive tendering (Davies, 2005) suggest that private operators can pursue profits at the expense of the public interest. Public service commissioners have introduced monitoring of contracts, which ironically adds to the costs of private contracting. Theoretically, it is possible to build stronger partnerships to ensure that practice is based on trust (see Coulson, 1998), but the profit motive is powerful and tends to override any pressures to commit to long-term relationships.

Partnership has also been undermined by the aggressive approach taken by government. PFI has been described as 'the only game in town' (Ruane, 2000). Franchising of NHS management was used as a punitive weapon against trusts deemed to have performed badly, but may have made the situation worse (*Hospital Doctor*, 2006), Some PCTs were forced to commission work from new private facilities, in particular the ISTCs (see Chapter Seven). Although the NHS may be compelled to create additional opportunities for business, this does not necessarily lead to better longer-term working relationships with the private sector.

Finally, a range of other concerns about private sector involvement make public service organisations reluctant to commit fully to partnerships (see IPPR, 2001; Pollock, 2004 Flinders, 2005). These include a lack of transparency and accountability, and inflexibility resulting from being tied into contracts (particularly with regard to hospital PFI projects). Notably, policies that aim to privatise public services actually create a more fragmented system, making it even more difficult to secure 'whole-system' approaches to policy problems.

Partnership with the voluntary sector

The voluntary sector has a long history of involvement in health and social care (Brenton, 1985). Although the creation of the NHS removed large areas of health care from the voluntary sector, the latter continued to play a significant role in providing care, information and support services, notably in areas such as maternity and childbirth, the care of the elderly and disabled people, long-term conditions, learning disabilities, mental health and palliative care. Voluntary organisations have been involved in public health issues through health promotion activities and by campaigning for policies to prevent illness. In addition, they can act as a voice for patients, service users, carers, vulnerable and disadvantaged groups and local communities (Baggott et al, 2005).

The voluntary sector has been described as 'a loose and baggy monster' (Kendall, 2003, p 127). It is highly differentiated and complex. The broadest definition of the voluntary sector (the broader 'non-profit sector') includes 'all entities which are formal organisations having an institutionalised character, constitutionally independent of the state and self-governing, non-profit distributing and involve some degree of voluntarism' (Kendall, 2003, p 21). On the basis of this definition, the contribution of the voluntary sector is significant: it accounts for 6 per cent of total employment and (if volunteer labour is included) just over 9 per cent of GDP.

In the post-war period, the voluntary sector was seen as useful in filling gaps in statutory provision. It was acknowledged as an innovator, developing new approaches to social problems that might in future become mainstream. It was also burdened with a persistent image of amateur 'do-gooders' dispensing to the needy, which reflected a lack of understanding about the sector.

Central government realised the importance of the voluntary sector, both as a contributor to services and as promoting health and well-being in a wider sense. In 1968, a central government grants scheme was introduced for voluntary organisations in the health and welfare field. In 1977, the government's NHS priorities document (DHSS, 1977) stressed the value of voluntary activities and urged greater collaboration between the statutory and voluntary sectors. Also, in the field of public health, urban and community development, projects were established with the involvement of voluntary groups (Brenton, 1985). Nonetheless, despite encouragement from central government, partnership working was highly variable at the local level (Wolfenden Committee, 1978), much depending on the history of collaboration in a particular locality or significant local figures who were effective in promoting joint working.

The Thatcher government saw the voluntary sector, along with the private sector, as a means of reducing the public sector. Yet it failed to develop a coherent strategy towards the voluntary sector (Kendall, 2003). Piecemeal changes were introduced, such as the introduction of new joint planning arrangements that required the inclusion of voluntary organisations on joint consultative committees, alongside NHS and local authority representatives. The Thatcher and Major governments did offer the voluntary sector greater opportunities, however, with regard to social care. For example, government policy increased the market for both voluntary and private service providers. Moreover, various policy documents and guidance urged greater collaboration between voluntary and statutory organisations, especially in service planning (Wyatt, 2002). Under the Major government, there was a greater recognition of the voluntary sector's role in public health (Sullivan and Skelcher, 2002; Wyatt, 2002). However, there remained an absence of strategic thinking about how to establish a framework within which the voluntary sector could develop, how its capacities and capabilities could be enhanced, or how it could play a fuller role as a partner in service planning. Rather the emphasis was upon how the state could get value for money by tying the sector more closely to the aims of government policy. Increasingly a 'contract culture' emerged, which had an impact on the aims and activities of voluntary groups and threatened their independence (Taylor, 1999; Sullivan and Skelcher, 2002).

In the 1990s, the voluntary sector pressed for a clear strategic framework. An independent commission established by voluntary sector groups, including their umbrella organisation, the National Council for Voluntary Organisations (NCVO), recommended among other things a concordat between government and the voluntary sector, setting out a core of good practice for future relations. This proposal was rejected by the Major government, but taken up by the Blair government. National compacts (that is, formal agreements) with the voluntary sector were introduced in each part of the UK, setting out key principles and undertakings (see Morison, 2000; Kendall, 2003). In addition, local-level compacts, to establish frameworks for partnership working at this level, were encouraged.

Sullivan and Skelcher (2002, p 91) describe the Blair government's agenda as 'a significant new phase in public–voluntary sector collaboration'. Indeed, the theme of partnership with the voluntary sector runs strongly through its policy initiatives in health and social care, public health and regeneration (Wyatt, 2002). More specifically, policy documents such as *Saving Lives* (1999), *Building on the Best* (2003) and *Our Health, Our Care, Our Say* (2006) explicitly mentioned the voluntary sector as a key partner. The latter document went further than previous documents in identifying a role for voluntary organisations (as well as social entrepreneurs and the private sector) to take over services deemed as underperforming. It announced the establishment of a social enterprise unit within the DoH to coordinate policy on the voluntary sector and social enterprise and a new fund to encourage developments. This built on previous actions to strengthen partnerships, including a strategic agreement between the DoH, the NHS and the voluntary and community sector, which set a framework for relationships between the various parties (DoH, 2004d). A National Strategic Partnership Forum was also established to take forward the initiative, including the promotion of local partnership agreements. This linked in with a further policy stream, that of patient and public involvement (PPI), where guidance explicitly recognised the role of voluntary organisations in service provision, health promotion and community representation (DoH, 2003b).

The government also established a Third Sector Commissioning Task Force to remove barriers to the involvement of voluntary and community organisations in the delivery of public services across government (see Third Sector Commissioning Task Force, 2006). With regard to wider public health issues, programmes such as Sure Start, New Deal for Communities, the Neighbourhood Renewal Fund and HAZs emphasised the importance of partnership with voluntary and community organisations (Sullivan and Skelcher, 2002). Furthermore, LSPs were expected to engage with voluntary groups (see Taylor, 2006).

The notion of partnership with the voluntary sector appealed strongly to the Blair government. It fitted neatly within its endorsement of the Third Way approach, and policies that combined market and state approaches (see Chapter One). It was also consistent with the government's communitarian ideals, based on individual responsibility, social inclusion, voluntarism and community empowerment.

What impact have these various initiatives had? First, the impact of compacts is difficult to judge. Where they reflect a genuine commitment on both sides, they appear to facilitate partnership. The process of negotiation is regarded as important as the product in building trust and good relations (Craig and Taylor,

2002; Osborne and McLaughlin, 2002). But there is a risk of compacts being tokenistic and consequently having little impact on the everyday relationship between statutory authorities and the voluntary sector (Alcock and Scott, 2002). Research on national voluntary groups representing patients, users and carers found the impact of the national compact on relations between this sector and the government was negligible (Baggott et al, 2005). Meanwhile at local level, the picture is rather patchy, with some areas showing improved relationships between statutory authorities and the voluntary sector (Craig and Taylor, 2002). However, further research has found that few local community strategies referred to compacts, and that the involvement of voluntary organisations in these plans was 'incredibly limited' (ODPM, 2006). This reflects wider concerns by voluntary organisations about the need for closer involvement in planning (Turning Point, 2004).

Second, despite the willingness of many voluntary organisations to engage in partnership activities such as planning, consultation and service development, there has been a failure by government to appreciate that these various roles impose significant costs on them. Financial support for the sector, to develop capacities and capabilities, and to compensate for the opportunity costs of participation has increased, but remains relatively low. Moreover, given the increasing demand for their involvement, one can understand how voluntary organisations get overloaded. 'Consultation fatigue' is a common complaint (Craig et al, 2004) and the proliferation of partnerships has undermined the capacity of organisations to get involved (Craig and Taylor, 2002). Much more could be done to integrate partnerships, reducing the need for multiple partnership arrangements (ODPM, 2006). Although, as noted, LSPs have been identified as a means of rationalising partnerships, research indicates that in spite of these efforts, voluntary and community representation in LSPs remains stretched and under-resourced (ODPM, 2006).

Third, the representative role of voluntary organisations is problematic (Alcock and Scott, 2002; Craig and Taylor, 2002; Baggott et al, 2005). There are major inequalities within the voluntary sector that mean that some voices are stronger and more influential than others. Genuine partnership means providing opportunities for weaker, marginalised and less well-resourced groups to participate. Otherwise, differences in the willingness and ability of groups to participate will, by default, advantage representatives of the better-resourced, politically astute, organisations. As a result, the diversity of views across the voluntary sector as a whole may not be captured.

Fourth, there are concerns that closer relations between the state and voluntary sector could compromise the autonomy and independence of the latter, a point made by voluntary sector interviewees. One stated that 'charities should not become simply an arm of government'. Another commented that 'voluntary organisations are not the same as the public sector, they represent as well as provide services. They are a critical voice which must not be quietened. The voluntary sector should be feisty and challenging.' Traditionally, public authorities have adopted a paternalistic approach to the voluntary sector (Allcock and Scott, 2002) and the power relationship between the state and voluntary sector has been unequal (Craig and Taylor, 2002). As voluntary groups work more closely with government, particularly providing services under contract, they could become even more dependent on their patronage, and could be more easily manipulated. Evidence that government has used funding to secure compliance from voluntary organisations is not new (Brenton, 1985). However, closer relationships with statutory bodies appear to have increased the potential for manipulation, raising a series of new dilemmas for voluntary organisations about how they seek to maintain their autonomy while working more closely with public authorities (Craig and Taylor, 2002). Moreover, the voluntary sector is still plagued by short-term funding and bureaucratic procedures that place it in a subservient position to local authorities and the NHS (Little, 2005b; National Audit Office, 2004b).

Conclusion

This chapter has shown that the implementation of health policies depends on effective working relationships between the NHS and other agencies, both statutory and independent. Ironically, health policies that seek to centralise the NHS, while at the same time opening up the health and social care market to non-public sector providers, have added to the difficulties of partnership working. This chapter has also shown that despite a more strategic approach to partnership and evidence of good examples of joint working, the picture remains one of limited success with a mixture of good and poor practice. In particular, it appears that the cultural aspects of partnership – the need to share vision and commitment – must be given greater weight, rather than simply concentrating on 'top-down' organisational structures and processes.

Summary

- Partnerships can contribute to better policies and improved services.
- Recent government policy has emphasised the importance of joined-up government and improved partnership working involving NHS organisations, local government and the private and voluntary sectors.
- There are several possible options for resolving the 'troubled' relationship between the NHS and local government social services. These include the NHS taking over social services, and local government acquiring health service responsibilities. Most initiatives, however, have attempted to improve coordination between the NHS and local government, with limited success.

- Local authorities have an important role to play in improving standards of health among their populations. Despite this, it is only recently that government health policy has begun to seriously acknowledge this role. There is still much to be done to coordinate the work of the NHS and local government in this field.
- Government policies to privatise health and social care have created additional challenges for partnership working, not least of which are the contrasting aims and principles of the private and public sectors.
- The voluntary sector is an important player in health and social care, and in public health. It is both an advocate of policy and a provider of services. Efforts to strengthen partnership with the sector must recognise this 'dual role'.

Key questions

1. What kinds of partnership exist in the health policy arena?
2. What factors facilitate a successful partnership?
3. What are the main reasons for working in partnership?
4. Should local government take over responsibility for health services? What might this mean in practice?
5. Discuss the various ways in which local government authorities may be able to improve the health of their population.
6. In what sense is the private sector now a partner in health policy and service provision?
7. Is the voluntary sector in danger of becoming merely an 'arm' of the state in health and social care?

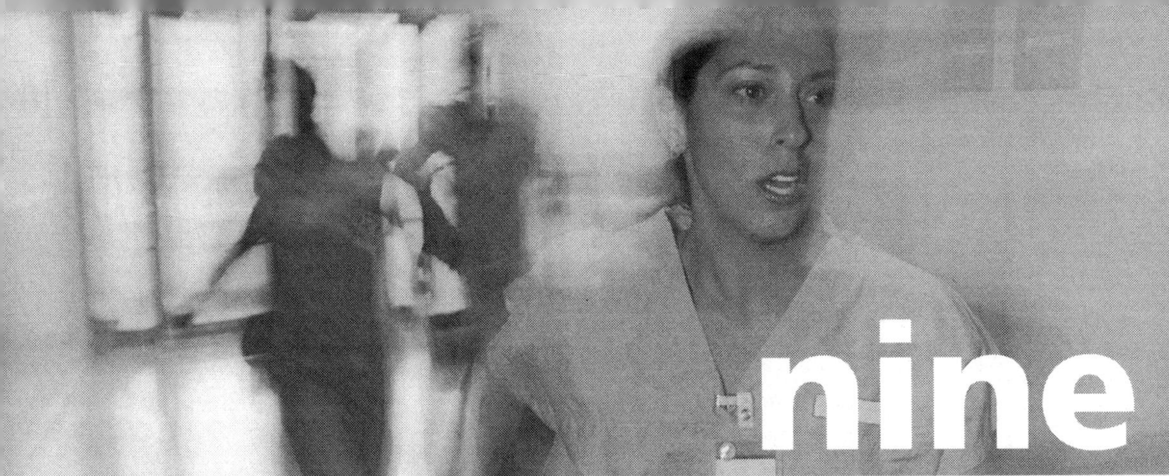

Health policy in other parts of the UK

Overview

Health policy may vary across different countries of the UK. New devolved governance arrangements have increased the scope for such policy variation. This chapter examines health policy processes in Scotland, Wales and Northern Ireland and also looks at the devolution of health policy at the regional level in England.

No study of UK health policy would be complete without acknowledging the differences in health policy between England, Scotland, Wales and Northern Ireland. These have become more pronounced since new devolved governance arrangements in the late 1990s. This chapter examines health policy making and implementation in these parts of the UK and also explores the implications for health policy of devolved regional government.

Health policy before devolution

Differences in health policy between different countries of the UK could be found before the recent devolutionary changes (see Levitt and Wall, 1984; Webster, 1996; Stewart, 2004; Woods, 2004). There were differences in NHS structure and organisation. The NHS in Scotland was governed by separate legislation and came within the responsibilities of the Secretary of State for Scotland and the Scottish Office. Although adopting the policies of the UK government, Scotland had some leeway in how it organised the NHS. For example, from the 1970s, Scotland had unified health boards responsible for family health services as well as hospital and community health services. England and Wales persisted with separate bodies for primary and secondary care until the 1990s. The NHS in Northern Ireland also evolved differently, introducing integrated health and social service boards in the 1970s (see Chapter Eight). Wales, meanwhile, began to enjoy a measure of administrative devolution for the NHS in the late 1960s, extended in 1974 when responsibility for all health services was delegated to the Secretary of State for Wales (Webster, 1996).

To some extent variations were shaped by political differences, even before political devolution. Scotland is regarded as having powerful medical elites (Greer, 2004). Scotland and Wales both have strong socialist traditions, embedded within their political culture. Such factors may explain discernible differences in policy implementation between the different countries of the UK in this period. Even so, there was little scope for policy variations in health, especially where the UK government was strongly committed (Woods, 2004). There was more room for a distinctive approach on issues where the UK government was disinterested. For example, in the 1980s, the Welsh NHS devised a public health improvement strategy, a markedly different approach from that taken in England (Baggott, 2000). Wales also adopted a pioneering approach to services for people with learning disabilities (Drakeford, 2006). Such deviations in policy exemplified new or different approaches, and provided important lessons for health policy makers in other parts of the UK. Similarly, Scotland's experience of managed clinical networks provided important insights into collaboration between health care professionals, while Northern Ireland's experience of joint boards, informed debates about the structural integration of health and social care.

Devolution

It is not possible to give a detailed account of the history and politics of devolution in the UK in this book (see Bogdanor, 2001; Pilkington, 2002). Briefly, both Scotland and Wales acquired devolved powers following the passage of legislation in 1998. Scotland established a Parliament and an Executive, and was granted wide competencies and powers, including the right to make primary legislation and to vary basic income tax levels by up to 3 per cent. Wales established an elected Assembly, although with less extensive powers. Initially at least, the Welsh Assembly operated within primary legislation passed by the UK Parliament, although clearer and more extensive legislative powers have been promised. In future, subject to the agreement of the Westminster Parliament, the Welsh Assembly will be able to pass its own laws in areas where it has devolved powers. Moreover, law-making powers of the Assembly may be extended to other policy areas, subject to a referendum. The Assembly was founded as a collective body. It has since moved to distinguish government and opposition functions by appointing a 'Welsh Assembly Government', which exercises executive power on its behalf (Jeffrey, 2006). Northern Ireland had its own Parliament until 1972, when it was suspended as a result of civil unrest and terrorism. Due to the peace process, devolved powers were restored. A new elected Assembly with primary legislative powers, and a Northern Ireland Executive were established in 1999, only to be suspended in 2002 amid continued acrimony between the sectarian political parties. The current situation is covered in ***Box 9.1***. Finally, there has been some devolution of powers to London, which has an elected Mayor and Assembly, and there has been a degree of administrative devolution to the English regions. The implications of devolved governance within England are discussed further in ***Box 9.2***.

It is not surprising that observers describe devolution in the UK as 'lopsided' (Jeffrey, 2006) or 'asymmetric' (Woods, 2004). Devolved governments vary, not only with regard to their powers, but in their politics. In contrast to the Westminster Parliament, the devolved assemblies are elected by various methods of proportional representation. Moreover, the way in which devolved governments and assemblies operate contrasts with each other and with the UK government and Parliament. It is therefore difficult to generalise about the impact of devolution, even in a specific policy area such as health.

Devolution and health

Health policy is an important arena for devolved governments (Woods, 2002, 2004; Jervis and Plowden, 2003). Health accounts for over a third of the devolved budgets of both Scotland and Wales. The NHS is the biggest single employer in both countries. Scotland and Wales (and Northern Ireland) also have much bigger health problems than England (as measured by rates of illness, mortality rates and other health indicators). In all, it is not surprising that health policy is important to the devolved assemblies and governments.

Ham (2004, p 111) has observed an 'increasing divergence in NHS structures and the political processes impacting on health policy'. Greer (2005), meanwhile, commented that the extent of policy divergence since devolution has been an uncomfortable surprise for the UK government. These observations were echoed in interviews with health policy actors, which included comments such as 'devolution is more and more important' (former DoH civil servant), and 'policies are diverging in different parts of the UK' (professional association spokesperson).

Observers of devolution have commented on the significant policy innovation that has occurred across many policy areas, including health (DCCP, 2005; IPPR, 2006). Some of this has taken the form of new departures in policy or services. The Scottish Executive decided to make personal care (such as help with washing, toileting and eating) free for elderly people, in contrast to the rest of the UK. The Welsh Assembly Government introduced free prescriptions for all in April 2007. However, much of the divergence between England and the rest of the UK has resulted not from 'positive' innovation but from decisions not to pursue the English health reforms in areas such as privatisation, patient choice and foundation trusts (Keating, 2005; IPPR, 2006).

Lessons can be learned from the different approaches taken. According to one observer of health policy, 'we have in effect a natural experiment or trial resulting from the different routes to reform taken in the various parts of the UK' (interview, think tank spokesperson). Others have noted that lessons can be learned from diversity, producing a 'virtuous circle' through policy-oriented learning. Although true in principle, the reality may be different. Some policy variation is rhetorical. Leaders of devolved governments and assemblies like to emphasise their differences from England, as reflected in the call of the Welsh First Minister, Rhodri Morgan (2003), for 'clear red water' to separate policies of the Welsh Assembly Government from Westminster. Actual policy differences may be smaller (see IPPR, 2006). Indeed, there are countervailing pressures that promote convergence across the UK, which have influenced the direction of policy in devolved governments.

Nonetheless, most attention has been on the scope for diversity following devolution. This is shaped by several factors (see Exworthy, 2001; Greer, 2004, 2005; Stewart, 2004; DCCP, 2005; IPPR, 2006; Jeffrey, 2006):

- *Different political cultures and parties* (IPPR, 2006). Other parts of the UK have contrasting political cultures. Scotland and Wales have a stronger socialist tradition, while Northern Ireland is dominated by sectarian political parties. In Wales and Scotland, the main opposition parties (the Scottish and Welsh nationalists) have been to the left of the governing parties, in contrast to England where the main competition is from the right. This means that political debate tends to be about the nature of state intervention rather than the classic 'state versus market' debate, producing great potential for policy differences with England.
- *Different electoral systems and coalition governments* (see Keating, 2005). The use of proportional representation in elections for the devolved assemblies has an additional impact. Without the exaggerated majorities usually produced by Westminster 'first past the post' elections, governing parties in Scotland and Wales are driven to adopt a consensual rather than adversarial approach to policy making. Given the left-oriented nature of party competition and political debate, this reinforces the potential for policy differences. Divergence is further encouraged where (as happened in Scotland, Northern Irelancd and Wales) parties enter into coalitions in order to form a government.

- *Different policy networks* (Greer, 2004, 2005). Differences in policy networks (the clusters of pressure groups that engage with government on policy) reinforce the impact of electoral and party factors. In both Scotland and Wales, policy networks have tended to promote consensus and stability. They have also advocated distinctive policy approaches, detailed in later sections of this chapter.
- *Constitutional autonomy*. Devolution in the UK has been unusual in placing few levers or controls in the hands of the UK government. The Scottish Parliament, for example, has one of the widest competences of any devolved government in Europe (Keating, 2005). The UK government has made little or no attempt to set minimum standards in areas that fall within the competence of the devolved governments (IPPR, 2006).
- *Financial discretion*. The devolved governments receive funds in the form of block grants from the UK government. Largely, this can be spent at the discretion of the devolved government. This gives the UK government little influence over how funds are spent and has been described as 'uniquely permissive' (DCCP, 2005).

But these factors are counterbalanced by others that produce convergence:

- Although the competences of devolved assemblies and governments are widely drawn, the UK government has reserved powers in a number of important areas, including health. These include medicines regulation and the regulation of professional standards. In addition, some professional contracts are negotiated at the national level, including those of hospital consultants and general practitioners. Furthermore, there are several key policy areas for which the UK government retains overall responsibility that have a significant impact on health policy. The most important of these is social security, which can restrict devolved governments' ability to devise policies for vulnerable groups such as the elderly, mentally ill people and those with learning disabilities (see DCCP, 2005; Fawcett, 2005). On top of this, it must be remembered that the UK still operates a common foreign policy, a unified tax system, a common market in goods and services and a single labour market, all of which promote convergence.
- The European Union (EU) is also a force for convergence (Greer, 2004; Woods, 2004; DCCP, 2005; see Chapter Ten). It can set a common regulatory framework across all member states, which affects devolved governments as well the UK government. As will become clear in the next chapter, EU institutions have taken an increasingly close interest in health policy, including public health, medicines regulation, professional regulation and the working

hours of health service employees. It has been noted that, on issues where the UK as a whole must negotiate on EU matters (especially on core EU issues, such as agriculture and fisheries), the devolved governments tend to liaise very closely with Whitehall in order to produce a common position (see Jeffrey, 2005).

- Inter-government coordination (IGC). Although IGC is formalised on EU matters, elsewhere it is weak (IPPR, 2006). Joint ministerial committees do exist to coordinate policy across the governments of the UK, including health policy, but these mechanisms are regarded as of marginal importance (Woods, 2004). For the most part, coordination and conflict resolution is undertaken informally through officials of the various devolved governments, or through political channels, via ministers. The latter approach has been relatively effective largely because the Labour Party, which introduced devolution, has so far simultaneously governed Wales (initially as a coalition partner with the Liberals and then as majority party), Scotland (in coalition with the Liberals) and the UK as a whole (Jeffrey, 2006).
- A further constraint on divergence is public opinion (Greer, 2005). Although public opinion in Scotland, Wales and Northern Ireland broadly supports devolved governance, it remains attached to notions of equality and solidarity (IPPR, 2006), which have strong resonance in the health field. Indeed (and despite some rebranding of the NHS in Scotland and Wales), the public and the media still regard the NHS as a national institution and will not tolerate inequities in services between the different parts of the UK. Hence, Scottish and Welsh governments have faced enormous public pressures to change policy in the light of waiting time targets adopted in England (Bevan and Hood, 2006; Drakeford, 2006).
- England continues to dominate policy development and debate. In part this is a legacy, reflecting stronger capacities for policy making in Whitehall prior to devolution. It is also a reflection of the power of the London-based media, and the pressure group system, which despite some refocusing on the devolved governments and assemblies, remains strongly oriented towards Whitehall and Westminster. Other factors underpinning this continued domination have been identified (DCCP, 2005; IPPR, 2006), including the fact that England still has the majority of the UK population (around 85 per cent) and remains the dominant economic power within the UK.
- The final source of convergence is that health systems across Europe, not just within the UK, are facing similar pressures and problems. Scotland, Wales and Northern Ireland have been forced to confront similar issues to England: public health problems and inequalities, service reorganisation, the quest for greater efficiency in health services, the coordination of health and social care, and so on. Although specific approaches adopted differ in style

and content, the menu of realistic policy options is fairly restricted, not least by public opinion, and inhibits divergence.

Devolution and health policy in Scotland

When looking at the differences in health policy between England and other parts of the UK, it is helpful to distinguish between policy processes, policy outputs and outcomes. This framework will now be used to examine the impact of devolution in Scotland.

Policy processes

In Scotland, health and social care falls within the responsibilities of the ministers for health and community care within the Scottish Executive. Ministers lead the Scottish Executive Health Department. They are accountable to the Scottish Parliament for the NHS in much the same way as the Secretary of State for Health is at Westminster. As in England there are a number of special health authorities and agencies for which ministers have responsibility. Ministers must answer PQs and respond to parliamentary debates. There is also a parliamentary Health Committee, which scrutinises policy and administration in health and social care. This committee has a wider remit and greater formal powers than its counterpart at Westminster. As well as investigating policy issues and commissioning its own research, the committee scrutinises legislation, and can bring forward its own legislative proposals. The committee can also consider petitions submitted by members of the public.

The Scottish Executive is smaller than the UK government and has fewer responsibilities, which has advantages. It facilitates a more 'joined-up' approach to policy making (Stewart, 2004). The smaller size of government in Scotland generally encourages a more informal policy style, a point discussed further in a moment. Small government can have disadvantages, however. Scottish government is said to lack capacity in policy making, partly due to the historical legacy of administrative devolution under the Scottish Office, which focused on implementation rather than policy formation (Keating, 2005).

Policy participants interviewed commented on the consensual and inclusive nature of the Scottish policy-making process. For example, a Westminster MP observed that 'policy is more considered and consensual', while a respondent from a health professional organisation stated that 'policy is made in a more open, consultative and informal way'. This is partly due to the nature of Scottish political debate, which, as noted, is to the left of England, and so debates are less ideologically polarised between left and right. It is reinforced by both electoral and party systems, which have so far produced coalition governments (Keating, 2005). However, there has also been conflict. Indeed, according to one interviewee, a former senior NHS manager, political rivalries in Scotland can be very bitter indeed. The conflict between the various parties of the left can be particularly intense.

Nonetheless, the dominant style is consultative and consensual. This is particularly noticeable in relationships between government and pressure groups, where in the words of one interviewee 'there is a genuine desire to work with stakeholders' (spokesperson, professional association). The limited policy-making capacity of Scottish government has placed value on constructive relationships with such groups with the knowledge and expertise to contribute to policy development and implementation (IPPR, 2006). Professional groups, and in particular the medical profession, enjoy a close relationship with government and exert great influence (Greer, 2004, 2005). However, as noted earlier, this dates back to long before devolution.

Devolution affected the pressure group system in Scotland. Groups responded by undertaking 'territorial differentiation'. They refocused their lobbying efforts towards the new devolved governing institutions, such as the Scottish Parliament and Executive (DCCP, 2005). In some cases they have reorganised or restructured their operations in order to focus their activities more effectively in this direction (Jeffrey, 2006). Notably, several groups representing health professionals and workers now have separate structures for dealing with devolved governments, including UNISON, the RCN and some medical Royal Colleges. Some health charities have also introduced changes to reflect devolution. For example, the Parkinson's Disease Society now has a full-time officer to work on Scottish issues (and a part-time post to deal with issues concerning Wales).

Policies

Devolution has affected the way policy is made in Scotland. It has also affected the content of health policy, distinguishing Scottish policies from other parts of the UK, notably England. Differences include the following (see Stewart, 2004):

- Free long-term personal care for the elderly. Scotland decided to use public funds to cover the cost of personal as well as nursing care, as recommended by the Royal Commission on Long Term Care (Cm 4192, 1999). This is a major departure from the policy pursued elsewhere in the UK, where only nursing care is funded by the government.
- Free eye and dental checks for all by 2007. This contrasts with the rest of the UK (although entitlements to free checks are wider in Wales than in England).

- Mental health reform. Scotland engaged in a root and branch reform of mental health legislation in 2003. These changes were broadly welcomed and introduced in a spirit of consensus (Darjee and Crichton, 2004). Attempts to change the law in England and Wales failed due to the opposition of professional bodies, patients' groups and mental health charities, which were concerned about the implications for patients' rights and civil liberties.
- Public health. Scottish health policy placed a much greater emphasis on health promotion than England (at least until the publication of the English public health White Paper, *Choosing Health*, in 2004). Specifically, Scotland was ahead of England in adopting a strategy on health inequalities, as well as programmes promoting healthy eating and physical exercise, introduced joint public health plans for the NHS and local government, and created a new public health practitioner role at local level to coordinate interventions. It also introduced a smoking ban in public places earlier than the rest of the UK.

The structure of the NHS in Scotland differs from England, although, as earlier noted, this happened to some extent before devolution. Scotland has its own special health boards. These include the Scottish Ambulance Service, NHS Quality Improvement Scotland (responsible for improving clinical standards) and NHS Health Scotland (responsible for health improvement). Another body, National Services Scotland, is responsible for a range of important national and regional services, including blood transfusion, information services, counter-fraud services, procurement, and ensuring that specialist health and screening services are in place.

At the local level, single health boards are responsible for a range of health services, including hospital services. NHS trusts and the purchaser–provider split have been abolished in Scotland and there are no foundation trusts. Community health partnerships have been established at local level to promote working across NHS organisations and between the NHS, local government and the voluntary sector.

Much policy variation has occurred as a result of not pursuing or discontinuing policies formulated in England (Stewart, 2004; Woods, 2004). The main emphasis of policy has been on integrating services (both within the NHS and across the health and social care divide) through collaborative professional networks and partnership bodies. Although a performance management regime was introduced for the Scottish NHS, unlike England this avoided giving institutions a simple 'star rating' based on performance (the English system has subsequently been reformed – see Chapter Seven). However, the Scottish Executive has used PFI for the NHS. It also decided to send NHS patients to private hospitals as a means of reducing waiting times and has used longer-term NHS contracts with the independent sector.

However, this pro-market approach was combined with the nationalisation of the largest private hospital in Scotland in 2002, as a means of increasing NHS capacity.

These policy variations are considerable, particularly given the short period of time since devolution. There are limits to divergence, however. Some policy innovations have faced difficulties. In particular the affordability and viability of funding long-term personal care has been an issue, with some local authorities operating waiting-lists. However, an initial assessment of the Scottish policy was broadly positive (Bell and Bowes, 2006). Meanwhile, pressure to adopt a policy of free prescriptions for all (as in Wales) has been fiercely resisted by the Scottish Executive on grounds of cost. There are also signs that the Scottish government has become more open-minded about English health reforms. The performance of the NHS in Scotland has attracted criticism, particularly in view of the relatively high level of funding it receives. The Scottish Executive (2004) responded with new waiting-time targets, including a maximum wait of six months for inpatient treatment and six months for first outpatient consultation by the end of 2005. Subsequently, an 18-week maximum waiting time from referral to treatment was introduced, to be achieved by December 2007. Targets for reducing delayed discharges and emergency inpatient admissions of elderly people were also introduced. An element of choice was also implemented; patients whose local hospital was unable to meet the waiting-time target were now offered a choice of alternative providers. Scotland also introduced a computerised booking scheme for outpatients, similar to 'Choose and Book' in England (Appleby, 2006a).

An official report set out the future direction for the Scottish NHS (Kerr, 2005), while affirming the distinctiveness of Scottish policies, in particular its ethos of collaboration and partnership. As well as urging steps towards closer collaboration, chiefly through the extension of managed clinical networks and community health partnerships, it suggested greater emphasis on shorter waiting times, improved access to services and clarification of policy on patient choice. Although rejecting the adoption of English policies such as foundation trusts and payment by results, it did raise the possibility of introducing internal competition and financial incentives within local health boards as a means of stimulating service improvement. The report also urged consideration of a system of fixed tariffs for treatment to encourage providers to find more cost-effective ways of delivering care, reflecting earlier moves in this direction by the Scottish Executive. Currently tariffs are only used to reimburse health boards for treating patients outside their boundaries (which represents around 5 per cent of hospitals' income), although it is possible in future that they may be used to compare costs and set hospital and clinical budgets (Appleby, 2006b).

Policy outcomes

Inevitably, comparisons of performance have been made between the various health care systems within the UK since devolution. Early evidence suggests that the Scottish NHS has not performed as well as England (see Audit Scotland, 2004; Talbot et al, 2004; Alvarez-Rosete et al, 2005). Although Scotland receives more funding per head of population, it has poorer levels of health and its people on average wait longer for treatment than in England. However, Scotland has done better in some specific areas, such as flu vaccinations of the elderly, MMR vaccination and breast cancer screening and, more recently, has significantly reduced waiting times for patients with a guaranteed waiting time (Audit Scotland, 2006). Meanwhile, the Scottish public's satisfaction with the NHS in general increased following devolution (1996/97 to 2002/03), but not as much as in England (Alvarez-Rosete et al, 2005). With regard to inpatient and GP services, satisfaction fell by slightly more than in England in this period. Satisfaction with outpatient care, which increased slightly in England, actually fell in Scotland.

However, such comparisons are based on limited information and, in some respects, poor-quality data (Alvarez-Rosete et al, 2005). They do not reflect that the Scottish reforms have focused on health improvement in the longer term, the outcomes of which can only be fairly judged in decades rather than years. As one interviewee observed, a much more comprehensive and sophisticated comparison is required. However, the reality is that simple indicators (waiting-lists, waiting times) generate media and public attention, and have created strong pressures for Scotland (and other parts of the UK) to conform to the English health care reform agenda (Bevan and Hood, 2006).

Box 9.1: Health policy in Northern Ireland

Health policy in Northern Ireland is the responsibility of the Department of Health, Social Services and Public Safety (DHSSPS), which also has responsibility for the fire service, food safety and emergency planning. For a brief period, between 1999-2002, health policy was within the remit of the devolved Northern Ireland Executive and Assembly. Currently, with devolution suspended, the DHSSPS is headed by a UK government minister within the Northern Ireland Office.

Under both direct rule and devolved arrangements, health policy making in the Province has been cautious and gradual (Greer, 2005). UK ministers have not wished to add further controversies, while the Province's politicians have been preoccupied with sectarian politics and have had little time for domestic reform (DCCP, 2005). A consequence is that Northern Ireland has tended to lag behind in introducing health reforms. For example, the NHS reforms of the Thatcher and Major governments were implemented later than elsewhere in the UK. By the same token, the Blair government's reforms, including the abolition of GP fund-holding, were also implemented at a later stage.

As already noted, Northern Ireland has adopted an integrated approach to health and social care. It established integrated regional health and social service boards in the 1970s (Heenan and Birrell, 2006). Under the Blair government these were supplemented by local health and social care groups. Northern Ireland has also pursued a more vigorous public health policy than in England, understandable perhaps given the higher levels of ill health in the Province and the role of socio-economic factors, such as poor housing, unemployment and social division. Public health interventions are explicitly linked to wider social welfare programmes in the Province, such as *Targeting Social Need and Promoting Social Inclusion* (www.ccruni.gov.uk/equality/docs/newstsn.htm). The Northern Ireland public health strategy, set out in *Investing for Health* (DHSSPS, 2002), and reiterated in subsequent policy documents (DHSSPS, 2004), emphasised stronger partnership working and joint planning arrangements between the NHS and local government. It introduced HAZs (which will continue until 2008). The strategy also set demanding targets for reducing health inequalities (aiming by 2010 to halve the gap in life expectancy between deprived areas and the average, as well as reducing the gap between levels of long-standing illness in the lowest and highest socio-economic groups by a fifth).

Important English policies, such as patient choice, foundation trusts and market-style reforms, have not been on the Northern Ireland agenda. With the exception of PFI, there has been little interest in working more closely with the private sector. Conscious of the initiatives on waiting times in England, Scotland and Wales, Northern Ireland has introduced targets. In 2005, health ministers introduced a 12-month maximum waiting time target for inpatient day case treatment to be achieved by April 2006, with shorter targets for hip and knee surgery (nine months), cardiac and cataract surgery (six months). Further targets followed including by March 2007, a maximum waiting time of six months for inpatient, day case and first outpatient appointments, and by March 2008, a 13-week waiting time for a first outpatient appointment, a 21-week wait for inpatient or day case treatment, a four-hour maximum wait in accident and emergency, a 48-hour access target for primary care services (24 hours by 2010), and a 72-hour maximum wait after being declared fit for discharge from hospital. The DHSSPS (2004) also set out a comprehensive range of objectives for policy and service development alongside a new planning system, with a stronger focus on performance management.

The NHS in Northern Ireland has undergone significant changes in recent years aimed at improving its effectiveness and efficiency. Following a review of public administration in the Province, reorganisation plans were announced in 2005. A strategic health and social services authority replaced the four regional boards, while taking on some of the functions of the DHSSPS. NHS trusts were reconfigured into five integrated acute and community health service trusts, covering specific geographical areas. Meanwhile, it was proposed that existing local health and social care groups be abolished and their role transferred to a smaller number of commissioning groups whose boundaries would be coterminous with local authorities.

Devolution and health policy in Wales

Policy process

The policy process in Wales bears some similarities to Scotland, but also exhibits important differences. Like Scotland, Welsh political debate is to the left of England and is similarly underpinned by competition between parties of the left rather than on a left-right axis (Drakeford, 2006). The electoral system for the Welsh Assembly also uses a form of proportional representation, which inhibits large governing majorities. This, coupled with the establishment of the Welsh Assembly as a corporate body, promoted an informal and consensual approach to policy making (although as noted there is now a clearer distinction between government and opposition). Informality is further encouraged by the small, close-knit nature of Welsh political culture and institutions (McLelland, 2002). A consultative approach is, as in Scotland, partly a consequence of the lack of policy-making capacity of Welsh institutions and their reliance on outside expertise.

Currently, the Labour Party governs, albeit with a small majority. However, it remains a more traditional 'old Labour' party than its counterpart in England (and to some extent, in Scotland) and its leaders have made great efforts to distinguish Welsh policy from that of England, as reflected by 'clear red water' rhetoric (DCCP, 2005). The Welsh Assembly lacks the powers of the Scottish Parliament, although these have recently been extended. Wales also lacks the strong policy communities of England and Scotland (Greer, 2005). Notably, medical elites are not as powerful as in Scotland, and this has allowed other players to exert influence, such as trade unions and local government.

Within the Welsh Assembly Government, the Minister of Health and Community Care is responsible for health policy and the NHS. The minister heads a Department of Health and Social Services, which manages and supports the delivery of health and social care services. The NHS in Wales is managed through three regional offices, which coordinate the activities of local health boards and NHS trusts. There are also a number of central bodies, including the Welsh National Public Health Service (providing advice and expertise on public health), the Wales Centre for Health (a centre for public health advice and information and research), Health Commission Wales (which is responsible for planning and commissioning highly specialised services), the National Leadership and Innovation Agency for Healthcare and a Healthcare Inspectorate.

Since devolution, parliamentary scrutiny of health and related matters has been undertaken by a Health and Social Services Committee, which is a subject committee of the Welsh Assembly. Its membership is drawn from all parties and includes the Assembly minister responsible for health policy. Its functions include scrutiny of legislation, securing accountability of ministers and health and social service bodies, and giving advice on budget allocations. It also undertakes policy reviews (see Health and Social Services Committee, 2005, for example) and makes recommendations on future policy and service development.

Policies

Traditionally, the Welsh and English NHS have shown strong similarities. However, the Welsh Assembly Government's efforts to pursue a distinctive approach to health policy has widened policy differences. The main variations can be summarised as follows (see Drakeford, 2006):

- Welsh health policy has prioritised public health, health inequalities and health promotion to a far greater degree than in England (although an English White Paper on this subject, as noted earlier, was introduced in 2004).
- The key local health care organisations in Wales (local health boards – LHBs) were reorganised, bringing them closer to local government. They are now coterminous with local authority boundaries in an effort to promote joint working between local government, the NHS and other partners, such as the voluntary sector. LHBs and local authorities are jointly responsible for planning of health, social care and well-being.
- Wales retained CHCs, the local patients' watchdogs in the NHS, which were abolished in England.
- A free eye-care service was introduced in Wales for groups at risk of developing serious eye diseases.
- Prescription charges were abolished for people under 25 and frozen for those who had to pay them. Free prescriptions were extended to all in April 2007.
- People under 25 and over 60 receive free dental checks.

Wales took a different approach to performance management in the NHS than England. It did not introduce star ratings. Targets were set for health services, but were not as demanding as in England or Scotland. For example, while the NHS Plan of 2000 set out to reduce waiting times to six months for inpatients, the corresponding Welsh target at the time was 18 months. However, criticism of the performance of the Welsh NHS with regard to waiting times led to a significant reorientation of policy (Welsh Assembly Government, 2005). New waiting-time targets were introduced including a 12-month maximum wait introduced in March 2005. The Welsh Assembly Government set an additional target of an eight-month maximum wait for outpatient appointments, day case treatment or inpatient treatment by 2007. This was augmented by a maximum 26-week waiting-time target from GP referral to treatment, to be achieved by December 2009. A new planning framework was introduced to achieve these and other targets, with measures to address poor performance, including development teams to improve local services and regional intervention to reconfigure hospital services. The Welsh Assembly Government also introduced changes to strengthen commissioning of services, while maintaining a commitment to promoting integrated health and social care through managed clinical networks and closer partnership with local government.

The Welsh government continued to reject some of the reforms being adopted in England, such as patient choice and foundation trusts. However, it adopted PFI and retained the purchaser–provider split, commissioning and NHS trusts. It also experimented with integrated models, as in Powys, where the LHB took over the services of the local NHS trust. Like Scotland, Wales has made greater use of the private sector to reduce waiting times. From April 2004, under the 'Second Offer Scheme', patients were guaranteed alternative treatment at another hospital if they were waiting for longer than the national target. Payment by results was resisted, reflecting the Welsh Assembly Government's dislike of market mechanisms, but it did endorse moves to create greater incentives in the health system, including the development of standard tariffs for services provided.

Policy outcomes

The overall performance of the health service in Wales since devolution has been described as poor (Wanless, 2003; Audit Commission, 2004; Talbot et al, 2004, Alvarez-Rosete et al, 2005; Auditor General for Wales, 2005). Measures have focused on waiting times, where Wales performed relatively badly following devolution, although it has done better in some areas, such as waiting times in accident and emergency. Some have argued that it is unfair to judge the Welsh NHS on English criteria (Drakeford, 2006). Nonetheless, the fundamental problems of the NHS in Wales have been identified. The Wanless (2003) review of the NHS in Wales concluded that the current system was unsustainable. The Audit Commission (2004) agreed, stating that health care in Wales was out of balance and unable to adapt to the needs of the future. These problems were reflected in public satisfaction levels. Overall satisfaction with the NHS in Wales actually fell following devolution (Alvarez-Rosete et al, 2005), while rising in Scotland and England. Satisfaction with general practice fell further than in England and Scotland. The drop in public satisfaction with inpatient care was slightly more in Wales and Scotland than in England. However, public satisfaction with outpatient services, which increased marginally in England, fell in Wales, and by more than in Scotland.

Health outcomes in Wales have remained poor, reflecting the legacy of long-term illness and underlying socio-economic factors, rather than current health policy or NHS performance (Wanless, 2003). Wales has invested in public health and focused on reducing health inequalities (see Townsend, 2001), but the impact of this strategy will take much longer to assess. It also placed much emphasis on improved joint working on public health and social care. But, in spite of these efforts, problems remained (Audit Commission, 2004), particularly associated with difficulties caused by the different structures and cultures of the NHS and local government (Health and Social Services Committee, 2005). More specifically, high emergency admissions and delayed transfers of care from hospital, both symptoms of poor joint working between health and social care, remained a key problem (Audit Commission, 2004; Auditor General for Wales, 2005).

As already mentioned, this produced a reorientation in policy, with a stronger focus on delivery. By March 2006, the number of people waiting for treatment in Wales had fallen substantially, with nobody waiting over 12 months for elective treatment and a very small number of people waiting for more than 12 months for a first outpatient appointment at a Welsh NHS trust (Wales Audit Office, 2006). Even so, the position still contrasted unfavourably with England and Scotland, which had tougher waiting-time targets.

Box 9.2: Regional government and health

Plans to devolve government to elected assemblies within England have been largely unsuccessful (Jeffrey, 2006). The negative verdict of the referendum in the North East in 2004 effectively ended efforts to create democratic regional assemblies. This left the Greater London Authority (GLA) as the only democratically elected devolved governing body in England (Pimlott and Rao, 2002; Rao, 2006). The GLA has a directly elected Mayor, currently Ken Livingstone, who has strategic powers and responsibilities across a range of areas, including housing, adult education, waste management, climate change, transport, economic development, the environment, policing and health. His powers are fairly limited, however, and depend on other bodies for implementation. The Mayor's strategies are scrutinised by an elected Assembly. The London Mayor has a specific duty in law to promote the health of Londoners (Ross and Tomaney, 2001) and has acquired responsibilities to prepare a health inequality strategy and to reduce health inequalities. He has no statutory powers, funding or functions with regard to health services, but is able to influence NHS and other bodies by forging partnerships and highlighting specific health problems and possible solutions. In 2000, the Mayor established a Health Commission for London, which includes representatives of the NHS, local government, the regional public health group, the London Development Agency and the King's Fund. He also appointed the Director of Public Health for London to his cabinet (Ross and Tomaney, 2001). The Mayor also has powers in some areas (such as transport and economic development), which can be used to improve public health. For the most part, the Mayor operates by exhortation, in particular by identifying problems, setting out strategies and providing a lead for other agencies (Hunter et al, 2005). The Mayor's Health Commission publishes annual reviews on the health of Londoners. Specific strategies have also been launched on issues such as food and air quality (Mayor of London, 2002; Mayor of London et al, 2006).

In other areas of England there has been some deconcentration and delegation in health. Greater responsibilities have been placed on local bodies (see Chapter Seven), within a framework of tight central control. There have also been some developments at the regional level. In the late 1990s, new regional institutions were established, including regional development agencies (RDAs) – which promote economic development. These bodies are appointed by ministers (except in London, where the Mayor appoints the development agency). Outside London, there are also regional chambers, consisting of councillors from local authorities within the region along with other stakeholders (such as representatives of other statutory service providers, business and voluntary organisations). Each regional chamber scrutinises the work of their RDA and must be consulted by it when drawing up plans. Regional chambers have additional powers and responsibilities, mainly in relation to strategic planning on issues such as sustainable development, transport and waste (ESRC, 2005). Regional chambers are also increasingly seen as a means of building cross-sectoral partnerships to coordinate public policy and services. In addition, there are government offices for the regions (GORs), which organise and coordinate the activities of 10 central government departments at the regional level (McMillan and Massey, 2001). These bodies, formed by the amalgamation of regional offices of the Departments of Trade and Industry, Education, Employment, Environment and Transport in 1994, subsequently incorporated regional functions of other departments, including public health. They also began to adopt a more strategic and integrated approach to policy implementation. More generally there has been an attempt to bring health matters more closely into regional policies and strategies (see Ross and Tomaney, 2001). Regeneration and planning is now expected to be more aware of the implications for health. Links between health inequalities and other socio-economic problems are increasingly acknowledged at the regional level. Moreover, since the abolition of NHS regional offices, regional public health teams have been incorporated in the GORs. They are now in closer proximity to those making strategic decisions that affect health in a wider sense, such as economic development, housing and transport (although more could be done to integrate health fully within regional-level decision making, see Hunter et al, 2005). In 2006, a step was taken in this direction when the DoH issued guidance to GORs and SHAs (eight out of ten of which now have coterminous boundaries) requesting them to agree specific aims for improved health and well-being, and establishing working arrangements to achieve this, within the context of national public health priorities (DoH, 2006b).

Conclusion

Devolution has made a difference to health policy across the UK. Clear policy differences have arisen, partly as a consequence of devolved powers, and partly as a result of differences in political cultures and political systems, some features of which preceded the devolution settlement. Policy variation has resulted from policy innovation and from a refusal to pursue particular English policies. Yet factors promoting policy convergence remain, and have become stronger of late. Criticism of health policy and the state of the NHS has led devolved governments to adopt English approaches, notably on waiting-time targets. However, important differences remain both in emphasis (for example, less extensive use of tariffs and limited patient choice) as well as outright rejection of policies (such as foundation trusts).

There is clearly much scope for learning from different policy experiences. Much can also be learned about the relative effectiveness of processes of policy making and implementation, given the different policy styles that exist across the countries of the UK. However, there are concerns that the value of lesson-drawing, about both policy and processes, is not being fully exploited. More needs to be done to ensure this occurs by, for example, providing comparative data across the four countries and thorough independent evaluation of policy initiatives and processes.

The final point is that there have been few overt disputes between UK and devolved governments. Conflicts, when they have arisen, have been resolved by informal rather than formal means. Moreover, the devolution settlement gives little leverage to the UK government to establish basic controls and minimum standards, so the scope for divergence is potentially wide. This is potentially problematic. Should different parties ever occupy UK and devolved governments, greater problems may arise in maintaining the coherence and consistency of health policy and the NHS across the UK as a whole.

Summary

- Differences in health policy between different countries of the UK preceded the recent devolutionary reforms.
- Devolution has given the different parts of the UK new opportunities to develop distinctive health policies.
- Considerable variation has been evident. This has resulted from devolved governments 'positively' introducing policies that differ from England. Divergence has also occurred as a result of 'negatively' refusing to pursue English policies.
- There are also forces that promote convergence. Different parts of the UK may learn from each other's experience and alter their policies. There are also constraints and pressures that promote convergence, such as public opinion and the media, common problems and dilemmas, EU regulations and the powers of the UK government.
- The policy processes in other parts of the UK contrast with England. Lessons can be learned about the relative effectiveness of policy processes as well as variations in policy.

Key questions

1. Why did aspects of health policy vary across the different countries of the UK prior to devolution?
2. What are the main differences in health policy between the different parts of the UK today?
3. How does the health policy process vary between the different countries of the UK?
4. To what extent have policies converged across the different countries of the UK since devolution?

Note: Elections for the Welsh Assembly and Scottish Parliament were held in May 2007, leading to significant changes in government. Elections for the Northern Ireland Assembly were held in March 2007, leading to a new power-sharing Executive and the restoration of devolved powers.

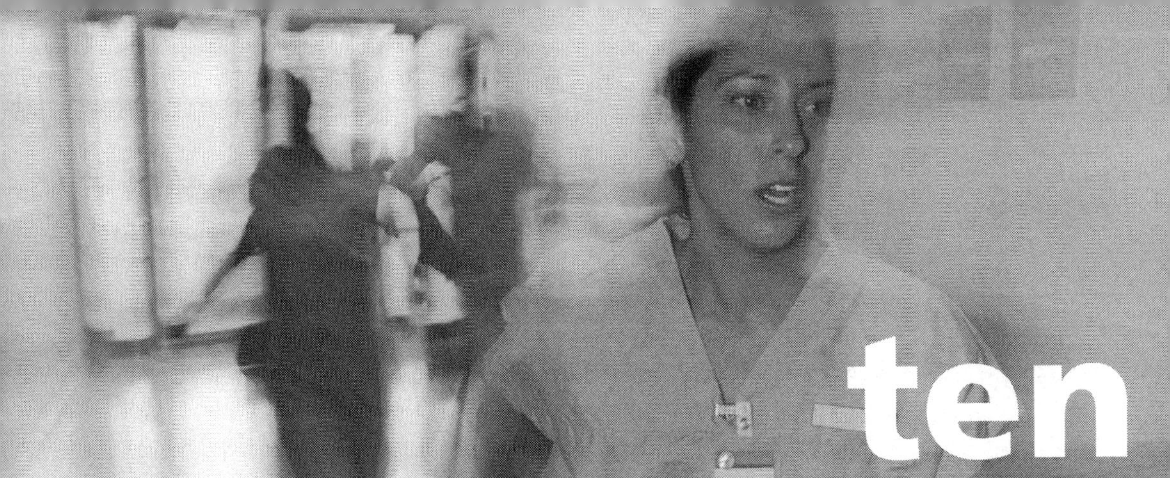

The international context of UK health policy

Overview

This chapter examines the global forces that impinge on UK health policies. It explores the impact of global trends and developments, and examines the activities of international institutions and organisations, such as the World Health Organisation (WHO), the World Bank, the World Trade Organisation (WTO), the Organisation for Economic Cooperation and Development (OECD) and multinational corporations. The chapter examines European influences on UK health policy including European Union (EU) institutions. It also explores how other countries' experiences have shaped UK health reforms.

UK health policy is shaped by forces outside its national boundaries. There are three main elements, all of which are examined in this chapter. Global influences, which include forces such as climate change and migration, as well as international institutions and organisations, such as WHO and multinational corporations. European influences, including those exerted through institutions such as the EU. Also, there is 'policy learning' from other health care systems, generated by their experiences of reform.

Global influences

Global influences on health policy can be seen as part of a broader process of 'globalisation'. Although the exact meaning of globalisation is disputed (see Lee and Collin, 2005; Koivusalo, 2006), it has been described in straightforward terms as 'a convenient way of describing the growing interconnectedness of the world's economies and societies' (Labonte and Schrecker, 2004, p 1662). Another basic definition is provided by Held et al (1999 – cited by Lee and Collin, 2005, p 4): 'a stretching of social, political and economic activities across frontiers such that events, decisions and activities in one region of the world can come to have significance for individuals and communities in distant regions of the globe'. However, these simple definitions should not obscure the intense debates over what exactly constitutes globalisation, whether or not it is an entirely new phenomenon, and whether it is a good or bad thing (see Redwood, 1994; Hirst and Thompson, 1996; Hertz, 2001; Robinson, 2003).

Health is part of the globalisation process in that it is affected by various international forces and trends from which individual countries cannot escape. This is not entirely new. Neither the transmission of epidemics across the world nor the globalisation of disease (that is, the spreading of the same clinical entities throughout the world) is unpredecented (Berlinguer, 1999). Rather it is the combination of globalising forces that is unique, bringing new pressures for change in many policy arenas. These forces are widely acknowledged (Lee, 2000; Lee and Collin, 2005) and include:

- climate and environmental changes, such as those linked to global warming;
- population displacement and migration, for example, due to war and economic inequalities;
- increase in international mobility, due to cheaper air travel, for example;
- the revolution in the media and electronic communications, such as the internet, mobile phone technology;
- other technological changes, notably with regard to health care, such as telemedicine and genetic-based technologies;
- war and terrorism;
- ageing populations and increasing levels of chronic disease, particularly in industrialised countries;
- the threat of new and resistant strains of disease;
- concentration of capital and economic power;
- the spread of Western consumer culture across the world;
- trade liberalisation, privatisation and deregulation;
- increasing inequalities both within and between countries.

This combination of forces has wide-ranging implications for health and health policy, including (Lee, 2000):

- Increased threats of infectious disease, as a result of emerging infections, increased travel and migration, climate change, over-use of antibiotics, war and bioterrorism.

- Rising levels of obesity, cancers and other chronic illnesses, resulting from ageing populations, Western consumerism and the market power of corporations whose products damage health (such as tobacco, alcohol and processed food).
- Rising levels of ill health related to poverty and social inequalities, caused by privatisation of public health care systems, reduction in access to health services, economic and social policies favouring the wealthy and undermining the welfare of poor people.
- Increased environmental health threats (food safety, transport safety, pollution – resulting from privatisation of public services, deregulation and trade liberalisation).

However, there are possible advantages from globalisation, including:

- pooled expertise to tackle health problems
- shared experiences of health reforms
- improved transfer of health technologies
- internationally coordinated action to combat the causes of ill health and alleviate the consequences of illness.

As will become clear, there is disagreement over the disadvantages and benefits of globalisation with regard to health, and about the capacity of international health bodies to improve health and reduce illness.

International health policy processes

Various international bodies are involved in the health policy process, including WHO, the World Bank and the WTO. Other players include the nation states and their alliances, the most powerful of which is the 'G8' group of nations (France, Germany, Italy, Japan, Canada, Russia, the USA and the UK). The health policy arena also includes a range of non-governmental organisations, multinational corporations and trade organisations.

The World Health Organisation

WHO was founded in 1948 as a specialist agency of the United Nations (Koivusalo and Ollila, 1997). Although not the first international health body, WHO heralded a more systematic and inclusive approach to cooperation on health policy and on improving standards of health at the global level. Its main functions were to provide scientific advice and set international standards (Lee et al, 1996). Notably, the organisation committed itself at the outset to health promotion as well as the reduction of disease. Its early efforts focused mainly on the prevention of infectious diseases, and included the formulation of international health regulations which required notification of certain diseases (plague, yellow fever and cholera). In 2005 these regulations were extended to combat any event that could constitute a public health emergency of international concern. Given the threat posed by new and emergent infectious diseases, such as SARS and avian flu, WHO has a major role in protecting health.

During the 1970s, WHO formulated a global *Health for All by the Year 2000* strategy that attempted to shift member states' policies towards disease prevention and health promotion (WHO/UNICEF, 1978; WHO, 1981). This emphasised: the need to address health and social inequalities, both between and within countries; the importance of primary health care in meeting people's needs, preventing illness and promoting health; the need to establish links between health and other sectors of policy, such as trade, housing and welfare, that have a bearing on health outcomes; and the importance of encouraging people to participate in health care planning and provision. Targets were set and countries reported back on their progress. *Health for All* was taken forward at both the international and regional level. The WHO European Region, for example, formulated its own targets. Its role is discussed later in this chapter.

Health for All (and other related initiatives, such as *Healthy Cities*, which emphasised the need to improve local environments and communities) helped to place public health back on the policy agenda. However, it could not compel governments to address such issues. In the UK, for example, the Thatcher and Major governments were hostile to many of the elements of the *Health for All* agenda and particularly opposed to WHO targets on health inequalities. The *Health for All* strategy and targets have since been revised by *Health 21* (WHO, 1998), and while they remain important as a framework, WHO has increasingly opted for action on specific 'priority areas', such as tobacco (where it formulated an international treaty on tobacco control). Other priorities include malaria, TB, HIV/AIDS, mental health, maternal health, cancer, heart disease and diabetes, food safety and safe blood products (see McCarthy, 2002a). WHO has also focused on health service reform and has undertaken comparative evaluations of the performance of different health systems (WHO, 2000), which may promote policy change (see ***Box 10.2***).

WHO has attracted criticism from friend and foe alike. Vested interests, such as the food, alcohol and tobacco industries, have criticised its approach to public health issues for obvious reasons. They have been joined by those governments that are heavily influenced by such interests (such as the US). In contrast, others believe that WHO has actually been subject to too much influence from commercial interests in health, including the drugs industry (Chowdhury and Rowson, 2000; McCarthy, 2002a). It has been criticised for lacking leadership, for being over-bureaucratic and over-politicised (Koivusalo and Ollila, 1997;

McCarthy, 2002b; Yamey, 2002a). Many also believe that WHO's leadership role in health has been ceded to other organisations, such as the World Bank (see later), and that it must do more to persuade other international bodies to acknowledge the health implications of their decisions (Horton, 2006). Some see WHO as increasingly disease- and treatment-oriented, and argue that it should reassert its role in integrating, coordinating and advancing the health agenda worldwide (Prah Ruger and Yach, 2005).

WHO underwent various reforms from the late 1990s. These included an internal reorganisation, a rationalisation of programmes and closer engagement with stakeholders, including commercial interests. There are mixed views on whether or not these have yielded improvements (Lerer and Matzopoulos, 2001; McCarthy, 2002b; Yamey, 2002b; Horton, 2006).

Other UN bodies

Although for many years WHO was regarded as the undisputed lead organisation on international health matters, other UN agencies have also been involved in this field (see Walt, 1994; Koivusalo and Ollila, 1997; Lee and Collin, 2005). These include the UN Educational, Scientific and Cultural Organisation (UNESCO), with interests in science and health education; the UN Children's Fund (UNICEF), which promotes child welfare, and the UN Food and Agriculture Organisation (FAO). Others also have an interest in health, such as the UN Development Programme (UNDP), the International Labour Organisation (ILO) (with regard to health and safety at work); the UN High Commission on Refugees (UNHCR); and the UN Conference on Trade and Development (UNCTAD). The UN Security Council has also considered health issues on occasion, such as HIV/AIDS for example (Lee and Collin, 2005). In addition special UN bodies have been established on health issues including HIV/AIDS (UNAIDS). The UN has also initiated action on the environment (the UN Environment Programme) and drugs (UN Drug Control Programme), both of which have implications for health. For example, the efforts of the UN to promote action on environmental issues led to the Rio Summit in 1992. This produced a declaration on the Environment and Development, a blueprint for sustainable development (*Agenda 21*), and a number of conventions on specific aspects of the environment. It also set the direction for future efforts to limit climate change. This has led to other interventions, including the 1997 Kyoto Protocol on reducing greenhouse gases, which have wide implications for public health.

In recent years the UN leadership has become more closely engaged with health and related issues. In 2000, the UN General Assembly adopted the Millennium Development goals, which included reducing child mortality; improving maternal health; eradicating extreme poverty and hunger;

combating HIV/AIDS, malaria and other diseases; and ensuring environmental sustainability (see www.un.org/millenniumgoals/). This strategy was supported by targets to be achieved by 2015 (for example, to reduce extreme poverty and hunger by half; reduce mortality of under fives by two thirds; reduce maternal mortality by three quarters; halt and reverse the spread of AIDS, HIV and TB; and halve the proportion of people without access to drinking water and sanitation).

WHO increasingly operates in a crowded policy environment, and with bodies that are larger and more powerful than itself. Indeed, many commentators believe that WHO has lost ground to these other players (Walt, 1994; Koivusalo and Ollila, 1997; Berlinguer, 1999; Yamey, 2002b; Ollila, 2005; Tudor-Hart, 2006). One interviewee, a former DoH civil servant, also recognised this, commenting that 'it is the non-health organisations that have the most implications for health'. Indeed, the leadership role in international health appears to have shifted decisively towards economic institutions, such as the World Bank, the International Monetary Fund (IMF), the OECD and the WTO. The World Bank is part of the financial system established after the Second World War (Walt, 1994; Koivusalo and Ollila, 1997; Lee and Collin, 2005). It is regarded as part of the UN system, although has considerable autonomy. Its initial role was to help rebuild economies in the post-war period by providing loans for infrastructure. Its attention later moved to developing countries and, along with the IMF (see below), the implementation of structural adjustment programmes (SAPs) to open their economies to foreign investment and competition. This entailed 'neo-liberal' policies such as reducing the public sector and liberalising markets in these countries, often with adverse health consequences. Subsequently, the World Bank has focused on cost-effectiveness of health interventions, poverty reduction and building social capital, although these continue to emphasise neo-liberal policies. The World Bank remains primarily focused on developing countries, but many of its policy prescriptions (such as the promotion of PPPs, for example) are also relevant to industrialised countries.

The IMF, like the World Bank, is an autonomous part of the UN system (Koivusalo and Ollila, 1997; Lee and Collin, 2005). It aims to expand international trade and lends short-term funds to countries with cash-flow problems. Like any 'banker' it imposes conditions, which usually entail prescriptions to reduce public spending, privatise public services and introduce deregulation. It also issues reports on the state of economies and economic policy, which can affect financial confidence and investment. These activities can affect health policy in a number of ways. Health and other public service budgets may be curtailed, as happened in the UK in the 1970s when the IMF imposed loan conditions during an economic crisis. More specifically, policies favoured by IMF (such as privatisation and deregulation) may be adopted to satisfy particular loan conditions or to build investor confidence in the economy.

The OECD is a member organisation that includes the main industrialised democracies (Koivusalo and Ollila, 1997). Its members account for three quarters of world trade. It too was established as part of post-war reconstruction plans. The OECD aims to promote economic growth, improved standards of living and world trade through economic cooperation. It does this by promoting agreements between members on issues of common concern, undertaking research into economic and social issues and disseminating ideas about policy and reform. Public services and health care fall within the OECD's remit and it has taken a greater interest in health care reform issues since the 1990s. It is seen by critics (for example, De Vos et al, 2004) as promoting the same kind of principles as the World Bank, the IMF and the WTO (see ***Box 10.1***), although is regarded as less powerful than these bodies in terms of direct influence. It has a more subtle role of facilitating reform through comparison, analysis and recommendation (Armingeon and Beyeler, 2004; Alasuutari, 2005). As one interviewee, a former DoH civil servant, commented 'OECD reports carry very considerable weight in government'.

Box 10.1: The World Trade Organisation

The WTO was created in 1995 to monitor and enforce trade agreements. Its 148 member states account for 90 per cent of world trade (Lee and Collin, 2005). The WTO aims to reduce barriers to trade between countries by negotiating new trade agreements and by settling disputes over existing agreements. Its rules and decisions are binding on members and it may bring sanctions against those that do not comply. Although WTO decisions are reached by consensus, the richer industrialised countries – the EU states, Japan, the USA and Canada – exert most influence (Ostry, 2001).

Liberalisation of trade is not necessarily good for health, although trade agreements do allow for a degree of protection on health grounds (Lee and Collin, 2005; Lee and Koivusalo, 2005; Waitzkin et al, 2005). Under WTO's 'sanitary and phytosanitary (SPS) agreement' trade in goods or services can be restricted 'to protect human, animal or plant life or health' (SPS, 1994). However, any restrictions must be based on clear scientific evidence. This may undermine the precautionary principle, which is based on risks that are often difficult to quantify. Moreover, any restrictions must not discriminate against particular countries or between domestic and foreign suppliers, but apply to all potential suppliers. The WTO rules also specify that any measures to protect health must place the least possible restraint on trade, implying that weaker forms of regulation (providing information to consumers, for example) will be chosen over stronger forms (such as punitive taxes or bans on products).

The WTO lacks in-house health expertise (Kimball, 2006). WHO has sought to influence some decisions on health grounds (WHO/WTO, 2002), while on food safety issues, international standards on labelling, content, additives, pesticides and drug residues are set by the Codex Alimentarius Commission (or Codex), a body established jointly by WHO and the FAO. Commercial interests are strongly represented on Codex committees, while consumers are under-represented, fuelling fears that commercial considerations prevail (Tansey and Worsley, 1995).

Critics of the WTO cite examples where they believe health standards have been ignored (Lee and Koivusalo, 2005). The dispute between the EU and the US over hormone-treated beef is one such case. The EU banned animal growth hormones in 1989 citing health grounds. This was opposed by the US and Canada on behalf of their cattle industry, which heavily used these drugs and faced the prospect of losing a large overseas market. Initially, retaliatory tariffs were imposed on European imports. Subsequently, the complainants took their cases to the WTO, which ruled in their favour on the grounds that the evidence of risk to health was insufficient to justify a ban. Despite losing an appeal, the EU refused to implement the WTO decision. In 2003, the EU agreed to comply with the WTO's ruling by specifying further scientific evidence on harm to health caused by one of the hormones and seeking a provisional prohibition for others where the scientific evidence was unclear. The US and Canada were not satisfied by this and sanctions, backed by the WTO, remained in place.

The extension of free-trade rules to services raises the prospects of further privatisation of health care, according to some commentators (Sexton, 2001; Price, 2002; Lee and Koivusalo, 2005; Koivusalo, 2006). Although trade agreements exempt 'services supplied in the exercise of government authority' (Lee and Collin, 2005, p 93), they apply to public services where there is already private sector provision. Currently, countries can exempt certain service areas, including health services, from the scope of trade agreements (Lipson, 2001). However, there are ways around this, notably in countries that have health insurance-based funding systems (which can be classified as financial services and therefore within the scope of WTO rules – see Laidlaw, 2002). Furthermore, future challenges to national health systems which allow private provision (including the NHS) are possible, forcing governments to open up even more areas of health care to competition from private operators (Ostry, 2001; Holden, 2005). All these changes are seen as especially in the interests of the US health care corporations, which are seeking to expand their businesses overseas (Price, 2002; Tudor-Hart, 2004; Holden, 2005).

Another consequence of the extension of trade rules to services is that trade restrictions are now deemed to include government measures that incidentally affect the supply of services. This extends the remit of the WTO beyond purely trade restrictions (such as tariffs) to other forms of government regulation in areas such as health, environment and safety, thereby restricting public policy options (Price, 2002). This could benefit multinational corporations whose activities can adversely affect health (such as the chemical, alcohol, tobacco and food industries).

Other WTO agreements have implications for health. The agreement on technical barriers to trade (TBT, 1994) prevents countries from restricting trade by imposing standards with regard to product characteristics and production, including packaging and labelling. It is permissible to use such standards to protect health, security and the environment, but they must not discriminate unfairly against foreign producers and must be evidence based. These requirements can operate against restrictions that are based on potential rather than actual risks to health and safety. Most health issues, however, are meant to be covered by the SPS agreement.

Also the WTO Agreement on Trade-related Aspects of Intellectual Property (TRIPS, 1994) has been criticised for undermining efforts to improve public health in developing countries (Pollock and Price, 2003). Although protection for public health and nutrition was written into the agreement, lack of clarity about the circumstances where states could depart from TRIPS rules produced widespread uncertainty. Controversy surrounded the extension of the intellectual property rights of drug companies to exploit their innovations, which raised concerns about poorer countries facing higher prices for essential drugs. In response to pressure from poorer countries and non-governmental organisations, the WTO stated that intellectual property rules could be over-ridden in this field, for example, by allowing countries to import generic copies of patented drugs to treat diseases such as HIV/AIDS, TB and malaria. Subsequently, the grounds for such action were clarified further, although critics remained unimpressed and continued to argue that TRIPS was not in the interests of the poorer countries.

According to Tudor-Hart (2006, p 211) 'effectively, bankers have replaced health professionals as directors of global health policy'. Although all these institutions claim to be neutral, their emphasis on economic, financial and trade priorities leads them to favour particular policy options, such as privatisation,

PPPs, cuts in taxation and public expenditure, deregulation, a greater role for markets, and more international trade (Lee and Collin, 2005; Waitzkin et al, 2005). They are opposed to policies that extend the public sector, redistribute income and diminish the role of markets and the private sector. As most health care systems have a strong public sector element, these international institutions regard them as inefficient and ripe for reform.

Commentators see institutions like the World Bank, the IMF, the WTO and the OECD as acting mainly in the interests of the richer countries of the world (although their activities impinge on industrialised countries as well as the less industrialised) (see, for example, De Vos et al, 2004). The US is particularly powerful within these international organisations and has a very strong pro-market or neo-liberal ideology, even in health care. This is counterbalanced to some extent by the EU, whose member states have a tradition of social protection, although neo-liberalism has also taken a stronger hold here too in recent years.

Added to their weight within these global institutions, the rich countries also dominate other international fora, such as summit meetings. In recent years the G8 summits have set the direction for health policy across the globe. They have made commitments on poverty reduction through aid and debt relief for the poorest countries, and have also supported efforts to tackle HIV/AIDS, TB and malaria (with the creation of a global fund to fight these diseases; see www.theglobalfund.org). The richer countries have also backed new public–private alliances to extend vaccination and improve nutrition (Ollila, 2005). Although these initiatives have been welcomed, they fall short of the stronger redistributive measures which many believe are needed to improve health in poorer countries (Fort et al, 2004; Labonte and Schrecker, 2004).

Other players

In addition to the UN agencies and institutions of global governance, a range of other organisations seek to influence international policies that impact on health. These include charities and trusts, some of which are engaged in funding or providing health care (such as the Gates Foundation, Oxfam and Médecins Sans Frontières). There are international alliances on specific health issues (such as the Framework Convention Alliance for Tobacco Control, which brought together anti-smoking campaigners across the world to press for a tobacco control treaty, and the Global Prevention Alliance, which promotes coordinated action on the WHO global strategy on diet, physical activity and health). There are also anti-globalisation, environmental and anti-poverty campaign groups, which oppose the current international order in view of what they see as its broader adverse consequences, including for health. The other players are powerful economic interests, the multinational corporations, which are either engaged in commercial activities that harm health (for example, the tobacco industry) or which produce health care products and services for profit (for example, the drugs industry).

It is acknowledged that multinational corporations are the dominant interests in global policy networks. In particular, they are very powerful in the global PPPs that have emerged in recent years (Lee and Collin, 2005; Ollila, 2005). However, there are occasions when such interests have been successfully challenged at the global level. One example was the tobacco control treaty, already mentioned. Another was the international code of practice on the promotion of breast milk substitutes of 1981, which resulted from a successful campaign by a range of organisations concerned about the health impacts of these products in less developed countries.

Reform

Health is increasingly on the agenda in international debates (Price-Smith, 2001; Labonte and Schrecker, 2004). It is increasingly recognised that 'there can be no global health without a global government' (Berlinguer, 1999, p 598). Moreover, better international governance is needed to overcome the fragmentation of roles and responsibilities at the global level, the duplication of efforts (on HIV/AIDS, for example) and the lack of openness and accountability of international decision-making processes (Kickbusch, 2000). There is also support for greater equity in international decision-making – to give more weight to weaker interests (poorer countries and disadvantaged people in richer countries) to counter the dominant players (the US, Europe and the multinational corporations).

Box 10.2: Health care reform

Health care systems face similar challenges, including ageing populations, changes in medical technology, and rising public expectations and demands (Saltman et al, 1998; Blank and Burau, 2004; OECD, 2004). In order to meet these, most countries have undertaken health care reform. These efforts have not occurred in isolation. Although each health care system is the product of a unique set of historical, cultural and political forces, changes have been influenced by the experience of other countries.

The UK is no exception. One can point to several key reforms imported from other health care systems. The creation of NHS foundation trusts was inspired by similar institutions in Spain, Sweden and Denmark. The introduction of commissioning into the British health care system was informed by countries that adopted a market-led approach to health care, notably the US. The increased use of the private sector as a supplier of state-funded health care was influenced by the experience of continental countries that adopt a pluralist approach (such as Germany and Holland).

Reform tends to arise from a distillation of other countries' experiences, rather than by simply drawing lessons from one country. Indeed, the spread of reform ideas across health care systems tends to happen multilaterally, rather than on a bilateral basis (an example is the growing interest in competition and contracting policies across health care systems since the 1980s). Also, the legacy of others' experiences is often diluted. Other countries' ideas and experiences may be imported, but they are usually implemented differently. For example, the GP fund-holding reform in the 1990s was based loosely on the experience of US health maintenance organisations (HMOs). But it was introduced in a way more compatible with the NHS: expensive procedures and areas of care were excluded (to discourage discrimination against 'high-cost' patients); there was less scope for patients to transfer between budget holders; and the system was highly regulated to minimise the adverse effects of competition (Glennerster et al, 1994).

Although the spread of reform ideas is complex, there are certain factors which appear to facilitate it. Academic research and other reports and investigations (by commissions, committees of inquiry; parliamentary committees, think tanks) often identify potential reforms from other systems, and these may be taken up by policy actors. Overseas visits by policy actors can generate new ideas for reform. An example was the NHS University – now disbanded – which was attributed to an influential UK policy actor, who was impressed by employer-led educational institutions during a visit to the US. Academics and policy experts visiting from other countries can also generate new ideas. For example, Professor Alain Enthoven, a US academic who visited the UK in the mid-1980s, provided important intellectual arguments for using market forces in the NHS (Enthoven, 1985), which were later taken up by politicians and think tanks. Improvements in international travel and communication have encouraged the spread of new policy ideas from abroad. It is now much easier to find out about experiences and reforms elsewhere. Finally, policy ideas are spread by global and international policy actors. These include institutions such as the OECD, the World Bank, the IMF, WHO, and the EU, as well as other organisations, such as multinational corporations and non-governmental organisations. Research bodies and think tanks also play a key role, including, for example, the European Observatory on Health Systems and Policies, which undertakes analysis of health care systems and reforms across Europe.

Health policy and Europe

A number of European institutions seek to influence health policy. These include WHO's Regional Office for Europe, which takes forward health initiatives often in collaboration with other European bodies. The European Region, in line with the *Health for All* strategy, and its successor, *Health 21*, introduced specific targets for the continent, tailored to its own particular priorities (WHO Regional Office for Europe, 1985, 1998). This set a policy framework for national strategies to improve public health and prevent disease. The WHO European Region has also developed strategies for particular health problems, such as alcohol misuse and smoking. Although it cannot compel member states to pursue policies, the Regional Office can create an environment where governments are pressured to take action by, for example, exemplifying effective strategies pursued in other states. It is also a partner in the European Observatory on Health Systems and Policies (see also ***Box 10.2***), which analyses reforms.

The Council of Europe was founded in 1949. It now has 46 member states, and therefore has a wider membership than the EU (which has 25). The Council of Europe aims to reinforce democracy, human rights and the rule of law. It develops common responses to various political, cultural, social and legal challenges facing European countries. It has introduced charters setting out citizens' rights, beginning with the 1950 European Convention on Human Rights. Signatories to this Convention – including the UK – are bound by its provisions. Individuals may pursue cases in the European Court of Human Rights and now in UK courts, following the 1998 Human Rights Act (Montgomery, 2003). The Convention has been used to challenge health care practices, the actions of health authorities, and decisions about access to care on grounds that they have breached human rights (such as the right to life, right to liberty, right to private and family life, prohibition of inhuman or degrading treatment and of discrimination on grounds of race or gender).

The UK is also a signatory to the European Social Charter (Council of Europe, 1996). This places several health responsibilities on states, which if not undertaken could provide a basis for legal challenge (Montgomery, 2003). These include the removal, as far as possible, of the causes of ill health; the provision of advisory and educational facilities for the promotion of health and encouragement of individual responsibility, and the prevention of infectious and other diseases as well as accidents. The Charter also requires states to ensure that ill people without resources can access care.

The Council of Europe also issues guidelines and standards in a variety of health and health care fields (such as the regulation of hazardous chemicals, including asbestos and pesticides, transplants and blood products, the mobility of health professionals, health service quality, citizen engagement in health services and the management of waiting-lists). It also promotes health in a number of areas, including better nutrition in schools. In addition, it encourages policies to help vulnerable groups, including people with HIV/AIDS, elderly people and those with chronic illness and disabilities.

Nonetheless, it is the EU that is regarded as the main player in European health policy. The remainder of this section is devoted to analysis of the role of EU institutions in developing Europe-wide approaches to health and health care.

The European Union

According to some commentators, the EU has had a significant impact on health policy (Randall, 2001; Duncan, 2002; Montgomery, 2003). As for the future, the European health policy agenda has been described as extensive (McKee, 2005) and EU involvement in this policy area is likely to increase (Mossialos and McKee, 2002; Greer, 2005; Koivusalo, 2005; Mahony, 2006). In contrast, interviewees from the UK health policy scene are less certain about the overall impact of the EU on domestic health policy. Some argued that the EU was influential on health policy issues such as the employment of health workers, health and safety, and public health. Others pointed to the limited powers of the EU in the health sphere and maintained that its influence has been overstated or exaggerated. However, there was more consensus about the potential for EU influence in future. Comments included: 'the EU has some influence over domestic policy and will increase' (MP); 'the EU will have an ever increasing role in relation to health' (respondent, health professional organisation); 'Europe has not had a major impact on UK health policy, though this may be beginning to change' (think tank spokesperson); and 'Europe's influence in the health arena will increase in future' (former DoH civil servant).

The development of European Union health policy

The EU derives its legal powers from the various treaties of the European Community, and from regulations and directives that derive from the 'competences' granted by these treaties. In addition, the judgments of the European Court of Justice (which is not the same body as the European Court of Human Rights, mentioned earlier), discussed further later, form a body of 'case law', which further delineates the powers of EU institutions (Montgomery, 2003).

Although the main focus of the European Community was economic cooperation and the creation of a 'common market', cooperation on social matters was acknowledged as important at the outset (Randall, 2001; Nugent,

2003). It was realised that unfettered competition could damage rather than improve living standards. Indeed, the protection of labour through occupational health and safety policies became one of the key areas of European Community (and later EU) activity, reflected in a large number of directives and regulations on issues such as dangerous substances and machinery, workers' rights and conditions of employment. There is now a European Agency for Safety and Health at Work, which takes forward the EU programme in this area.

According to several interviewees from the UK health policy process, one of the most important worker protection issues affecting UK health policy in recent years was the European Working Time Directive. This directive has already reduced junior doctors' working hours to 58 hours per week and introduced new provisions for rest periods. Under the directive, maximum working hours per week for junior doctors are set to fall to 58 hours from 2007 and to 48 hours by 2009. This is having a major impact on the organisation of health care and on medical training, both of which have depended on long working hours for junior doctors.

The 1957 Treaty of Rome, which established the European Economic Community (EEC), allowed for the development of a social policy by cooperation between states and through a European Social Fund (Nugent, 2003, pp 313-14). A number of initiatives flowed from this, including activities to help disabled people and the elderly (Hantrais, 1995). Then, in 1989, to counterbalance the move towards a single European market, a Charter of Fundamental Rights for Workers was agreed. This covered issues such as improvement of living and working conditions, equal treatment of workers in access to employment and social protection, protection of children and adolescents, and health and safety at work. It formed the basis for the Social Chapter attached to the Maastricht Treaty of 1992, which the UK refused at first to endorse.

In 2000, a charter of fundamental rights for all EU citizens was introduced, which included many aspects of social policy. With regard to health, the new charter states that 'everyone has the right of access to preventive health care and the right to benefit from medical treatment under the conditions established by national laws and practices. A high level of human health protection shall be ensured in the definition and implementation of all Union policies and activities' (Charter of Fundamental Rights of the European Union, 2000, Article 35). The legal status of the charter is currently uncertain, however. Initially launched as a statement of principles, it later formed part of the EU constitutional treaty of 2004. This was agreed by member states, but has not yet been ratified by all – see discussion later.

The agenda of the European Community has impinged on health policy and health care in many other ways. One of the main aims of the European Community was to increase the mobility of labour (Randall, 2001). Initially, this had a limited impact on health care, in view of differences in professional qualifications and training requirements between countries, as well as cultural and language barriers. However, as a result of legal challenges to domestic barriers, and a greater willingness to employ doctors from elsewhere in Europe, significant changes have occurred. Notably, in the 1990s the UK had to reform its entire system of medical training in order to comply with European law.

By the late 1980s, the European Community had turned its attention to tackling particular diseases (Randall, 2001). The 'Europe Against Cancer' programme was launched, to strengthen collaboration in research and to promote awareness of causal factors, particularly those linked to lifestyle such as smoking. Similar programmes were later launched for heart disease and HIV/AIDS. A European drug abuse programme was also established, along with a European Monitoring Centre. These various programmes did not directly challenge the sovereignty of member states with regard to health policy, but nonetheless encouraged action through health promotion, research, and efforts to promote collaboration.

Furthermore, health care products, such as drugs and medical equipment, were increasingly subject to European Community harmonisation and regulation (Randall, 2001; Mossialos et al, 2004). The drugs industry was subjected to several directives – the first in 1965 – aimed at improving competition and protecting public health. However, these twin objectives have been in conflict, and this caused considerable difficulties for the European Community and now the EU (Randall, 2001). Added to this, the drugs industry is a powerful political actor, both internationally and within individual member states (see Chapter Six) and has resisted efforts to control its commercial activities (Abraham, 2002; Health Committee, 2005). Even so, the European regulatory system is increasingly important. A European Medicines Agency was established in 1995 to undertake key monitoring and regulatory roles and to provide expert advice to the European Commission and EU member states.

The impact of Economic Union

The process of creating a common market in goods, services, capital and labour, accelerated after the passage of the Single European Act (SEA) in 1987. The SEA attempted to create a more competitive market for goods across the European Community. This economic imperative was again balanced by social considerations. The SEA stated that harmonisation must be based on regulations that offer a high level of health protection. This provided a foundation for many health initiatives, notably the specification of health warnings on tobacco products (O'Connor, 1991). Another area of activity was food policy, not surprising given its proximity to the health agenda. Specific actions included directives on food labelling and food safety, a nutrition programme and the creation of a European Food Safety Authority.

The SEA also extended the activities of the European Community institutions with regard to the environment. Community environmental legislation had been introduced in the 1970s (Nugent, 2003) covering issues such as air and water pollution, disposal of chemicals and waste management. A European Environmental Agency was established in 1994 to implement programmes in this field. Although the environment is a separate policy area, it has important implications for health. There have been some efforts to bring these arenas closer together in recent years with the publication of the European Environment and Health Action Plan, which focuses on issues such as chemical contamination, water pollution, air quality and noise levels (European Commission, 2003).

The SEA was followed by efforts to create a more closely integrated 'European Union', enshrined in the 1992 Maastricht Treaty (Treaty on European Union, 1992; Nugent, 2003; Booker and North, 2005). Article 129 of this treaty created a new responsibility for public health, stating that 'the community shall contribute towards ensuring a high level of human health protection by encouraging cooperation between member states and, if necessary, lending support to their action' (Treaty on European Union, 1992) and that 'health protection requirements shall form a constituent part of the community's other policies'. Another key clause stated that 'the Community and member states shall foster cooperation with third countries and the competent international organisations in the sphere of public health'. Decisions were to be made by qualified majority (see discussion later) but specifically excluded 'harmonisation of the laws and regulations of the member states'. In other words, the EU had no direct means of producing convergence in the health care systems of member states.

This was seen as a major weakness. Nonetheless, in the years that followed, the EU developed a framework for action on public health. A network for the control and surveillance of communicable diseases was established and programmes initiated in cancer prevention, HIV/AIDS and drug addiction. Approval was also granted for four further programmes – health monitoring, pollution-related disease, injury prevention; and rare diseases – but these were slow to develop (Randall, 2001).

Several developments since Maastricht extended the EU's role in relation to health policy. First the Treaty of Amsterdam strengthened public health provisions by stating that 'a high level of human health protection shall be ensured in the definition and implementation of all EC policies and activities' (European Union, 1997, Article 129). The scope for community action was extended from 'the prevention of diseases and in particular the major health scourges' to 'improving public health, preventing human illness and diseases and obviating sources of danger to human health'. The Treaty extended the scope of the EU to set minimum standards for the quality and safety of organs, substances of human origin, and blood products used in treatment. It also allowed for intervention in animal and plant health in situations where the direct objective was the protection of public health. Other than this, the powers of EU institutions remained confined to promoting research, health information and education, and coordination between member states. Only incentive measures could be pursued and 'harmonisation of laws and regulations of member states' was again specifically excluded.

One reason behind the stronger public health provisions in the Treaty of Amsterdam was the fierce criticism of the EU's mis-handling of the BSE/CJD crisis (Baggott, 1998). This prompted a sharper focus on health policy and a reorganisation of responsibilities within the European Commission (Randall, 2001). A new Directorate of Health and Consumer Protection was created, with a much stronger focus on public health matters. Subsequently, concern about the threats of new, emerging and resurgent infections, such as SARS, influenza and drug-resistant forms of TB and AIDS, bolstered the case for a European-wide approach to communicable disease, leading to the establishment of a European Centre for Disease Prevention and Control in 2004. Its mission is to identify, assess and communicate about the threats of communicable disease to human health.

Other developments

The EU's role in health was further encouraged by the accession of economically poorer countries (such as former communist bloc countries of Eastern Europe) and by immigration from poverty-stricken and war-torn countries of the world. This raised the prospects of greater socio-economic inequality within the EU, which not only made it more difficult to achieve social objectives, but threatened its economic goals by undermining the capacity of goods, services, people and capital to move freely between richer and poorer member states. This led to interest in policies that might reduce health and social inequalities both across Europe and within member states (McCarthy, 2002b; McKee et al, 2004; Neroth, 2004; McKee, 2005).

Meanwhile, Europe's leaders acknowledged the importance of health and other social policies (such as education, for example) in strengthening the economic competitiveness of the EU, especially against the North American and South East Asian economies. This approach, which was part of the 'Lisbon Agenda', highlighted the contribution of health policy and health care reform in improving economic efficiency and competitiveness (Nugent, 2003; Byrne, 2004; Koivusalo, 2005; McKee, 2005). Another factor was the increase in patients' mobility between European health care systems. Several

ECJ judgments supported the right of patients to seek treatment in other member states, reimbursed by their insurer or member state (McCarthy, 2003b). This increased the prospect of increased cross-border flows and a consumer market in health care. It also underlined the need for adequate regulation of health care standards to ensure fair competition.

Gradually, EU health policy began to develop a sharper focus. A six-year public health strategy was introduced in 2002 (for the period 2003-8) with a budget of €353m (Decision of the European Parliament and of the Council, 2001). This programme had three aspects: improving health information and knowledge for the development of public health; enhancing the capability of responding rapidly to threats to health; and addressing health determinants.

In 2004, the creation of a constitution for the EU, in the form of a new treaty, appeared to provide further opportunities to extend the role of its institutions in health policy. The constitution included the EU's Charter of Fundamental Rights of 2000, discussed earlier. The treaty's article on public health reiterated that a high level of human health protection be ensured in EU policies and set out new areas for intervention including monitoring, early warnings and combating serious cross-border threats to health; encouraging cooperation between member states to improve complementarity of their services in cross-border areas; and measures setting high standards of quality and safety for medical products and devices; and measures to tackle alcohol and tobacco-related health problems. The treaty also reiterated that the EU would respect the responsibilities of member states for 'the definition of their health policy and for the organisation and delivery of health services and medical care', including 'the management of health services and medical care and the allocation of resources assigned to them' (Treaty Establishing a Constitution for Europe, 2004; Article III-278).

A new European Union programme for health

Following the agreement of the treaty the Director General for Health and Consumer Protection, David Byrne (2004), published a non-official paper that called for health to be put at the centre of EU policy making. His view, reflecting the Lisbon agenda, was that efforts to improve health must be seen as an economic priority. Byrne emphasised the importance of health promotion and prevention; a robust EU-wide knowledge base; the need to foster partnerships (with citizens and other stakeholders) the need to enhance the EU's international role in health; and its role in promoting cooperation between health care systems to achieve 'synergies and savings'.

This eventually led to a new EU programme for health in 2006 (Decision of the European Parliament and of the Council, 2006), which had three objectives: to improve citizen's health security; to promote health for prosperity and solidarity; to generate and disseminate health knowledge. More specifically, this included responses to communicable disease threats, action on patient safety, efforts to address health inequalities, and the fostering of cooperation on cross-border issues such as patient and professional mobility. Action on health determinants such as alcohol, tobacco and illicit drug consumption, as well as social and physical environments, also formed part of the EU's proposals. With regard to disseminating health knowledge, the EU proposed action with regard to rare diseases, cross-border issues, gender, mental health and children's health. This also included EU-wide health monitoring, the development of tools and indicators, and better health information for citizens.

Although initially ambitious, the programme finally agreed by the EU institutions was actually scaled down. The number of programme objectives was reduced. Three strands of work additional to those included in the 2002 programme (delivering an efficient response to health threats; helping prevent diseases; fostering cooperation between health systems) were dropped. However, the European Commission claimed that the programme objectives (see discussion earlier) were broad enough to include action in these specific areas. More damaging perhaps was the decision – backed by the UK government – to cut the budget for the programme by two thirds (Martin, 2005).

The EU role in health policy continues to develop. However, there are a number of obstacles. First, the 2004 Treaty of Rome, which established the EU constitution and represented a much stronger drive towards integration in health and other policy areas, has not yet been ratified by all member states. Until this happens, it is difficult (although not impossible, as some have noted – see Booker and North, 2005) to advance the provisions of the treaty, including those relating to health. Second, even if the treaty comes into force, the EU remains a relatively weak player in health policy, underlined by the continued commitment to retain health policy and health care systems as a member state responsibility. Furthermore, the EU has relatively few resources (McCarthy, 2002b; European Health Policy Forum, 2003) – less than one per cent of its budget is allocated to health, which limits its influence. Third, the EU is still regarded as poorly organised in relation to health policy. Since the creation of the Directorate on Health and Consumer Protection, calls to restructure the European Commission have continued. For example, there have been recommendations for a dedicated Directorate for Health with its own Commissioner (ie, separating health from consumer protection) (see European Parliament, 1999; European Health Policy Forum, 2003).

Fourth, health remains a relatively low priority for the most powerful EU institutions, such as the Council of Ministers and the European Commission. Not only is the health budget small (and attempts to increase it substantially have been rebuffed), but health considerations continue to weigh less heavily than economic issues, despite the EU's commitment to a high level of health protection in all policies (Baeten and Jorens, 2006). In practice, where there is conflict between the two, economic considerations prevail. This is nowhere more evident than in the Common Agricultural Policy, where subsidies for tobacco, alcohol and high-fat food products continue to encourage production (Lobstein, 1998; Randall, 2001; Neroth, 2004).

Nonetheless, the ability of the EU to influence health policy should not be judged wholly in terms of its formal powers. In many policy areas, the EU has been adept in influencing policy 'through the backdoor'. This is done in several ways. First, ECJ decisions can lead to a reinterpretation of EU legislation in such a way that extends the power of EU organisations. This happened in the BSE crisis during the 1990s when the court upheld the worldwide ban on British beef imposed by the European Commission (Randall, 2001). ECJ judgments can also promote a more active role for EU institutions in particular policy areas. For example, the various decisions on patients' mobility, mentioned earlier, have prompted EU institutions to take a closer interest in issues such as patient safety and quality of service across Europe.

The EU's activities on economic and trade issues can also influence health policy. Its activities on the mobility of health care professionals and health care products have been noted. Its potential to influence health through regulation of industries such as food, alcohol and tobacco has also been mentioned. However, any extension of European market rules to health services will have wide implications for the organisation and delivery of health care in member states. Such an extension was in fact proposed as part of a European Directive in 2004. This was seen as part of an attempt to create an internal market in health services that would fundamentally alter the character of individual health care systems and shift them significantly away from the state model (De Vos et al, 2004; Koivusalo, 2005; Neroth, 2005). After much lobbying, its opponents won the day, and health care was excluded.

The EU will continue to exert influence through the spread of ideas about health policy and reform. This role has already been identified by some academics (Randall, 2001) and European health actors (Byrne, 2004). By encouraging the spread of ideas, EU institutions could facilitate policy transfer (see ***Box 10.3***). Indeed, according to one UK think tank spokesperson, 'the influence of Europe may be more subtle than operating via EU directives. There has been an increase in policy tourism, where policy makers borrow ideas from other countries.'

Finally, the EU can influence the domestic health policies of member states through its role as an international player. The EU is active in international policy debates on health and health-related issues (including those connected with environment and trade). These can lead to international-level policies or standards with which EU member states are expected to comply. These include health treaties and regulations, such as the framework convention on tobacco or international health regulations, and WTO decisions, which, as noted earlier, can have a significant impact on health.

Box 10.3: European Union decision-making process

The EU decision-making process is complex. Essentially there are a number of key institutions that influence policy. The *European Commission* is often regarded as the 'civil service' of the EU. It seeks to implement and enforce EU law by monitoring member state compliance and, if necessary, brings cases before the ECJ. It also has an important legislative role, drafting proposals for consideration by other EU institutions. The European Commission consists of permanent officials (and seconded staff) divided into directorates, each of which is headed by a commissioner drawn from a different member state. Each directorate has a specific area of responsibility. Health comes under the portfolio of the Commissioner and Directorate General of Health and Consumer Protection. These portfolios are allocated by the President of the European Commission, who is responsible for strategic direction, central administrative functions, coordination, and is the main representative of the European Commission in its dealings with institutions both in and outside the EU.

The *Council of Ministers* comprises the ministers of member states dealing with a particular issue (such as health). The composition of the Council therefore varies according to the issue being discussed. The Council coordinates policy and, along with the European Parliament, legislates and sets budgets for EU programmes. Decisions in the Council are increasingly made by qualified majority, so that member states cannot veto proposals alone. The Council of Ministers has a 'presidency' which is held for six months by each member state on a rotating basis. This provides an opportunity for this member state to raise particular issues on the EU agenda. Below the Council of Ministers are coordinating committees of civil servants and advisers drawn from the member states. These prepare the ground for discussions and decisions. They also help to identify possible solutions where there is disagreement within the Council or between the Council and other EU institutions. A General Secretariat provides administrative support, information and policy analysis for the Council. In addition, the heads of government of the member states meet four times a year as the *European Council*. This sets strategic direction, deals with major concerns, and attempts to resolve the major conflicts and tensions between governments. The European Council also has a six-monthly presidency, held concurrently with the presidency of the Council of Ministers.

The European Parliament comprises directly elected members (MEPs) drawn from all members states in five-yearly elections. The Parliament has powers of scrutiny and legislation. Most legislation is now subject to a 'co-decision' procedure that involves Parliament. In addition, the Parliament can veto the budget and appointments to the European Commission, but these are 'all or nothing' powers (specific budget items or particular commissioners cannot be rejected). In undertaking its roles, the Parliament has created committees of MEPs that specialise in particular policy areas. The Environment, Public Health and Food Safety Committee scrutinises EU health policy and activities in this field and makes recommendations about reform.

These formal institutions are surrounded by a range of informal bodies and networks. The EU system is relatively open to pressure groups, business organisations and professional bodies seeking to influence policy. Increasingly, these organisations operate through pan-European lobby groups to express their views. Examples include the European Disability Forum, the Standing Committee of European Doctors, the Association of European Cancer Leagues and European Federation of Pharmaceutical Industries and Associations. The European Parliament is very accessible to pressure groups. The European Commission is also relatively open, partly because it lacks technical expertise and other information essential for policy development and is heavily dependent on outside advice and information. The European Commission tends to proceed by consensus and usually canvasses views before proceeding, giving outside bodies an opportunity to comment. The EU has established various stakeholder fora in the health policy field. The most significant is the health policy forum, established in 2001 to act as a two-way process of communication between EU institutions and outside organisations. Its members include a range of groups representing patients, health care industries, health care professions and workers, and public health advocates.

The European Court of Justice (ECJ) considers cases brought before it under European law. It has increasingly made judgments on health issues, including decisions affecting greater patient mobility across Europe. The ECJ ruled that insurers (including, in the case of the NHS, PCTs as commissioners of health care) must in particular circumstances reimburse patients who have been treated in other member states. The ECJ has also made judgments on public health issues, endorsing the British beef ban imposed by the EU in the 1990s. Other key judgments include rulings against the European Commission's ban on tobacco advertising and against the ban on alcohol advertising and private imports imposed by Sweden's state alcohol retail monopoly.

Sources: Randall (2001); Nugent (2003); Jones (2007)

Conclusion

This chapter has shown that UK health policy cannot be examined in isolation from broader international and global forces. Indeed, many of the policies developed in the UK are in some way connected to events, decisions and ideas originating from outside its borders. These include international health threats and global commercial pressures. Decisions by global and supranational bodies, particularly those on trade and environment issues, also shape domestic health policy.

Summary

- UK health policy must not be seen in isolation from global forces and institutions.
- A range of international bodies influence health policy, including WHO, the WTO, the OECD, the IMF, the World Bank, multinational corporations, non-governmental organisations and alliances.
- Increasingly, domestic health policies are being influenced by developments in other health systems. The UK is no exception.
- European institutions, particularly EU institutions, have taken a great interest in health policy in recent years. They have influenced health policy in member states in many ways, despite having no direct powers over health care systems.

Key questions

1. Which key global institutions and organisations are the most powerful influences on health policy?
2. Give examples of UK health policies that have been derived, at least in part, from the experience of other health care systems.
3. How has the EU extended its influence over health policy?
4. What would the extension of free-trade principles to health care mean for the NHS?

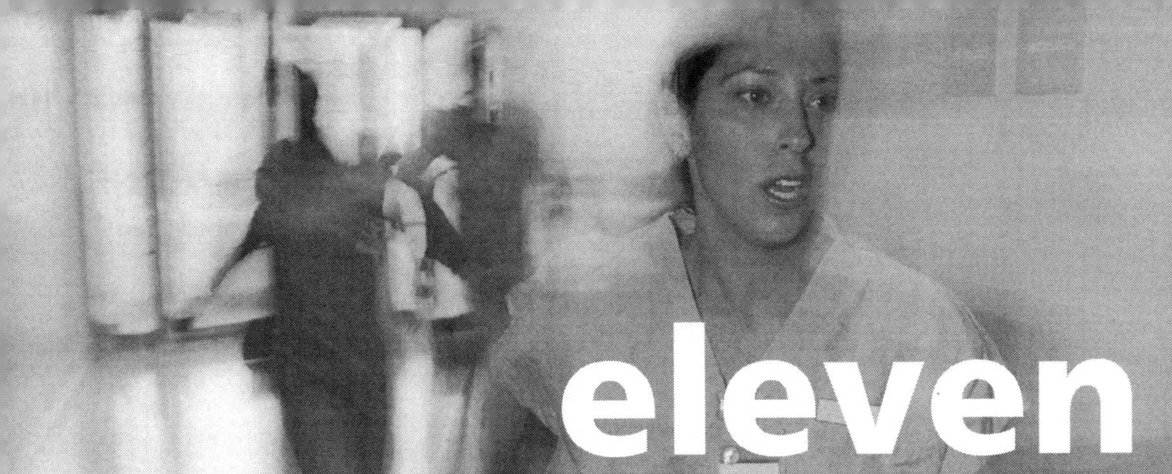

Conclusion

Overview

This chapter sets out the main conclusions of the book and makes a number of recommendations about how the health policy process might be improved.

Who makes health policy?

By exploring the role of key institutions and organisations and their involvement in various processes (such as agenda setting, consultation, policy advice, implementation) it has been possible to draw some broad conclusions. However, a word of caution is perhaps needed. The analysis has been performed at a level of generality, although illustrated by particular cases. In any specific circumstance the balance of the institutions and forces described in this book will differ. The policy process is difficult to predict in advance and one cannot simply 'read off' likely outputs or outcomes from a list of policy participants or the characteristics of a policy issue. What has been achieved here is a broad framework of analysis, which may be used by those investigating how specific policies have emerged and developed.

As shown in Chapter Two, party politics is important in setting the parameters and direction of health policy. However, there is considerable continuity between governments, irrespective of the party in power. There is also substantial policy change under governments of the same party. So party ideology does not automatically always dictate what will happen in government. In practice, governments are more pragmatic than their rhetoric would suggest. Policy is shaped by party competition and the borrowing of ideas from other parties. Ideological policies may be discarded on grounds of ineffectiveness or impracticality, to be replaced by more pragmatic approaches. There is also a certain amount of path dependency in health, which limits the impact of new ideological policies. Political circumstances, internal party conflict and pressure group lobbying may also dilute parties' ideological policies.

But this is not to say that ideology had no impact on policy. On the contrary, ideologies such as neo-liberalism and to some extent more recently, communitarian ideas, have driven policy development. The parties have been vehicles for these ideologies, but they have also been expressed through other political and social institutions, such as international agencies, government bodies, the media, think tanks and pressure groups.

Health policy making is dominated by central government. Moreover, the core executive institutions (Number Ten/Cabinet Office/Treasury) appear to have a much stronger grip on the policy-making process than before. In general, the health policy agenda has been driven by the Prime Minister and his advisers, who play a key role in pushing particular policy ideas. The Treasury has acted as a counterweight to some of these ideas, as well as pursuing its own agenda. The involvement of these core executive institutions in health policy is not new, but is more overt and systematic than before.

Within central government key changes have taken place in the way in which policies are made. The most important developments have been the rise of special advisers and the decline of the traditional civil service role in policy formation. The genesis of most key health policies in recent years can be traced back to special advisers. Prime ministerial advisers have been particularly influential. In general, the influence of civil servants with a health professional background has waned, offset to some extent by the appointment of the health 'czars' who have exerted strong influence over policy in specific condition areas.

Parliament has only a marginal impact on health policy, largely because of its weakness in relation to central government. Its influence over policy is limited by party discipline and by restrictions on its ability to initiate, amend and veto legislation. Parliament can play a valuable role in scrutinising central government and highlighting failures of public administration, but even these functions are hamstrung by limited powers. However, there are certain circumstances when Parliament can make a difference – on non-partisan issues, when the governing party is internally divided, or when the government cannot command a majority in the House of Commons. MPs retain an important role in redress of grievances and can bring cases to public attention, which may propel wider issues on to the political agenda. Also, in conjunction with others, such as the media and pressure groups, Parliament can shape agendas and contribute to policy change, particularly in the longer term.

The media has a very significant role in health policy. As has been shown, health issues attract media attention, and the reporting of health issues shapes perceptions of both the public and policy makers. The media can influence the policy agenda in a positive way, by raising awareness about particular issues or policy options. However, it is mainly a negative force, blocking policies. The importance of the media is borne out by the efforts of other policy actors to influence it (notably, government and pressure groups) and reflects the importance of symbolic politics in health policy.

Pressure groups are extremely diverse, and it is therefore difficult to assess their overall impact on policy. Traditionally, the medical profession has been regarded as the most influential interest in the health field. Although organisations representing the profession have been challenged by non-medical groups and have faced a more difficult political environment, they still exert more influence than any other single interest. The health policy network, however, is more crowded than it once was. Some groups have become more influential, notably some private health care interests, think tanks and health consumer and patients' organisations. However, there are considerable inequalities in influence within as well as between the various interest blocs.

Access to key personnel within government is important for policy influence. Groups have responded to changes in policy processes within government (such as the rise of special advisers, the appointment of czars, and the tightening grip of the core executive institutions over health policy) by altering the focus of their lobbying. Although central government remains an important target for pressure groups, access does not guarantee influence. Groups are aware that they need to maintain good relationships with other political institutions (such as Parliament and the media) in order to influence policy. Influence often depends greatly on building alliances within and across the different interest groups (professional, commercial and the voluntary sector) and producing a coherent lobbying effort. Increasingly, these alliances have coalesced around specific diseases and conditions (such as breast cancer, childbirth and mental health), which can be seen as competing with each other for resources and status.

Although most emphasis has been on the interaction between pressure groups and policy-making institutions, one should not forget that influence is often exerted through control of routine processes and practices, and the dominance of values and ideas within such systems. Indeed, it is acknowledged that the influence of the medical profession over policy has depended to a large extent on its hegemony within the health care system. This has enabled it to influence the agenda. Commercial interests today exercise power in a similar way. Meanwhile, challenging these dominant interests, diffuse and amorphous social forces, such as social movements (the childbirth and mental health movement, for example), can exert influence over the health policy agenda in the longer term, by challenging dominant values and ideas in health care practice, as well as through the use of both direct action and conventional lobbying in the policy arena.

Turning to the implementation of health policy, it is clear that the political salience of health and health care has encouraged centralisation. Somewhat paradoxically, this has been accompanied by some decentralisation of functions and an attempt to shift responsibility on to local managers and professionals. The centralisation process has intensified in recent years. A raft of new central regulatory bodies has been created, performance management has been strengthened and centrally imposed priorities and targets have predominated. Even where autonomy is granted, it must be 'earned' by compliance with central priorities. More recently, attempts to decentralise have gone beyond rhetoric and led to reforms that, if implemented fully, could lead to the devolution of power to local communities, managers and professionals. For the moment, however, such reforms (which include foundation trusts) remain controlled by central government regulatory frameworks.

Dissatisfaction with top-down models of decision making, and concern that they are particularly inappropriate to complex policy areas such as health, has led to a growing interest in alternative approaches. These rely more on promoting cultural change, collaboration, networking and organisational learning rather than 'command and control' hierarchies. They may improve policy implementation, by engaging more closely with both clinicians and users and offers potential to develop better policies from the 'bottom up', by encouraging innovation and experimentation. Although several policy initiatives in recent years have sought to promote cultural change in the NHS, they do not sit easily with the dominant culture of policy making.

It is now acknowledged that health policy implementation is contingent on other institutions outside the NHS. Increasingly, health policy and health services depend on a range of providers, statutory, voluntary and private sector. Indeed, the traditional problems of coordination have multiplied partly as a result of government policy, which has encouraged competition, pluralism and privatisation in health and social care service provision. There are other challenges too, such as the rising numbers of people with complex needs (for example, among elderly people) and the new public health agenda, which requires 'joined-up working' across a range of public and private sector organisations. In the past, the main emphasis has been on securing cooperation by financial incentives, planning arrangements, joint bodies, co-location and structural reorganisation. While these remain important, it is important that future efforts to improve collaboration give greater weight to the cultural aspects of partnership and in particular need the promotion of a common vision and commitment among partners.

The devolution of powers to Scotland, Wales and Northern Ireland means that health policy in these parts of the UK is generated by different processes and contrasting political cultures compared to England. Consequently, policy differences have emerged between the four nations, in some cases resulting from a deliberate effort to set a new direction (such as free prescriptions in Wales and free personal care in Scotland) or a refusal to follow England's lead (for example, foundation trusts). Such variations offer the possibility of learning from different policy experiences, although as noted this is not fully exploited. In addition, there are factors that encourage convergence, not least the way in which health care systems in Northern Ireland, Wales and Scotland are judged by the public and the media on criteria set for the English NHS. There has also been some devolution of health policy within the UK in the form of the London government, which has responsibilities in relation to health inequalities, for example. Regional governance arrangements for the rest of England have placed health alongside other important functions such as regeneration, transport and planning, increasing the potential for joined-up working at this level.

Health policy is shaped by broader international and global forces. These include threats to health from communicable disease and the health implications of economic pressures. Also, decisions made by international and supranational organisations, such as the institutions of the UN and the EU, have a bearing on health, including bodies with an economic remit, such as the WTO and the OECD. Health is therefore subject to multiple levels of governance. There has been a process of 'hollowing out' as international-level bodies have a taken on a greater role in shaping domestic policies, while national government functions have been transferred to new arm's-length agencies and to the private and voluntary sectors (Rhodes, 1997). The reality is that a wide range of institutions, at various levels, shape policy. However, this does not appear to have quenched the enthusiasm of UK central government, which continues to drive policy in a top-down fashion.

How can health policy making be improved?

When writing about any field of public policy, it is difficult to resist making suggestions about how the process might be improved, with a hope that more effective policies might emerge. This risks overstepping the boundary between academic analysis and policy advocacy. Yet to avoid making any recommendations would surely be too reticent.

A number of critical issues regarding the policy process have been raised during this analysis, and the following are recommended for further consideration:

- Strengthen Parliament's powers of scrutiny over health policy (for example, by giving the relevant select committees stronger powers of investigation

and recommendation, and increasing Parliament's powers over secondary legislation).
- Clarify accountability for health policy at all levels (including national arm's-length agencies, which should all be directly accountable to Parliament).
- Increase the powers of the Ombudsmen to investigate cases of maladministration and maltreatment and to recommend redress.
- Clarify further the role of special advisers and make them accountable to Parliament
- Introduce greater openness within central government about how policies are made and the evidence on which they are based.
- Improve consultation processes to provide more time for comments and better feedback to participants, and include all potential stakeholders in consultations.
- Introduce more openness into the relationship between government and commercial interests in health.
- Implement a moratorium on large-scale reorganisation in the NHS.
- Clarify and rationalise the roles of central health monitoring and regulatory bodies. Avoid creating new regulators that duplicate the functions of existing bodies. Ensure that all regulators are accountable primarily to Parliament.
- Strengthen the 'regional tier' of the NHS, integrating health more closely with other regional government functions and making regional government bodies more democratic and accountable to the people.
- Improve the accountability of local partnerships (especially local strategic partnerships) to local people.
- Place greater emphasis on culture, networks and social learning approaches in policy formation, implementation and partnership working.
- Encourage more accurate reporting by the media of health risks, health issues and health policies.
- Improve policy learning through independent evaluation of reforms and policies and sharing of experiences (especially between different parts of the UK and also internationally).
- Increase the democratic accountability of international institutions that shape domestic health policy.

There is one final thing. A notable omission from this list is the creation of a separate NHS agency, urged by some as a means of taking health policy out of politics. The creation of another unaccountable central agency would, in my view, be a disaster. The creation of a politically sterile NHS agency is not only a forlorn hope, given the political profile and importance of health issues, but of itself would do nothing to improve openness, accountability or responsiveness of policy makers to the public.

Key questions

1. What are the main features of the contemporary health policy process?
2. Examine the reforms suggested in this chapter in terms of their feasibility.

Bibliography

Abraham, J. (2002) 'The Pharmaceutical Industry as a Political Player', *The Lancet*, vol 360, pp 1498-502.

Addicott, R., McGivern, G. and Ferlie, E. (2006) 'Networks, Organisational Learning and Knowledge Management: NHS Cancer Networks', *Public Money and Management*, vol 26, no 2, pp 87-94.

Addison, P. (1975) *The Road to 1945*, London: Cape.

Aggleton, P. (1990) *Health*, London: Routledge.

Alasuutari, P. (2005) 'The Governmentality of Consultancy and Competition: The Influence of the OECD', Paper Presented at the 31st World Congress of the International Institute of Sociology, Stockholm, 5-9 July.

Alcock, P. and Scott, D. (2002) 'Partnerships and the Voluntary Sector: Can Compacts Work?', in Glendinning, C., Powell, M. and Rummery, K. (eds) *Partnerships, New Labour and Governance*, Bristol: The Policy Press, pp 113-30.

Alcohol Concern (2005) *Health Select Committee on the Public Health White Paper: A Response from Alcohol Concern*, London: Alcohol Concern.

Alford, R. (1975) *Health Care Politics*, Chicago, IL: University of Chicago Press.

Ali, N., Thoebe, L., Auvache, V. and White, P. (2001) 'Bad Press for Doctors: 21 Year Survey of Three National Newspapers', *British Medical Journal*, vol 323, pp 782-3.

All Party Group on Cancer (2004) *Meeting National Targets: Setting Local Priorities. The Future of Cancer Services in England*, London: APG on Cancer.

Allison, C., Rolzen, J. and Olivier, P. (1997) 'The 1995 Pill Scare: Women's Perceptions of Risk and Sources of Information', *British Journal of Family Planning*, vol 23, no 3, pp 79-82.

Allsop, J. (1984) *Health Policy and the NHS*, Harlow: Longman.

Allsop, J. and Baggott, R. (2004) 'The NHS in England: From Modernisation to Marketisation?', in Ellison, N., Bauld, L. and Powell, M. (eds) *Social Policy Review 16*, Bristol: The Policy Press, pp 29-44.

Allsop, J. and Saks, M. (eds) (2002) *Regulating the Health Professions*, London: Sage.

Alvarez-Rosete, A., Bevan, G., Mays, N. and Dixon, J. (2005) 'Effect of Diverging Policy across the NHS', *British Medical Journal*, vol 331, pp 946-50.

Appleby, J. (2006a) 'Choice a Right in England – But what about Scotland's Patients?', *The Scotsman*, 3 June (www.kingsfund.com/news/articles/choice_a_right.html), accessed 3 July 2006.

Appleby, J. (2006b) 'Scottish Tariffs', *Health Service Journal*, vol 116, 22 June, p 21.

Appleby, J. and Coote, A. (2002) *Five Year Health Check: A Review of Government Health Policy 1997-2000*, London: King's Fund.

Armingeon, K. and Beyeler, M. (2004) *The OECD and European Welfare States*, Cheltenham: Edward Elgar.

Arrowsmith, J. and Sisson, K. (2002) 'Decentralisation in the Public Sector: The Case of the UK National Health Service', *Industrial Relations*, vol 57, no 2, pp 354-79.

Ashley, J. (1992) *Acts of Defiance*, Harmondsworth: Penguin.

Atkinson, D. (1994) *A Common Sense of Community*, London: Demos.

Audit Commission (1997) *The Coming of Age*, London: Audit Commission.

Audit Commission (1998) *Effective Partnership Working*, London: Audit Commission.

Audit Commission (2002) *Integrated Services for Older People*, London: Audit Commission.

Audit Commission (2003) *Targets in the Public Sector*, London: Audit Commission.

Audit Commission (2004) *Transforming Health and Social Care in Wales*, London: Audit Commission.

Audit Commission (2005) *Governing Partnerships*, London: Audit Commission.

Audit Scotland (2004) *An Overview of the Performance of the NHS in Scotland*, Edinburgh: Audit Scotland.

Audit Scotland (2006) *Tackling Waiting Times in the NHS in Scotland*, Edinburgh: Audit Scotland.

Auditor General for Wales (2005) *NHS Waiting Times in Wales: Executive Summary*, Cardiff, National Assembly for Wales.

Babor, T., et al (2003) *Alcohol: No Ordinary Commodity. Research and Public Policy*, Oxford: Oxford University Press.

Bachrach, P. and Baratz, M. (1962) 'Two Faces of Power', *American Political Science Review*, vol 56, no 4, pp 1947-52.

Baeten, R. and Jorens, Y. (2006) 'The Impact of EU Law and Policy', in Dubois, C-A., McKee, M. and Nolte, E. (eds) *Human Resources for Health in Europe*, Maidenhead: Open University Press, pp 214-34.

Baggott, R. (1990) *Alcohol, Politics and Social Policy*, Aldershot: Avebury.

Baggott, R. (1994a) *Health and Health Care in Britain* (1st edn), Basingstoke: Macmillan.

Baggott, R. (1994b) 'Getting Politics Out of Health? Ministers, Managers and the Market', *Public Policy and Administration*, vol 9, no 3, pp 33-51.

Baggott, R. (1995a) *Pressure Groups Today*, Manchester: Manchester University Press.

Baggott, R. (1995b) 'From Confrontation to Consultation: Pressure Group Relations from Thatcher to Major', *Parliamentary Affairs*, vol 48, no 3, pp 484-502.

Baggott, R. (1998) 'The BSE Crisis: Public Health and the Risk Society', in Gray, P. and t'Hart, P. (eds) *Public Policy Disasters in Western Europe*, London: Routledge, pp 61-78.

Baggott, R. (2000) *Public Health: Policy and Politics*, Basingstoke: Palgrave.

Baggott, R. (2004) *Health and Health Care in Britain* (3rd edn), Basingstoke: Palgrave.

Baggott, R. (2005) 'A Funny Thing Happened on the Way to the Forum? Reforming Patient and Public Involvement in the NHS in England', *Public Administration*, vol 83, no 3, pp 533-54.

Baggott, R. (2006) *Alcohol Strategy and the Drinks Industry: A Partnership for Prevention*, York: York Publishing Services.

Baggott, R. and McGregor-Riley, V. (1999) 'Renewed Consultation or Continued Exclusion? Organised Interests and the Major Governments', in Dorey, P. (ed) *The Major Premiership: Politics and Policies under John Major 1990-97*, Basingstoke: Macmillan, pp 68-86.

Baggott, R., Allsop, J. and Jones, K. (2005) *Speaking for Patients and Carers*, Basingstoke: Palgrave.

Balloch, S. and Taylor, M. (2001) *Partnership Working: Policy and Practice*, Bristol: The Policy Press.

Banks, P. (2002) *Partnerships Under Pressure*, London: King's Fund.

Bara, J. and Budge, I. (2001) 'Party Policy and Ideology: Still New Labour', *Parliamentary Affairs*, vol 54, no 4, pp 590-606.

Barker, A. and Peters, B.G. (1993) *The Politics of Expert Advice: Creating, Using and Manipulating Scientific Knowledge for Public Policy*, Edinburgh: Edinburgh University Press.

Barnes, M., Bauld, L., Benzeval, M., Judge, K., Mackenzie, M. and Sullivan, H. (2005) *Health Action Zones: Partnerships for Health Equity*, Abingdon: Routledge.

Barnes, M., Harrison, S., Mort, M. and Shardlow, P. (1999) *Unequal Partners: User Groups and Community Care*, Bristol: The Policy Press.

Barrett, S. (2004) 'Implementation Studies: Time for a Revival? Personal Reflections on 20 Years of Implementation Studies', *Public Administration*, vol 82, no 2, pp 249-62.

Barrett, S. and Fudge, C. (eds) (1981) *Policy and Action*, London: Methuen.

Bate, P. (2000) 'Changing the Culture of a Hospital from Hierarchy to Networked Community', *Public Administration*, vol 78, no 3, pp 485-512.

Batty, D. (2001) 'The Perils of Celebrity Endorsements', *The Guardian*, 3 August.

Baumgartner, F. and Jones, B. (1993) *Agendas and Instability in American Politics*, Chicago, IL: University of Chicago Press.

BBC (2006) 'Cameron wants "Independent" NHS', *BBC News Online*, news.bbc.co.uk/1/hi/uk_politics/6032473.stm, accessed 11 December 2006.

BBC TV (2000) 'Spin Doctors', *Panorama*, 13 March.

Beckett, M. and Brown, N. (1994) *The Maples Report: the National Health 'Secret Service'*, London: Labour Party.

Beer, S. (1965) *Modern British Politics*, London: Faber and Faber.

Begg, N., Ramsay, M., White, J. and Bozoky, Z. (1998) 'Media Dents Confidence in MMR Vaccine', *British Medical Journal*, vol 316, p 561.

Bell, D. and Bowes, A. (2006) *Financial Care Models in Scotland the UK*, York: Joseph Rowntree Foundation.

Bell, I. (1991) *The Language of News Media*, Oxford: Blackwell.

Bennett, C. (1991) 'What is Policy Convergence and What Causes It?', *British Journal of Political Science*, vol 21, no 4, pp 215-33.

Benson, L., Boyd, A. and Walshe, K. (2004) *Learning from CHI: The Impact of Healthcare Regulation*, Manchester: University of Manchester.

Bentley, A. (1967) (Odegard, P. (ed)) *The Process of Government*, Cambridge, MA: Belknap.

Berlinguer, G. (1999) 'Globalisation and Global Health', *International Journal of Health Services*, vol 29, no 3, pp 579-95.

Berman, S. (1998) 'Path Dependency and Political Action: Re-examining Responses to the Depression', *Comparative Politics*, vol 20, no 4, pp 379-400.

Berridge, V. (1991) 'AIDS, the Media and Health Policy', *Health Education Journal*, vol 50, no 4, pp 179-85.

Berridge, V. (1996) *AIDS in the UK: The Making of Policy 1981-1994*, Oxford: Oxford University Press.

Bevan, G. and Hood, C. (2006) 'Have Targets Improved Performance in the English NHS?', *British Medical Journal*, vol 332, pp 419-22.

Birch, A.H. (1964) *Representative and Responsible Government*, London: George Allen and Unwin.

Black, D. (1987) *Recollections and Reflections*, London: BMJ.

Blackstone, T. and Plowden, W. (1988) *Inside the Think Tank*, London: Heinemann.

Blake, R. (1985) *The Conservative Party from Peel to Thatcher*, London: Fontana.

Blank, R. and Burau, V. (2004) *Comparative Health Policy*, Basingstoke: Palgrave Macmillan.

Blaxter, M. (2004) *Health*, Oxford: Polity Press.

Bochel, C. and Bochel, H. (2004) *The UK Social Policy Process*, Basingstoke: Palgrave.

Bogdanor, V. (2001) *Devolution in the United Kingdom*, Oxford: Oxford University Press.

Booker, C. and North, R. (2005) *The Great Deception: Can the European Union Survive?*, London: Continuum.

Boudioni, M., Mossman, J., Jones, A., Leydon, G. and McPherson, K. (1998) 'Celebrity Death from Cancer Resulted in Increased Calls to CancerBACUP', *British Medical Journal*, vol 317, 10 October, p 1016.

Bovens, M. and t'Hart, P. (1996) *Understanding Policy Fiascoes*, New Brunswick: Transaction.

Brenton, M. (1985) *The Voluntary Sector in British Social Services*, London: Longman.

Brindle, D. (1999) 'Media Coverage of Social Policy: A Journalist's Perspective', in Franklin, B. (ed) *Social Policy, the Media and Misrepresentation*, London: Routledge, pp 39-50.

Bristol Royal Infirmary Inquiry, The (2001) *The Inquiry into the Management of Care of Children Receiving Complex Heart Surgery at the Bristol Royal Infirmary – final report*, London: The Stationery Office.

Brown, C. (1989) 'Pluralism: A Lost Perspective', *Talking Politics*, vol 1, no 3, pp 95-100.

Brown, P. and Zavestoski, S. (eds) (2004) *Sociology of Health and Illness*, vol 26, no 6, Special issue: Social Movements in Health.

Brown, R. (1979) *Reorganising the NHS*, Blackwell: Robinson.

BSE Inquiry, The (2000) *Report* (the Phillips Report), London: The Stationery Office.

Burch, M. and Holliday, I. (1996) *The British Cabinet System*, Hemel Hempstead: Prentice Hall.

Burch, M. and Holliday, I. (2004) 'The Blair Government and the Core Executive', *Government and Opposition*, vol 39, no 1, pp 1-21.

Burke, S., Gray, I., Patterson, K. and Meyrick, J. (2002) *Environmental Health 2012: A Key Partner in Delivering the Public Health Agenda*, London: Health Development Agency.

Burns, H. (2004) 'Health Tsars', *British Medical Journal*, vol 328, pp 117-18.

Bury, M. and Gabe, J. (1994) 'Television and Medicine: Medical Dominance or Trial by Media?', in Gabe, J., Kelleher, D. and Williams, G. (eds) *Challenging Medicine*, London: Routledge, pp 64-83.

Buse, K., Mays, N. and Walt, G. (2005) *Making Health Policy*, Maidenhead: Open University Press.

Butcher, T. (1995) *Delivering Welfare: The Governance of Social Services in the 1980s*, Buckingham: Open University Press.

Butler, I. and Drakeford, M. (2005) *Scandal, Social Policy and Social Welfare* (2nd edn), Bristol: The Policy Press.

Butler, J. (1992) *Patients, Policies and Politics: Before and After Working for Patients*, Buckingham: Open University Press.

Byrne, D. (2004) *Partnerships for Health in Europe* (Non-paper), Brussels: European Commission.

Byrne, P. (1997) *Social Movements in Britain*, London: Routledge.

Cabinet Office (2004) *Code of Practice on Consultation*, London: Cabinet Office.

Campbell, A. and Zeichner, D. (2001) 'Partners in Power?', *Fabian Review*, Winter, pp 16-19.

Campbell, F. (2002) *Health and the New Political Structures in Local Government*, London: Local Government Information Unit.

Cancer Research UK (2006) 'Kylie Effect can Confuse Women over Breast Cancer Risk', *Press Release*, 23 October (info.cancerresearchuk.org/news/pressreleases/2006/October/235144).

Carvel, J. (2000) 'NHS Chief Executive Says Centralisation is Deterring Local Initiative', *The Guardian*, 29 June.

Carvel, J. (2004) 'NHS Trusts Bullied into Private Contracts', *The Guardian*, 1 June, p 5.

Cawson, A. (1982) *Corporatism and Welfare: Social Policy and State Intervention in Britain*, London: Heinemann.

Challis, L., Klein, R. and Webb, A. (1988) *Joint Approaches to Social Policy: Rationality and Practice*, Cambridge: Cambridge University Press.

Chapman, J. (2002) *System Failure: Why Governments Must Learn to Think Differently*, London: Demos.

Charter of Fundamental Rights of the European Union (2000) *Official Journal of European Communities*, C364 1, December 7th (http://eur-lex.europa.eu/LexUriServ/site/en/oj/2000/c_364/c_36420001218en00010022.pdf).

CHI (Commission for Health Improvement) (2002) *Emerging Themes From 175 Clinical Governance Reviews*, London: CHI.

CHI (2003) *Getting Better? A Report on the NHS*, London: CHI.

CHI/Audit Commission (2001) *National Service Frameworks No.1*, London: CHI.

Chowdhury, Z. and Rowson, M. (2000) 'The People's Health Assembly', *British Medical Journal*, vol 321, pp 1361-2.

Clarke, J. (1999) 'Breast Cancer in Mass Circulating Magazines in the USA and Canada 1974-1995', *Women and Health*, vol 8, no 4, pp 113-30.

Clarke, J. (2004) 'A Comparison of Breast, Testicular and Prostate Cancer in Mass Print Media (1996-2001)', *Social Science and Medicine*, vol 59, pp 541-51.

Clarke, J. and Everest, M. (2006) 'Cancer in the Mass Print Media: Fear Uncertainty and the Medical Model', *Social Science and Medicine*, vol 62, pp 2591-600.

Clarke, J. and Glendinning, C. (2002) 'Partnership and the Remaking of Welfare Governance', in Glendinning, C., Powell, M. and Rummery, K. (eds) *Partnerships, New Labour and Governance*, Bristol: The Policy Press, pp 33-50.

Clarke, J. and Newman, J. (1997) *The Managerial State*, London: Sage.

Clinical Standards Advisory Group (1998) *Community Health Care for Elderly People*, London: DoH.

Cm 555 (1989) *Working for Patients*, London: HMSO.
Cm 1523 (1991) *Health of the Nation: A Consultative Document for Health in England*, London: HMSO.
Cm 1986 (1992) *The Health of the Nation: A Strategy for Health in England*, London: The Stationery Office.
Cm 3807 (1997) *The NHS: Modern, Dependable*, London: The Stationery Office.
Cm 4014 (1998) *Modern Local Government – In Touch with the People*, London: The Stationery Office.
Cm 4169 (1998) *Modernising Social Services: Promoting Independence, Improving Protection, Raising Standards*, London: The Stationery Office.
Cm 4192 (1999) *With Respect to Old Age. Long Term Care – Rights and Responsibilities. A Report by the Royal Commission on Long Term Care*, London: The Stationery Office.
Cm 4310 (1999) *Modernising Government*, London: The Stationery Office.
Cm 4386 (1999) *Saving Lives*, London: The Stationery Office.
Cm 4818 (2000) *The NHS Plan: A Plan for Investment – A Plan for Reform*, London: The Stationery Office.
Cm 5503 (2002) *Delivering the NHS Plan: Next Steps on Investment, Next Steps on Reform*, London: The Stationery Office.
Cm 5730 (2003) *The Victoria Climbié Inquiry*, London: The Stationery Office.
Cm 6079 (2003) *Building on the Best: Choice, Responsiveness and Equity in the NHS*, London: The Stationery Office.
Cm 6268 (2004) *The NHS Improvement Plan*, London: The Stationery Office.
Cm 6374 (2004) *Choosing Health*, London: The Stationery Office.
Cm 6499 (2005) *Independence, Well-being and Choice: Our Vision for the Future of Social Care for Adults in England*, London: The Stationery Office.
Cm 6737 (2006) *Our Health, Our Care, Our Say; A New Direction for Community Services*, London: The Stationery Office.
Cm 6939 (2006) *Strong and Prosperous Communities: The Local Government White Paper*, London: The Stationery Office.
Cmd 9663 (1956) *Report of the Committee of Inquiry into the Cost of the National Health Service*, London: HMSO.
Cmnd 7615 (1979) *Report of the Royal Commission on the National Health Service*, London: HMSO.
Coaffee, J. (2005) 'Shock of the New: Complexity and Emerging Rationales for Partnership Working', *Public Policy and Administration*, vol 20, no 3, pp 23-41.
Cobb, R. and Elder, C. (1972) *Participation in American Politics: The Dynamics of Agenda-Building*, Baltimore, MD: Johns Hopkins Press.
Cocker, P. and Jones, A. (2002) *Contemporary British Politics and Government*, (3rd edn), Liverpool: Academic Press.

Colebatch, H. (2002) *Policy* (2nd edn), Buckingham: Open University Press.
Coleman, A. (2004) 'Local Authority Scrutiny of Health: Making the Views of the Community Count?', *Health Expectations*, *vol* 7, pp 29-39.
Collier, J. (1989) *The Health Conspiracy – How Doctors, the Drug Industry and Government Undermine our Health*, London: Century Hutchinson.
Collingridge, D. and Reeve, C. (1986) *Science Speaks to Power: The Role of Experts in Policy Making*, London: Pinter.
Commission to Strengthen Parliament (2000) *Report of the Commission*, London: Conservative Party.
Committee on Standards in Public Life (2003) *9th Report: Defining the Boundaries within the Executive: Ministers, Special Advisors and the Permanent Civil Service* (Cm 5775), London: The Stationery Office.
Community Charter of the Fundamental Social Rights of Workers (1989) (www.psi.org.uk/publications/archivepdfs/trade%20unions/TUAPPI.pdf).
Consumers' Association (2001) *The National Institute for Clinical Excellence: A Patient-centred Inquiry*, London: Which?.
Cope, J. (2002) 'Cause Celebre', *The Guardian*, 4 April.
Cottle, S. (2001) 'Television News and Citizenship: Packaging the Public Sphere', in Bromley, M. (ed) *No News is Bad News: Radio, Television and the Public*, London: Longman, pp 61-79.
Coulson, A. (1998) *Trust and Contracts: Relationships in Local Government, Health and Public Services*, Bristol: The Policy Press.
Council of Europe (1996) *European Social Charter* (www.conventions.coe.int/treaty/en/Treaties/html/163.htm).
Cox, J. (2001) 'Appointed Czars, Elected Presidents and Windows of Opportunity', *British Journal of Psychiatry*, vol 178, pp 292-93.
Coxall, W. (2001) *Pressure Groups in British Politics*, London: Longman.
Craig, F.W.S. (1975) *British General Election Manifestos 1900-74*, Basingstoke: Macmillan.
Craig, F.W.S. (1990) *British General Election Manifestos 1959-87*, Basingstoke: Macmillan.
Craig G. and Taylor, M. (2002) 'Dangerous Liaisons: Local Government and the Voluntary and Community Sectors', in Glendinning, C., Powell, M. and Rummery, K. (eds) *Partnerships, New Labour and Governance*, Bristol: The Policy Press, pp 131-48.
Craig, G., Taylor, M. and Parkes, T. (2004) 'Protest or Partnership? The Voluntary and Community Sectors in the Policy Process', *Social Policy and Administration*, vol 38, no 3, pp 221-39.
Crayford, T., Hooper, R. and Evans, S. (1997) 'Death Rates of Characters in Soap Operas on British Television: Is a Government Health Warning Required?', *British Medical Journal*, vol 315, pp 1649-52.

Crossley, N. (2006) 'The Field of Psychiatric Contention in the UK, 1960-2000', *Social Science and Medicine*, vol 62, pp 552-63.

Crossman, R. (1972) *Inside View: Three Lectures on Prime Ministerial Government*, London: Jonathan Cape.

CSCI (Commission for Social Care Inspection), Audit Commission and the Healthcare Commission (2006) *Living Well in Later Life*, London: CSCI and Audit Commission.

Currie, E. (1989) *Life Lines: Politics and Health 1986-1988*, London: Pan.

Dahl, R. (1961) *Who Governs?*, New Haven, CT: Yale University Press.

Darjee, R. and Crichton, J. (2004) 'New Mental Health Legislation', *British Medical Journal*, vol 329, pp 634-35.

David, P. (1985) 'Clio and the Economics of Qwerty', *American Economic Review*, vol 75, no 2, pp 332-7.

Davies, A. (2000) 'Don't Trust Me, I'm a Doctor – Medical Regulation and the 1999 NHS Reforms', *Oxford Journal of Legal Studies*, vol 20, pp 437-56.

Davies, S. (2005) *Hospital Contract Cleaning and Infection Control*, London: UNISON.

Davis, S. (2005) 'Public Medicine: The Reception of a Medical Drama', in King, M. and Watson, K. (2005) *Representing Health: Discourses of Health and Illness in the Media*, Basingstoke: Palgrave, pp 27-46.

Day, P. and Klein, R. (1989) 'Interpreting the Unexpected: The Case of AIDS Policy Making in Britain', *Journal of Public Policy*, vol 9, no 3, pp 337-53.

Day, P. and Klein, R. (1992) 'Constitutional and Distributional Conflict in British Medical Politics: The Case of General Practice, 1911-1991', *Political Studies*, vol XL, pp 462-78.

Day, P. and Klein, R. (1997) *Steering but not Rowing: The Transformation of the Department of Health*, Bristol: The Policy Press.

Day, P. and Klein, R. (2004) *The NHS Improvers: A Study of the Commission for Health Improvement*, London: King's Fund.

DCCP (Devolution and Constitutional Change Programme) (2005) *Final Report*, www.devolution.ac.uk/final_report.htm, accessed 21 June 2006.

De Vos, P., Dewitte, H. and Van der Stuyft, P. (2004) 'Unhealthy European Policy', *International Journal of Health Services*, vol 34, no 2, pp 255-69.

Deacon, D. (1999) 'The Construction of Voluntary Sector News', in Franklin, B. (ed) *Social Policy, the Media and Misrepresentation*, London: Routledge, pp 51-68.

Deakin, N. and Parry, R. (2000) *The Treasury and Social Policy*, London: Macmillan.

Deakin, N. and Walsh, K. (1996) 'The Enabling State: The Role of Markets and Contracts', *Public Administration*, vol 74, no 1, pp 33-48.

Decision of the European Parliament and of the Council (2001) *Adopting a Programme of Community Action in the field of Public Health (2001-6)*, amended proposal, 2000/0119 (COD).

Decision of the European Parliament and of the Council (2006) *Establishing a Second Programme of Community Action in the Field of Health (2007-13)*, amended proposal, 2004/0042 A (COD).

Declerq, E. (1998) 'Changing Childbirth in the United Kingdom: Lessons for US Health Policy', *Journal of Health Politics, Policy and Law*, vol 23, no 5, pp 833-59.

Deeming, C. (2004) 'Decentring the NHS: A Case Study of Resource Allocation Decisions within a Health District', *Social Policy and Administration*, vol 38, no 1, pp 57-72.

Degeling, P., Kennedy, J. and Hill, M. (1998) 'Do Professional Subcultures Set the Limits of Hospital Reform', *Clinicians in Management*, vol 7, pp 89-98.

DHSS (Department of Health and Social Security) (1970) *National Health Service: The Future Structure of the National Health Service*, London: HMSO.

DHSS (1976a) *Priorities for Health and Personal Social Services in England: A Consultative Document*, London: HMSO.

DHSS (1976b) *Report of the Regional Chairmen's Inquiry into the Working of the DHSS, in Relation to Regional Health Authorities*, London: DHSS.

DHSS (1977) *The Way Forward*, London: HMSO.

DHSS (1981) *Care in Action*, London: DHSS.

DHSS (1983) *NHS Management Inquiry* (Griffiths Management Report), London: DoH.

DHSS (1988) *Community Care: Agenda for Action* (Griffiths Community Care Report), London: HMSO.

DHSSPS (Department of Health, Social Services and Public Safety) (2002) *Investing for Health*, Belfast: DHSSPNI.

DHSSPS (2004) *A Healthier Future: A Twenty Year Vision for Health and Wellbeing in Northern Ireland*, Belfast: DHSSPNI.

Dinsdale, P. (2004) 'The Wheels go Round', *Health Service Journal*, 1 April, pp 36-7.

Dixon, J. (2001) 'Health Care: Modernising the Leviathan', *Political Quarterly*, vol 72, no 1, pp 30-8.

DoH (Department of Health) (1991) *The Patient's Charter*, London: DoH.

DoH (1998a) *Partnership in Action: New Opportunities for Joint Working between Health and Social Services: A discussion document*, London: DoH.

DoH (1998b) *Modernising Health and Social Services: National Priorities Guidance 1999-2000/2001-2*, London: DoH.

DoH (1998c) *The Health of the Nation: A Policy Assessed*, London: The Stationery Office.

DoH (2001a) *Shifting the Balance of Power within the NHS: Securing Delivery*, London: DoH.
DoH (2001b) *National Service Framework for Older People*, London: DoH.
DoH (2002) *Preventing Accidental Injury – Priorities for Action. Report of the Accidental Injury Task Force*, London: DoH.
DoH (2003a) *Tackling Health Inequalities: A Programme for Action*, London: DoH.
DoH (2003b) *Strengthening Accountability: Involving Patients and the Public. Practice Guidance Section 11 of the Health and Social Care Act 2001*, London: DoH.
DoH (2004a) *Reconfiguring the Department of Health's Arm's Length Bodies*, London: DoH.
DoH (2004b) *Government and Industry Launch Joint Report Encouraging Innovations in NHS and Healthcare*, DoH Press Release, 2004/0412.
DoH (2004c) *Better Health in Old Age*, London: DoH.
DoH (2004d) *Making Partnership Work for Patients, Carers and Service Users: A Strategic Agreement between the Department of Health, the NHS and the Voluntary and Community Sector*, London: DoH.
DoH (2005) *Creating a Patient Led NHS: Delivering the NHS Improvement Plan*, London: DoH.
DoH (2006a) *Good Doctors, Safer Patients: A Report by the Chief Medical Officer*, London: DoH.
DoH (2006b) *Strengthening Regional Partnerships for Health and Wellbeing*, London: DoH.
DoH (2006c) *Department of Health Business Plan 2006-07*, London: DoH.
Dolowitz, D. and Marsh, D. (1996) 'Who Learns What from Whom: A Review of the Policy Transfer Literature', *Political Studies*, vol 44, no 2, pp 343-57.
Dopson, S. and Fitzgerald, L. (2006) *Knowledge to Action? Evidence-based healthcare in context*, Oxford: Oxford University Press.
Dopson, S., Locock, L. and Stewart, R. (1999) 'Regional Offices in the New NHS: An Analysis of the Effects and Significance of Recent Changes', *Public Administration*, vol 77, no 1, pp 91-110.
Dorey, P. (2005) *Policy Making in Britain: An Introduction*, London: Sage.
Dowling, B. (1997) 'Effect of Fundholding on Waiting Times: A Database Study', *British Medical Journal*, vol 315, pp 290-2.
Dowling, B., Powell, M. and Glendinning, C. (2004) 'Conceptualising Successful Partnerships', *Health and Social Care in the Community*, vol 12, no 4, pp 309-17.
Downs, A. (1972) 'Up and Down with Ecology: The Issue Attention Cycle', *Public Interest*, vol 28, no 1, pp 38-50.
Doyal, L. (1979) *The Political Economy of Health*, London: Pluto.

Doyle, H. (2000) 'Health Scares, Media Hype, Policy Making', in Hann, A. (ed) *Analysing Health Policy*, Aldershot: Ashgate, pp 147-64.

Drakeford, M. (2006) 'Health Policy in Wales: Making a Difference in Conditions of Difficulty', *Critical Social Policy*, vol 26, no 3, pp 543-61.

Driver, S. and Martell, L. (2002) *Blair's Britain*, Cambridge: Polity Press.

Drummond, C. (2004) 'An Alcohol Strategy for England: The Good, the Bad and the Ugly', *Alcohol and Alcoholism*, vol 39, no 5, pp 377-9.

Dubs, A (1989) *Lobbying: An Insiders' Guide*, London: Pluto.

Duncan, B. (2002) 'Health Policy in the European Union: How it's Made and How to Influence it', *British Medical Journal*, vol 324, pp 1027-30.

Dunleavy, P. (1981) 'Professions and Policy Change: Notes towards a Model of Ideological Corporatism', *Public Administration Bulletin*, vol 36, pp 3-16.

Dunsire, A. (1978) *Implementation in a Bureaucracy*, Oxford: Martin Robinson.

Durham, M. (1991) *Sex and Politics: The Family and Morality in the Thatcher Years*, Basingstoke: Macmillan.

Durward, L. and Evans, R. (1990) 'Pressure Groups and Maternity Care', in Kilpatrick, R. and Richards, M. (eds) *The Politics of Maternity Care*, Oxford: Oxford University Press, pp 256-73.

Dye, T. (1992) *Understanding Public Policy* (7th edn), Englewood Cliffs, CO: Prentice Hall.

Eckstein, H. (1960) *Pressure Group Politics: The Case of the BMA*, London: George Allen and Unwin.

Edelman, M. (1964) *The Symbolic Uses of Politics*, Urbana, IL: University of Illinois Press.

Edelman, M. (1971) *Politics as Symbolic Action*, New York, NY: Academic Press.

Edelman, M. (1977) *Political Language: Words that Succeed and Policies that Fail*, New York, NY: Institute for the Study of Poverty.

Edelman, M. (1985) *The Symbolic Uses of Politics*, Urbana, IL: University of Illinois Press.

Edwards, B. (1993) *The National Health Service: A Manager's Tale 1946-92*, London: Nuffield Provincial Hospitals Trust.

Edwards, B. and Fall, M. (2005) *The Executive Years of the NHS; The England Account 1985-2003*, Oxford: Radcliffe.

Edwards, N. (2006) 'Scrutiny and the Bounty', *Health Service Journal*, vol 161, 1 June, pp 18-19.

Elcock, H. and Haywood, S. (1980) 'The Centre Cannot Hold: Accountability and Control in the National Health Service', *Public Administration Bulletin*, vol 36, pp 53-62.

Eldridge, J., Kitzinger, J. and Williams, K. (1999) *The Mass Media and Power in Modern Britain*, Oxford: Oxford University Press, pp 160-80.

Ellmore, R. (1980) 'Backward Mapping: Implementation Research and Policy Decisions', *Political Science Quarterly*, vol 94, no 4, pp 601-16.

Ennew, C., Whynes, D., Jolleys, J. and Robinson, P. (1998) 'Entrepreneurship and Innovation Among GP Fundholders', *Public Money and Management*, vol 18, no 1, pp 59-68.

Enthoven, A. (1985) *Reflections on the Management of the NHS*, London: Nuffield Provincial Hospitals Trust.

Entwhistle, T. and Downe, J. (2005) 'Picking Winners to Define and Disseminate Best Practice', *Public Policy and Administration*, vol 20, no 4, pp 25-37.

Entwhistle, V. (1995) 'Reporting Research in Medical Journals and Newspapers', *British Medical Journal*, vol 310, pp 920-3.

Entwhistle, V. and Beaulieu-Hancock, M. (1992) 'Health and Medical Coverage in the UK National Press', *Public Understanding of Science*, vol 1, no 4, pp 367-82.

Entwhistle, V. and Sheldon, T. (1999) 'The Picture of Health? Media Coverage of the Health Service', in Franklin, B. (ed) *Social Policy, the Media and Misrepresentation*, London: Routledge, pp 118-34.

Entwhistle, V., Watt, I., Bradbury, R. and Pehl, L. (1996) 'Media Coverage of the Child B Case', *British Medical Journal*, vol 312, pp 1587-91.

ESRC (Economic and Social Research Council) (2005) *Devolution is a Process not a Policy: The New Governance of the English Regions*, ESRC Programme on Devolution and Constitutional Change Briefing no 18, www.devolution.ac.uk/Briefing_papers.htm, accessed 21 June 2006.

Etzioni, A. (1993) *The Spirit of Community*, New York, NY: Random House.

European Commission (2003) *European Environment and Health Action Plan 2004-2010*, Brussels: European Commission.

European Health Policy Forum (2003) *Recommendations on Health and EU Social Policy*, EHPF: Brussels.

European Parliament (1999) *Report 0082/99* (the Needle report), February, Luxembourg: Office for Official Publications of the European Communities.

European Union (1997) *Treaty of Amsterdam*, available at www.eurotreaties.com/amsterdamtext.html, accessed 24 January 2006.

Exworthy, M. (2001) 'Primary Care in the UK: Understanding the Dynamics of Devolution', *Health and Social Care in the Community*, vol 9, no 5, pp 266-78.

Fairclough, N. (2000) *New Labour, New Language?*, London: Routledge.

Fawcett, H. (2005) *Social Exclusion in Scotland and the UK: Devolution and the Welfare State Briefing 22*, www.devolution.ac.uk/Briefing_papers.htm, accessed 21 June 2006.

Ferlie, E., Ashburner, L., Fitzgerald, L. and Pettigrew, A. (1996) *The New Public Management*, Oxford: Oxford University Press.

Ferner, R. (2005) 'The Influence of Big Pharma', *British Medical Journal*, vol 330, pp 857-8.

Ferner, R. and McDowell, S. (2006) 'How NICE may be Outflanked', *British Medical Journal*, vol 332, pp 1268-71.

Finlayson, B. (1999) 'Third Way Theory', *Political Quarterly*, vol 70, no 3, pp 42-51.

Fischer, F. (1990) *Technocracy and the Politics of Expertise*, Newbury Park: Sage.

Fitzgerald, L. and Dufour, Y. (1997) 'Clinical Management as Boundary Management: Comparative Analysis of Canadian and UK Health Institutions', *International Journal of Public Sector Management*, vol 10, no 1/2, pp 5-10.

Fitzgerald, L. and Reeves, S. (1999) *An Exploratory Examination of the Management of Four Clinical Directorates*, London: City University and St Bartholomew's School of Nursing and Midwifery.

Fleurke, F. and Willemse, R. (2006) 'Measuring Local Autonomy: A Decision-making approach', *Local Government Studies*, vol 32, no 1, pp 71-87.

Flinders, M. (2005) 'The Politics of Public-Private Partnerships', *British Journal of Political Science*, vol 7, no 2, pp 215-39.

Foot, M. (1975) *Aneurin Bevan: A Biography, vol 2 1945-60*, London: Paladin.

Foote, C. and Stanners, C. (2003) *Integrating Care for Older People. New Care for Old – A Systems Approach*, London: Jessica Kingsley.

Fort, M., Mercer, M. and Gish, O. (eds) (2004) *Sickness and Wealth: The Corporate Assault on Global Health*, Cambridge, MA: South End Press.

Fowler, N. (1991) *Ministers Decide: A Personal Memoir of the Thatcher Years*, London: Chapman.

Fox, M.J. (2002) *Lucky Man: A Memoir*, London: Ebury Press.

Franklin, B. (ed) (1999) *Social Policy, the Media and Misrepresentation*, London: Routledge.

Friedman, M. (1962) *Capitalism and Freedom*, Chicago, IL: University of Chicago Press.

Frye, M. and Webb, A. (2002) *Working Together: Effective Partnership Working on the Ground*, London: Treasury.

Gabe, J., Gustaffson, U. and Bury, M. (1991) 'Mediating Illness: Newspaper Coverage of Tranquilliser Dependence', *Sociology of Health and Illness*, vol 13, pp 332-53.

Gamble, A. (1994) *The Free Economy and the Strong State: The Politics of Thatcherism* (2nd edn), London: Macmillan.

Garcia, J., Redshaw, M., Fitzsimmons, B. and Keene, J. (1998) *First Class Delivery: A National Survey of Women's Views of Maternity Care*, London: Audit Commission/NPEU.

Gard, M. and Wright, J. (2005) *The Obesity Epidemic: Science, Morality and Ideology*, London: Routledge.

Garfield, S. (1994) *Britain in the time of AIDS*, London: Faber and Faber.

Garner, R and Kelly, R. (1998) *British Political Parties Today* (2nd edn), Manchester: Manchester University Press.

Giddens, A. (1998) *The Third Way: The Renewal of Social Democracy*, Cambridge: Polity.

Gilbert, B. (1970) *British Social Policy 1914-1939*, London: Batsford.

Gillam, S., Abbott, S. and Banks-Smith, J. (2001) 'Can Primary Care Groups and Trusts Improve Health?', *British Medical Journal*, vol 323, pp 89-92.

Glasby, J. and Littlechild, R. (2004) *The Health and Social Care Divide: The Experiences of Older People* (2nd edn), Bristol: The Policy Press.

Glasby, J. and Peck, E. (2003) *Care Trusts: Partnership Working in Action*, Abingdon: Radcliffe Medical Press.

Glasby, J., Smith, J. and Dickinson, H. (2006) *Creating NHS Local: A New Relationship between PCTs and Local Government*, Birmingham: Health Services Management Centre.

Glendinning, C., Abbott, S. and Coleman, A. (2001) 'Bridging the Gap: New Relationships between Primary Care Groups and Local Authorities', *Social Policy and Administration*, vol 35, no 4, pp 411-25.

Glendinning, C., Coleman, A. and Rummery, K. (2003) 'Looking Outwards; Primary Care Organisations and Local Partnerships', in Dowling, B. and Glendinning, C. (eds) *The New Primary Care*, Maidenhead: Open University Press, pp 196-216.

Glendinning, C., Hudson, B. and Means, R. (2005) 'Under Strain? Exploring the Troubled Relationship between Health and Social Care', *Public Money and Management*, vol 25, no 4, August, pp 245-51.

Glennerster, H., Owens, P. and Matsaganis, M. (1994) *Implementing GP Fundholding: Wild Card or Winning Hand?*, Buckingham: Open University Press.

Goddard, M., Mannion, R. and Smith, P. (2000) 'The Performance Framework: Taking Account of Economic Behaviour', in Smith, P. (ed) *Reforming Markets in Health Care*, Buckingham: Open University Press, pp 139-61.

Grant, W. (2000) *Pressure Groups and British Politics*, Basingstoke: Macmillan.

Grant, W. (2005) 'Pressure Politics: A Politics of Collective Consumption?', *Parliamentary Affairs*, vol 58, no 2, pp 366-79.

Gray, A. and Harrison, S. (2004) *Governing Medicine*, Maidenhead: Open University Press.

Gray, A. and Jenkins, W. (1985) *Administrative Politics in British Government*, Brighton: Wheatsheaf.

Gray, P. and t'Hart, P. (eds) (1998) *Public Policy Disasters in Western Europe*, London: Routledge.

Green, D.S. (1987) *The New Right: The Counter Revolution in Political Economic and Social Thought*, Brighton: Wheatsheaf.

Green, J. and Thorogood, N. (1998) *Analysing Health Policy*, London: Longman.

Greenaway, J. (2003) *Drink and British Politics since 1830: A Study in Policy-Making*, Basingstoke: Palgrave.

Greener, I. (2004a) 'Path Dependency and the Creation and Reform of the NHS', in Smythe, N. (ed) *Healthcare in Transition, vol 3*, Hauppage, NY: Novascience.

Greener, I. (2004b) 'The Political Economy of Health Service Organisation', *Public Administration*, vol 82, no 3, pp 657-76.

Greener, I. (2004c) 'Three Moments of Labour's Health Policy Discourse', *Policy and Politics*, vol 32, no 3, pp 303-16.

Greener, I. (2004d) 'The New Political Economy of the NHS', *Critical Public Health*, vol 14, no 3, pp 239-50.

Greener, I. and Powell, M. (2003) 'Health Authorities' Priority-Setting and Resource Allocation', *Social Policy and Administration*, vol 37, no 1, pp 39-48.

Greer, S. (2004) *Territorial Politics and Health Policy: UK Health Policy in Comparative Perspective*, Manchester: Manchester University Press.

Greer, S. (2005) 'The Territorial Bases of Health Policy Making in the UK after devolution', *Regional and Federal Studies*, vol 15, no 4, pp 501-18.

Gregory, P. and Giddings, P. (2002) *The Ombudsman, the Citizen and Parliament*, London: Politicos.

The Guardian (2000) 'The 15 Most Powerful People in Health', www.society.guardian.co.uk /health/story/0,7890,397769,00.html, accessed 15 December 2005.

Gustaffson, U. (2002) 'School Meals Policy: The Problem with Governing Children', *Social Policy and Administration*, vol 26, no 6, pp 685-97.

Gwyn, R. (1999) 'Killer Bugs, Silly Buggers, Politically Correct Pals, Competing Discourses in Health Care Reporting', *Health*, vol 3, no 3, pp 335-45.

Habermas, J. (1976) *Legitimation Crisis*, London: Heinemann.

Habermas, J. (1987) *The Theory of Communicative Action*, vol 2, Cambridge: Polity.

Hain, P. (2004) 'Reclaim the Party', *The Guardian*, 10 March, available at http://politics.guardian.co.uk, accessed 7 February 2005.

Hallam, J. (2000) *Nursing the Image: Media, Culture and Professional Identity*, London: Routledge.

Ham, C. (1981) *Policy-Making in the National Health Service*, London: Macmillan.

Ham, C. (2000) *The Politics of the NHS Reform 1988-97: Metaphor or Reality?*, London: King's Fund.

Ham, C. (2004) *Health Policy in Britain* (5th edn), Basingstoke: Palgrave Macmillan.

Ham, C. and Hill, M. (1984) *The Policy Process in the Modern Capitalist State*, Brighton: Wheatsheaf.

Hambleton, R. (1983) 'Health Planning – A Second Chance', *Policy and Politics*, vol 11, no 2, pp 198-201.

Hamer, L. and Easton, N. (2002) *Planning Across the LSP: Case Studies of Integrating Community Strategies and Health Improvement*, London: Health Development Agency.

Hansard Society Commission on Parliamentary Scrutiny (2001) *The Challenge for Parliament: Making Government Accountable*, London: Vacher Dod Publishing.

Hantrais, L. (1995) *Social Policy in the European Union*, Basingstoke: Palgrave.

Harrabin, R., Coote, A. and Allen, J. (2003) *Health in the News: Risk Reporting and Media Influence*, London: King's Fund.

Harrison, S. (1988) *Managing the National Health Service: Shifting the Frontier?*, London: Chapman and Hall.

Harrison, S. (2001) 'Reforming the Medical Profession in the United Kingdom 1989-97: Structural Interests in Health Care', in Bovens, M., Peters. B.G. and t'Hart, P. (eds) *Success and Failure in Public Governance*, Aldershot: Edward Elgar, pp 277-92.

Harrison, S. and Ahmad, W. (2000) 'Medical Autonomy and the UK State 1975-2005', *Sociology*, vol 34, no 1, pp 129-46.

Harrison, S. and Pollitt, C. (1994) *Controlling Health Professionals*, Buckingham: Open University Press.

Harrison, S. and Wood, B. (1998) 'Designing Health Service Organisation in the UK, 1968 to 1998: From Blueprint to Bright Idea and Manipulated Emergence', *Public Administration*, vol 77, no 4, pp 751-68.

Harrison, S., Hunter, D., Marnoch, G. and Pollitt, C. (1992) *Just Managing: Culture and Power in the National Health Service*, Basingstoke: Macmillan.

Hart, C. (2004) *Nurses and Politics: The Impact of Power and Practice*, Basingstoke: Palgrave.

Hartley, H. (2002) 'The System of Alignment Challenging Physicians' Professional Dominance: An Elaborated Theory of Countervailing Powers', *Sociology of Health and Illness*, vol 24, pp 178-207.

Hattersley, R. (2002) 'The Perils of Plain Speaking', *The Guardian*, 20 May, p 21.

Hayek, F. (1976) *The Road to Serfdom*, London: Routledge and Kegan Paul.

Haywood, S. and Alaszewski, A. (1980) *Crisis in the Health Service*, London: Croom Helm.

Haywood, S. and Hunter, D. (1982) 'Consultative Processes in Health Policy in the UK', *Public Administration*, vol 60, no 2, pp 143-62.

Health and Social Services Committee (2005) *Report of Review of the Interface between Health and Social Care*, Cardiff: National Assembly for Wales.

Health Committee (1999) *The Relationship between Health and Social Services*, HC 74-I, 1st report, 1998/99, London: HMSO.

Health Committee (2001) *The National Institute for Clinical Excellence*, 2nd report, 2001/2, London: The Stationery Office.

Health Committee (2003) *Minutes of Evidence*, 30 October 2003, London: The Stationery Office.

Health Committee (2004) *Obesity*, HC 23, 3rd Report, 2003/4, London: The Stationery Office.

Health Committee (2005) *The Influence of the Pharmaceutical Industry*, HC 42, 4th Report, vol 1, 2004/5, London: The Stationery Office.

Health Committee (2006) *Changes to Primary Care Trusts*, HC 646, 2nd Report, 2005/6, London: The Stationery Office.

Health Service Journal (2005) 'Staff Sick to Death of Change', 9 June, p 7.

Health Service Journal (2006) 'Proud to Introduce the NHS Top Table', 14 September, pp 40-54.

Healthcare Commission (2004) *State of Healthcare Report*, London: Healthcare Commission.

Heclo, H. and Wildavsky, A. (1974) *The Private Government of Public Money*, London: Macmillan.

Heenan, D. and Birrell, D. (2006) 'The Integration of Health and Social Care: The Lessons from Northern Ireland', *Social Policy and Administration*, vol 40, no 1, pp 47-66.

Heinz, J., Laumann, E., Nelson, R. and Salisbury, R. (1993) *The Hollow Core: Private Interests in National Policy Making*, Cambridge, MA: Harvard University Press.

Held, D., McGrew, A., Goldblatt, D. and Perraton, J. (1999) *Global Transformations: Politics, Economics and Culture*, Palo Alto, CA: Stanford University Press.

Henderson, L. (1999) 'Producing Serious Soaps', in Philo, G. (ed), *Messages Received,* Glasgow Media Group Research 1993-98, London: Longman, pp 62-81.

Henderson, L. and Kitzinger, J. (1999) 'The Human Drama of Genetics: "Hard" and "Soft" Media Representations of Inherited Breast Cancer', *Sociology of Health and Illness*, vol 21, no 5, pp 560-78.

Hennessy, P. (1998) 'The Blair Style of Government', *Government and Opposition*, vol 33, no 1, pp 3-20.

Hertz, N. (2001) *The Silent Takeover: Global Capitalism and the Death of Democracy*, London: Heinemann.

Heywood, A. (1994) *Political Ideas and Concepts: An Introduction*, Basingstoke: Macmillan.

Hickson, K. (2004) 'The Postwar Consensus Revisited', *Political Quarterly*, vol 75, pp 142-53.

Hilder, P. (2005) *Open Parties? A Map of 21st Century Democracy*, www.opendemocracy.net//democracy-open-politics/article_2312.jsp, accessed 7 February 2005.

Hill, M. (1997) 'Implementation Theory: Yesterday's Issue?', *Policy & Politics*, vol 25, no 4, pp 375-85.

Hill, M. and Hupe, P. (2002) *Implementing Public Policy*, London: Sage.

Hirst, P. and Thompson, G. (1996) *Globalisation in Question: The International Economy and the Possibilities*, Cambridge: Polity.

HM Treasury (2005) *Public Expenditure Statistical Analyses*, Cm 6521, London: The Stationery Office.

HM Treasury/Department of Health (DoH) (2002) *Tackling Health Inequalities: Summary of the 2002 Cross-Cutting Review*, London: DoH.

Hogg, C. (1999) *Patients, Power and Politics*, London: Sage.

Hogg, C. (2002) *National Service Frameworks: Involving Patients and the Public*, London: The Patients Forum.

Hoggett, P. (1996) 'New Modes of Control in the Public Service', *Public Administration*, vol 74, no 1, pp 9-32.

Hogwood, B. and Gunn, L. (1984) *Policy Analysis for the Real World*, Oxford: Oxford University Press.

Hogwood, B. and Peters, B.G. (1983) *Policy Dynamics*, Brighton: Wheatsheaf.

Holden, C. (2005) 'Privatisation and Trade in Health Services: A Review of the Evidence', *International Journal of Health Services*, vol 35, no 4, pp 675-89.

Honigsbaum, F. (1970) *The Struggle for the Ministry of Health*, London: Social Administration Research Trust.

Hood, C. (1976) *The Limits of Administration*, London: John Wiley.

Hopkins, J. (2000) 'Celebrity Illnesses Raise Awareness but Can Give the Wrong Message', *British Medical Journal*, vol 321, p 1099.

Hoque, K., Davis, S. and Humphreys, M. (2004) 'Freedom to Do What You are Told: Senior Management Autonomy in an NHS Acute Trust', *Public Administration*, vol 82, no 2, pp 355-75.

Horton, R. (2004) *MMR: Science and Fiction*, London: Granta.

Horton, R. (2006) 'WHO: Strengthening the Road to Renewal', www.thelancet.com, vol 367, pp 1793-5.

Hospital Doctor (2006) 'Hopes Dashed', 18 May, www.hospital-doctor.net/hd_news, accessed 12 June 2006.

Howie, J., Heaney, D. and Maxwell, M. (1995) *General Practitioner Fundholding Shadow Project and Evaluation*, Edinburgh: University of Edinburgh.

Hudson, B. (1998) 'Circumstances Change: Local Government and the NHS', *Social Policy and Administration*, vol 32, no 1, pp 71-86.

Hudson, B. (2002) 'Interprofessionality in Health and Social Care: the Achilles' Heel of Partnership?', *Journal of Interprofessional Care*, vol 6, no 1, pp 7-15.

Hudson, B. and Hardy, B. (2002) 'What is a Successful Partnership and How can it be Measured?', in Glendinning, C., Powell, M. and Rummery, K. (eds) *Partnerships, New Labour and Governance*, Bristol: The Policy Press, pp 51-66.

Hudson, B. and Henwood, M. (2002) 'The NHS and Social Care: The Final Countdown', *Policy and Politics*, vol 30, no 2, pp 153-66.

Hudson, J. and Lowe, S. (2004) *Understanding the Policy Process*, Bristol: The Policy Press.

Hudson, B., Hardy, B., Henwood, M. and Wistow, G. (1997) 'Working Across Professional Boundaries: Primary Health Care and Social Care', *Public Money and Management*, vol 17, no 4, pp 25-30.

Hughes, D. and Griffiths, L. (1999) 'On Penalties and the Patient's Charter: Centralism v Decentralised Governance in the NHS', *Sociology of Health and Illness*, vol 2, no 1, 71-94.

Hughes, C. and Wintour, P. (1990) *Labour Rebuilt: The New Model Party*, London: Fourth Estate.

Hultberg, E.-L., Glendinning, C., Allebeck, P. and Lönnroth, K. (2005) 'Using Pooled Budgets to Integrate Health and Welfare Services: A Comparison of Experiments in England and Sweden', *Health and Social Care in the Community*, vol 13, no 6, pp 531-41.

Hunter, D. (2000) 'Managing the NHS', in Appleby, J. and Harrison, A. (eds) *Health Care UK*, Winter, pp 69-76.

Hunter, D., Wilkinson, J. and Coyle, E. (2005) 'Would Regional Government have been Good for your Health?', *British Medical Journal*, vol 330, pp 159-60.

Hutton, W. (2000) *New Life for Health: The Commission on the New NHS*, London: Vintage.

Immergut, E. (1992) *Health Politics, Interests and Institutions in Western Europe*, Cambridge: Cambridge University Press.

Independent Healthcare Association and the Department of Health (2000) *For the Benefit of Patients: A Concordat with the Private and Voluntary Health Providers*, London: IHA/DOH.

Independent Inquiry into Inequalities in Health (1998) *Report*, London: The Stationery Office.

Ingle, S. (1999) *The British Party System* (3rd edn), Oxford: Blackwell.

Ingle, S. and Tether, P. (1981) *Parliament and Health Policy: The Role of MPs 1970-5*, Farnborough: Gower.

IPPR (Institute for Public Policy Research) (2001) *Building Better Partnerships: The final report of the Commission on Public–Private Partnerships*, London: IPPR.

IPPR (2006) (Adams, J. and Schmuecker, K. (eds)) *Devolution in Practice 2006: Public Policy Differences within the UK*, London: IPPR.

Irvine, D. (2003) *The Doctor's Tale: Professionalism and Public Trust*, Oxford: Radcliffe Medical Press.

James, S. (1992) *British Cabinet Government*, London: Routledge.

Jeffrey, C. (2005) 'Devolution and the European Union: Trajectories and Futures', in Trench, A. (ed) *The Dynamics of Devolution: The State of Nations 2005*, Thoverton: Imprint Academic.

Jeffrey, C. (2006) 'Devolution and the Lopsided State', in Dunleavy, P., Heffernan, R., Cowley, P. and Hay, C. (eds) *Developments in British Politics*, Basingstoke: Palgrave, pp 138-58.

Jenkins-Smith, H. and Sabatier, P. (1994) 'Evaluating the Advocacy Coalition Framework', *Journal of Public Policy*, vol 14, no 2, pp 175-203.

Jennings, M.K. (1999) 'Political Responses to Pain and Loss: Presidential Address, American Political Science Association, 1998', *American Political Science Review*, vol 93, no 1, pp 1-15.

Jervis, P. and Plowden, W. (2003) *The Impact of Political Devolution on the UK's Health Services*, London: Nuffield Trust.

Jessop, B. (1999) 'The Changing Governance of Welfare: Recent Trends in its Primary Functions, Scale and Modes of Coordination', *Social Policy and Administration*, vol 33, no 4, pp 348-59.

John, P. (1998) *Analysing Public Policy*, London: Pinter.

Johnson, T. (1995) 'Governmentality and the Institutionalisation of Expertise', in Johnson, T., Larkin, G. and Saks, M. (eds) *Health Professions and the State in Europe*, London: Routledge, pp 7-24.

Johnstone, D. (1984) *The Middle of Whitehall*, Bath: School of Humanities and Social Science.

Jones, A. (2007) *Britain and the EU*, Edinburgh: Edinburgh University Press.

Jones, J. (1990) 'Party Committees and All Party Groups', in Rush, M. (ed) *Parliament and Pressure Politics*, Oxford: Clarendon, pp 112-36.

Jones, N. (1995) *Soundbites and Spin Doctors: How Politicians Manipulate the Media and Vice Versa*, London: Cassell.

Jones, N. (2002) *The Control Freaks: How New Labour Gets Its Own Way*, London; Politicos.

Jones, T. (1996) *Remaking the Labour Party*, London: Routledge.

Jordan, G. (1990) 'Policy Community Realism v "New" Institutionalist Ambiguity', *Political Studies*, vol 38, pp 470-84.

Jordan, G. and Maloney, W. (1997) *The Protest Business: Mobilising Campaign Groups*, Manchester: Manchester University Press.

Judge, D. (1993) *The Parliamentary State*, London: Sage.

Kammerling, R. and Kinnear, A. (1996) 'The Extent of the Two Tier Service for Fundholders', *British Medical Journal*, vol 312, pp 1399-401.

Karpf, A. (1988) *Doctoring the Media: The Reporting of Health and Medicine*, London: Routledge.

Kavanagh, D. and Seldon, A. (2000) 'Support for the Prime Minister: The Hidden Influence of No. 10', in Rhodes, R. (ed) *Transforming British Government*, vol 2, *Changing Roles and Relationships*, Basingstoke: Macmillan, pp 63-78.

Kay, A. (2001) 'New Labour on Drugs: The Changing Relationship between Government and the Pharmaceutical Industry', *Political Quarterly*, vol 72, pp 322-8.

Keane, J. (1991) *The Media and Democracy*, Cambridge: Polity.

Keating, M. (2005) *Policy Making and Policy Divergence in Scotland after Devolution*, ESRC Briefings on Devolution and Constitutional Change, no 21, available at www.devolution.ac.uk, accessed 21 June 2006.

Keefe, R., Lane, S. and Swarts, H. (2006) 'From the Bottom Up: Tracing the Impact of Four Health-Based Social Movements on Health and Social Policies', *Journal of Health and Social Policy*, vol 21, no 3, pp 55-69.

Kendall, J. (2003) *The Voluntary Sector*, London: Routledge.

Kerr, D. (2005) *Building a Health Service Fit for the Future: A National Framework for Service Change in the NHS in Scotland*, Edinburgh: Scottish Executive.

Kewell, B., Hawkins, C. and Ferlie, E. (2002) 'From Market Umpires to Relationship Managers?: The Future of NHS Regional Offices in a Time of Transition', *Public Management Review*, vol 4, no 1, pp 3-22.

Kickbusch, I. (2000) 'The Development of International Health Policies – Accountability Intact?', *Social Science and Medicine*, vol 51, pp 979-89.

Kimball, A. (2006) 'The Health of Nations: Happy Birthday WTO', www.thelancet.com, vol 367, pp 188-9.

King, M. and Street, C. (2005) 'Mad Cows and Mad Scientists', in King, M. and Watson, K. (eds) *Representing Health: Discourses of Health and Illness in the Media*, Basingstoke: Palgrave, pp 115-32.

King, M. and Watson, K. (2005) *Representing Health: Discourses of Health and Illness in the Media*, Basingstoke: Palgrave.

King's Fund (2002) *The Future of the NHS: A Framework for Debate*, London: King's Fund.

Kingdon, J. (1984) *Agendas, Alternatives and Public Policy*, Boston, MA: Little Brown.

Kingsley, H. (1993) *Casualty: The Inside Story*, London: BBC.

Kitzinger, J. (2000) 'Media Templates: Patterns of Association and the (Re)construction of Meaning over Time', *Media, Culture and Society*, vol 22, no 1, pp 61-84.

Klein, R. (1990) 'The State and the Profession: The Politics of the Double-Bed', *British Medical Journal*, vol 301, pp 700-2.

Klein, R. (1995) *The New Politics of the NHS* (3rd edn), London: Longman.

Klein, R. (1999) 'Has the NHS a Future?', in Appleby, J. and Harrison, A. (eds) *Health Care UK*, London: King's Fund, pp 1-5.

Klein, R. (2000) *The New Politics of the NHS* (4th edn), London: Prentice Hall.

Klein, R. (2001) 'First Past the Post', *Health Service Journal*, 12 April, pp 26-7.

Klein, R., Day, P. and Redmayne, S. (1996) *Managing Scarcity: Priority Setting and Rationing in the National Health Service*, Buckingham: Open University Press.

Koivusalo, M. (2005) 'The Future of European Health Policies', *International Journal of Health Services*, vol 35, no 2, pp 325-42.

Koivusalo, M. (2006) 'The Impact of Economic Globalisation on Health', *Theoretical Medicine and Bioethics*, vol 27, no 1, pp 1-34.

Koivusalo, M. and Ollila, E. (1997) *Making a Healthy World*, London: Zed.

Labonte, R. and Schrecker, T. (2004) 'Committed to Health for All?: How the G7/G8 rate', *Social Science and Medicine*, vol 59, pp 1661-76.

Labour Party (1990) *A Fresh Start for Health*, London: Labour Party.

Labour Party (1992) *Your Good Health: A White Paper for a Labour Government*, London: Labour Party.

Labour Party (1994) *Health 2000: The Health and Wealth of the Nation in the 21st Century*, London: Labour Party.

Labour Party (1995) *Renewing the NHS*, London: Labour Party.

Labour Party (1997) *New Labour because Britain Deserves Better. Britain will win with New Labour*, London: Labour Party (www.labour-party.org.uk/manifestos/1997/1997-labour-manifesto.shtml, accessed 9 March 2007).

Labour Party (2001) *Ambitions for Britain*, London: Labour Party (www.labour-party.org.uk/manifestos/2001/2001-labour-manifesto.shtml, accessed 19 March 2007).

Laidlaw, S. (2002) 'World Trade Organisation Targets Canadian health care system', *Toronto Star*, www.commondreams.org/cgi-bin/print.cgi?file=/views01/0328-03.htm, accessed 22 August 2006.

Larson, R., Woloshin, S., Schwartz, L. and Welsh, H. (2005) 'Celebrity Endorsements of Cancer Screening', *Journal of the National Cancer Institute*, vol 97, no 9, pp 693-5.

Latham, E. (1965) *The Group Basis of Politics*, Ithaca, NY: Cornell University Press.

Laurance, J. and Grice, A. (2000) 'Campbell Accuses BBC of NHS Bias', *Independent*, 2 November, p 10.

Lawrie, S. (2000) 'Newspaper Coverage of Psychiatric and Physical Illness', *Psychiatric Bulletin*, vol 24, pp 104-6.

Le Grand, J., Mays, N. and Mulligan, J. (eds) (1998) *Learning from the NHS Internal Market: A Review of Evidence*, London: King's Fund.

Leatherman, S. and Sutherland, K. (2003) *The Quest for Quality in the NHS*, London: Nuffield Trust.

Lee, K. (2000) 'The impact of globalisation on public health: implications for the UK Faculty of Public Health Medicine', *Journal of Public Health Medicine*, vol 22, no 3, pp 253-62.

Lee, K. and Collin, J. (eds) (2005) *Global Change and Health*, Maidenhead: Open University Press.

Lee, K. and Koivusalo, M. (2005) 'Trade and Health: Is the Community Ready for Action', *Public Library of Science (PLoS) Medicine*, vol 2, no 1, p 8.

Lee, K., Collinson, S., Walt, G. and Gilson, L. (1996) 'Who Should be Doing What in International Health: A Confusion of Mandates in the United Nations?', *British Medical Journal*, vol 312, pp 302-7.

Lee-Potter, J. (1997) *A Damn Bad Business: The NHS Deformed*, London: Indigo.

Lerer, L. and Matzopoulos, R. (2001) 'The Worst of both Worlds?: The Management Reform of the World Health Organisation', *International Journal of Health Services*, vol 31, no 2, pp 415-38.

Levitt, R. and Wall, A. (1984) *The Reorganised National Health Service* (3rd edn), London: Croom Helm.

Liberal Democrats (1992) *Restoring the Nation's Health*, London: Liberal Democrats.

Likierman, A. (1988) *Public Expenditure*, London: Penguin.

Lindblom, C. (1959) 'The Science of Muddling Through', *Public Administration Review*, vol 19, no 2, pp 78-88.

Lindblom, C. (1965) *The Intelligence of Democracy*, New York, NY: Free Press.

Ling, T. (2000) 'Unpacking Partnership: The Case of Health Care', in Clarke, J., Gewirtz, S. and McLaughlin, E. (eds) *New Managerialism, New Welfare*, London: Sage, pp 82-101.

Lipsky, M. (1979) *Street-Level Bureaucracy*, New York, NY: Russell Sage.

Lipson, D. (2001) 'The World Trade Organisation's Health Agenda', *British Medical Journal*, vol 329, pp 1139-40.

Lister, J. (2006) 'Simons Stevens and his Amazing Dancing Balance Sheet', *Red Pepper*, March, p 10.

Little, W. (2005a) 'Councils and Trusts – A Winning Partnership', *Health Service Journal*, 23 June, pp 30-1.

Little, W. (2005b) 'Charities Ready to Play with the Big Boys but Say: Let's be Fair', *Health Service Journal*, 27 January, pp 14-15.

Lloyd, G. and Norris, C. (1999) 'Including ADHD?', *Disability and Society*, vol 14, no 4, pp 505-17.

Lloyd, J. (2001) *The Third Sector and the Fourth Estate*, Hinton Lecture, available at www.ncvo-vol.org.uk/events/speeches/hinton/index.asp?id=1154, accessed 24 January 2007.

Lobstein, T. (1998) 'The Common Agriculture Policy: A Dietary Disaster', *Consumer Policy Review*, vol 8, no 2, pp 83-7.

Local Government Association (LGA) (2000) *Partnership with Health: A Survey of Local Authorities*, London: LGA.

Lowe, R. (1993) *The Welfare State in Britain Since 1945*, Basingstoke: Macmillan.

Lowndes, V. and Skelcher, C. (1998) 'The Dynamics of Multi-organisational Partnerships: An Analysis of Changing Modes of Governance', *Public Administration*, vol 76, no 2, pp 313-33.

Lukes, S. (1974) *Power: A Radical View*, London: Macmillan.

Lupton, D. (1994) 'Femininity, Responsibility and the Technological Imperative: Discourses on Breast Care in the Australian Press', *International Journal of Health Services*, vol 24, no 1, pp 73-89.

Maddock, S. and Morgan, G. (2000) *Conditions for Partnership*, Manchester: Manchester Business School.

Mahony, H. (2006) 'The Creep Towards an EU Health Policy', Eurobserver. com/867/21628, accessed 22 August 2006.

Majone, G. (1989) *Evidence, Argument and Persuasion in the Policy Processes*, New Haven, CT: Yale University Press.

Maloney, W., Jordan, A.G. and McLaughlin, A. (1994) 'Interest Groups and the Policy Process: The Insider/Outsider Model Revisited', *Journal of Public Policy*, vol 14, no 1, pp 17-38.

Mandelstam, M. (2006) *Betraying the NHS: Health Abandoned*, London: Jessica Kingsley Publishers.

Maniadakis, M., Hollingsworth, B. and Thanassoulis, E. (1999) 'The Impact of the Internal Market on Hospitals Efficiency, Productivity and Service Quality', *Health Care Management Science*, vol 2, no 2, pp 75-85.

Mannion, R., Davies, H. and Marshall, M. (2005a) 'Impact of Star Performance Ratings in English Acute Hospital Trusts', *Journal of Health Service Research and Policy*, vol 10, no 1, pp 18-24.

Mannion, R., Davies, H. and Marshall, M. (2005b) *Cultures for Performance in Health Care*, Maidenhead: Open University Press.

Mannion, R., Goddard, M., Kuhn, M. and Bate, A. (2005c) 'Decentralisation Strategies and Provider Incentives in Healthcare: Evidence from the English National Health Service', *Applied Health Economics and Health Policy*, vol 4, no 1, pp 47-54.

March, J. and Olsen, J. (1984) The New Institutionalism: Organisational Factors in Political Life', *American Political Science Review*, vol 78, no 3, pp 734-48.

Marinetto, M. (1998) *Studies of the Policy Process*, Hemel Hempstead: Prentice Hall.

Marsh, D. and Rhodes, R. (eds) (1992a) *Implementing Thatcherite Policies*, Buckingham: Open University Press.

Marsh, D. and Rhodes, R. (eds) (1992b) *Policy Networks in British Government*, Oxford: Clarendon.

Marsh, D. and Smith, M. (2000) 'Understanding Policy Networks: Towards a Dialectic Approach', *Political Studies*, vol 48, no 4, pp 4-21.

Martin, D. (2005) 'EU Budget Cuts Sought by Blair put Public Health at Risk', *Health Service Journal*, 15 December, p 5.

Martin, G. (2001) 'Social Movements, Welfare and Social Policy', *Critical Social Policy*, vol 21, no 3, pp 361-83.

Matka, E., Barnes, M. and Sullivan, H. (2002) 'Health Action Zones: Creating Alliances to Achieve Change', *Policy Studies*, vol 23, no 2, pp 97-106.

May, J. and Wildavsky, A. (eds) (1978) *The Policy Cycle*, Beverly Hills, CA: Sage.

Mayor of London (2002) *Cleaning London's Air: The Mayor's Air Quality Strategy*, London: Mayor of London.

Mayor of London, London Food, London Development Agency (2006) *Health and Sustainable Food for London: The Mayor's Food Strategy*, London: London Development Agency.

Mays, N., Mulligan, J. and Goodwin, N. (2000) 'The British Quasi Market in Health Care: A Balance Sheet of the Evidence', *Journal of Health Services Research and Policy*, vol 5, pp 49-58.

McCarthy, M. (2002a) 'What's going on at the World Health Organisation?', *The Lancet*, vol 360, pp 1108-12.

McCarthy, M. (2002b) 'Regulating Health in Europe', *Journal of Public Health Medicine*, vol 25, no 4, pp 279-80.

McGregor-Riley, V. (1997a) *The Politics of Medical Representation: The Care of the BMA from 1979-1995*, Leicester: De Montfort University, unpublished.

McGregor-Riley, V. (1997b) 'The Declining Political Influence of the British Medical Association: Fact or Fiction?', *PSA conference*, Belfast, April 1997.

McKee, M. (2005) 'European Health Policy: Where Now?', *European Journal of Public Health*, vol 15, no 6, pp 557-8.

McKee, M., Dubois, C.-A. and Sibbald, B. (2006) 'Changing "Professional Boundaries"', in Dubois, C.-A., McKee, M. and Nolte, E. (eds) *Human Resources for Health in Europe*, Maidenhead: Open University, pp 63-78.

McKee, M., MacLehose, L. and Nolte, E. (2004) *Health Policy and European Union Enlargement*, Maidenhead: Open University.

McLachlan, G. (1990) *What Price Quality?: The NHS in Review*, London: Nuffield Provincial Hospitals Trust.

McLelland, S. (2002) 'Health Policy in Wales: Distinctive or Derivative?', *Social Policy and Society*, vol 1, no 4, pp 325-33.

McMillan, J. and Massey, A. (2001) 'A Regional Future for the UK Civil Service? The Government Offices for the English Regions and the Civil Service in Scotland', *Public Money and Management*, vol 25, no 2, April-June, pp 25-31.

McNulty, T. and Ferlie, E. (2002) *Re-Engineering Health Care*, Oxford: Oxford University Press.

Mechanic, D. (1991) 'Sources of Countervailing Power in Medicine', *Journal of Health Policy, Politics and Law*, vol 16, no 3, pp 485-98.

Melucci, A. (1989) *The Nomads of the Present*, London: Radius.

Milburn, A. (2001) *Reforming Public Services: Reconciling Equity with Choice*, London: Fabian Society.

Miliband, R. (1982) *Capitalist Democracy in Britain*, Oxford: Oxford University Press.

Millar, B. (2000) 'The Director's Cut', *Health Service Journal*, 20 April, pp 22-5.

Miller, C. (1990) *Lobbying Government: Understanding and Influencing the Corridors of Power*, Oxford: Blackwell.

Miller, D. (1998) 'Public Relations and Journalism: Promotional Strategies and Media Power', in Briggs, A. and Cobley, P. (eds) *The Media: An Introduction*, London: Longman, pp 65-80.

Miller, D. and Reilly, J. (1994) *Food Scares in the Media*, London: Routledge.

Miller, D., Kitzinger, J., Williams, K. and Beharrell, P. (1998) *The Circuit of Mass Communication. Media Strategies, Representation and Audience Reception in the AIDS Crisis*, London: Sage.

Millward Brown (2004) *National Media Coverage of Public Health Issues and the NHS*, London: DoH.

Ministry of Health (1968) *National Health Service: The Administrative Structure of the Medical and Related Services in England and Wales*, London: HMSO.

Mohan, J. (1995) *A National Health Service?*, Basingstoke: Macmillan.

Mohan, J. (2002) *Planning, Markets and Hospitals*, London: Routledge.

Montgomery, J. (2003) *Health Care Law* (2nd edn), Oxford: Oxford University Press.

Moran, M. (1999) *Governing the Health Care State: A Comparative Study of the United Kingdom, the United States and Germany*, Manchester: Manchester University Press.

Moran, M. (2000) 'Understanding the Welfare State: The Case of Health', *British Journal of Politics and International Relations*, vol 92, June, pp 135-60.

Moran, M. and Wood, B. (1992) *States, Regulation and the Medical Profession*, Buckingham: Open University Press.

Morgan, R. (2003) 'Clear Red Water', *Agenda*, Spring, Cardiff: Insititute of Welsh Affairs.

Morison, J. (2000) 'The Government–Voluntary Sector Compacts: Governance, Governmentality and Civil Society', *Journal of Law and Society*, vol 27, no 1, pp 98-132.

Morley, A. and Campbell, F. (2003) *People Power and Health: A Green Paper on Democratising the NHS*, London: Democratic Health Network.

Mosca, I. (2006) 'Is Decentralisation The Real Solution? A Three Country Study', *Health Policy*, vol 77, no 1, pp 113-20.

Mossialos, E. and McKee, M. (2002) 'Health Care and the European Union', *British Medical Journal*, vol 324, pp 991-2.

Mossialos, E., Walley, T. and Mrazek, M. (2004) 'Regulating Pharmaceuticals in Europe: An Overview', in Mossialos, E., Walley, T. and Mrazek, M. (eds) *Regulating Pharmaceuticals in Europe: Striving for Efficiency, Equity and Quality*, Maidenhead: Open University Press.

Moynihan, R. (1998) *Too Much Medicine: The Business of Health and Its Risks for You*, Sydney: ABC Books.

Moynihan, R., Heath, I. and Henry, D. (2002) 'Selling Sickness: The Pharmaceutical Industry and Disease-mongering', *British Medical Journal*, vol 324, pp 886-91.

Mui, L. (1997) *Developing Medical Directors in Clinical Directorates*, http://groups.csail.mit.edu/medg/people/lmui/MedicalDirectors/index.html.

Mulligan, J. and Appleby, J. (2001) 'The NHS and Labour's Battle for Public Opinion', in Park, A., Curtice, J., Thomson, K., Jarvis, L. and Bramley, C. (eds) *British Social Attitudes: The 18th Report – Public Policy, Social Ties*, London: Sage.

Nairne, P. (1983) 'Managing the DHSS Elephant: Reflections on a Giant Department', *Political Quarterly*, vol 54, pp 243-56.

Nairne, P. (1984) 'Parliamentary Control and Accountability', in Maxwell, R. and Weaver, N. (eds) *Public Participation in Health*, London: King Edwards Fund for London, pp 33-51.

National Audit Office (2003) *Achieving Improvement through Clinical Governance: A Progress Report*, London: The Stationery Office.

National Audit Office (2004a) *Improving Emergency Care in England*, HC 1075, 2003/4, London: The Stationery Office.

National Audit Office (2004b) *Home Office: Working with the Third Sector*, HC 75, 2005/6, London: The Stationery Office.

National Audit Office (2005) *The Refinancing of the Norfolk and Norwich PFI Hospital: How the Deal can be Viewed in the Light of Refinancing*, HC 78, 2004/5, London: The Stationery Office.

Nattinger, A., Hoffmann, R., Howell-Pelz, A. and Goodwin, J. (1998) 'Effect of Nancy Reagan's Mastectomy on Choice of Surgery for Breast Cancer by US Women', *Journal of the American Medical Association*, vol 279, pp 762-6.

Naughtie, J. (2002) *The Rivals: The Inside Story of a Political Marriage*, London: Fourth Estate.

Navarro, V. (1978) *Class Struggle, the State and Medicine*, Oxford: Martin Robertson.

Negrine, R. (1994) *Politics of the Mass Media in Britain*, London: Routlegde.

Neroth, P. (2004) 'Fat of the Land', www.thelancet.com, vol 364, pp 651-2.

Neroth, P. (2005) 'Can Health Survive the Single Market?', www.thelancet.com, vol 365, pp 461-5.

Nestle, M. (2003) *Food Politics*, Berkeley, CA: University of California Press.

Newman, J. (2001) *Modernising Governance: New Labour Policy and Society*, London: Sage.

Newton, K. (2001) 'The Transformation of Governance?', in Axford, B. and Huggins, R. (eds) *New Media and Politics*, London: Sage, pp 151-71.

NHS Alliance (2002) *The Vision in Practice*, Retford: NHS Alliance.

Nicoll, A., Jones, J., Aavitsland, P. and Giesecke, J. (2005) 'Proposed New International Health Regulations', *British Medical Journal*, vol 330, pp 321-22.

North, N. and Peckham, S. (2001) 'Analysing Structural Interests in Primary Care Groups', *Social Policy and Administration*, vol 35, no 4, pp 426-40.

Norton, P. (1981) *The Commons in Perspective*, Oxford: Martin Robertson.

Nozick, R. (1974) *Anarchy, State and Utopia*, London: Blackwell.

NPCRDC (National Primary Care Research and Development Centre) (2006) *The Implementation of Local Authority Scrutiny of Primary Health Care 2002-2005*, Manchester: NPCRDC.

Nugent, N. (2003) *The Government and Politics of the European Union* (5th edn), Basingstoke: Palgrave.

O'Connor, J. (1973) *The Fiscal Crisis of the State*, New York, NY: St Martin's Press.

O'Connor, M. (1991) 'Public Health and the European Community', *Health Education Journal*, vol 50, no 4, pp 200-3.

O'Donovan, O. (2005) 'Time to weed out the astroturf from the grassroots? Exploring the implications of pharmaceutical industry funding of "patient" advocacy organisations', Paper presented at *Concepts of the Third Sector: The European Debate*, ISTR/EMES Conference, Paris, 27-29 April 2005.

O'Donovan, O. and Glavanis-Grantham, K. (2003) 'Researching the Political and Cultural Influence of the Transnational Pharmaceutical Industry in Ireland', *Administration*, vol 52, no 3, pp 21-42.

O'Neill, F. (2000) 'Health, the Internal Market and Reform of the NHS', in Dolowitz, D., *Policy Transfer and British Social Policy*, Buckingham: Open University Press, pp 59-76.

Oborne, P. and Walters, S. (2004) *Alistair Campbell*, London: Aurum.

ODPM (Office of the Deputy Prime Minister) (2003) *Evaluation of Local Strategic Partnerships*, London: ODPM.

ODPM (2005a) *Process Evaluation of Plan Rationalisation. Formative Evaluation of Community Strategies*, London: ODPM.

ODPM (2005b) *Formative Evaluation of the Take-up and Implementation of the Well-being Power 2003-6*, London: ODPM.

ODPM (2005c) *A Process Evaluation of the Negotiation of Local Area Agreements*, London: ODPM.

ODPM (2006) *National Evaluation of Local Strategic Partnerships: Formative Evaluation and Action Research Programme 2002-2005*, London: ODPM.

Offe, C. (1984) *The Contradictions of the Welfare State*, London: Hutchinson.

Ollila, E. (2005) 'Global Health Priorities: Priorities of the Wealthy?', *Globalisation and Health*, vol 1, no 6, pp 1-6.

Olson, M. (1965) *The Logic of Collective Action*, Cambridge, MA: Harvard University Press.

Organisation for Economic and Cooperation and Development (OECD) (2004) *Towards High Performing Health Systems*, Paris: OECD.

Osborne, S. and McLaughlin, K. (2002) 'Trends and Issues in the Implementation of Local Voluntary Sector Compacts in England', *Public Money and Management*, vol 22, no 1, pp 55-63.

Ostry, A. (2001) 'International Trade Regulation and Publicly Funded Health Care in Canada', *International Journal of Health Services*, vol 31, no 3, pp 475-80.

Parliament First (2003) *Parliament's Last Chance*, London: Parliament First.

Parsons, W. (1995) *Public Policy*, Aldershot: Edward Elgar.

Paton, C. (1993) 'Devolution and Centralism in the National Health Service', *Social Policy and Administration*, vol 27, no 2, pp 8-107.

Peckham, S. (2003) 'Improving Local Health', in Dowling, B. and Glendinning, C. (eds) *The New Primary Care*, Maidenhead: Open University Press, pp 159-78.

Peckham, S., Exworthy, M., Powell, M. and Greener, I. (2005) *Decentralisation as an Organisational Model for Health Care in England*, London: NHS Coordinating Centre for Service Delivery and Organisation.

Performance and Innovation Unit (2000) *Reaching Out: The Role of Central Government at Regional and Local Level*, London: Cabinet Office.

Perri 6., Leat, D., Seltzer, K. and Stoker, G. (2002) *Towards Holistic Governance: The New Reform Agenda*, Basingstoke: Palgrave.

Peston, R. (2005) *Brown's Britain*, London: Short Books.

Pharmaceutical Industry Competitiveness Task Force (2001) *Final Report*, London: DoH and ABPI.

Philo, G. (ed) (1996) *Media and Mental Distress*, London: Longman.

Philo, G. (1999) 'Media and Mental Illness', in Philo, G. (ed) *Message Received, Glasgow Media Group Research 1993-98*, London: Longman, pp 54-61.

Pilkington, C. (2002) *Devolution in Britain Today*, Manchester: Manchester University Press.

Pimlott, B. and Rao, N. (2002) *Governing London*, Oxford: Oxford University Press.

Platt, S. (1998) *Government by Task Force*, London: Catalyst.

Pollitt, C., Birchall, J. and Putman, K. (1998) *Decentralising Public Service Management*, Basingstoke: Macmillan.

Pollock, A. (2004) *NHS PLC: The Privatisation of our Health Care*, London: Verso.

Pollock, A. and Price, D. (2003) 'New Deal from the World Trade Organisation', *British Medical Journal*, vol 327, pp 571-2.

Powell, M. (1997) *Evaluating the NHS*, Buckingham: Open University Press.

Powell, M. and Glendinning, C. (2002) 'Introduction', in Glendinning, C., Powell, M. and Rummery, K. (eds) *Partnerships, New Labour and Governance*, Bristol: The Policy Press, pp 1-15.

Powell, M. and Moon, G. (2001) 'Health Action Zones: The Third Way of a New Area-based Policy', *Health and Social Care in the Community*, vol 9, no 1, pp 43-50.

Prah Ruger, J. and Yach, D. (2005) 'Global Functions at the World Health Organisation', *British Medical Journal*, vol 330, pp 1099-1100.

Pressman, J. and Wildavsky, A. (1973) *Implementation*, Berkeley, CA: University of California Press.

Price, D. (2002) 'How the WTO Extends the Rights of Private Property', *Critical Public Health*, vol 12, no 1, pp 55-63.

Price-Smith, A. (2001) *The Health of Nations: Infectious Disease, Environmental Change and their Effects on National Security and Development*, Cambridge, MA: MIT Press.

Prime Minister's Strategy Unit (2003) *Alcohol Harm Reduction Project: Interim Analytical Report*, London: Cabinet Office.

Prime Minister's Strategy Unit (2004) *Alcohol Harm Reduction Strategy for England*, London: Cabinet Office.

Public Accounts Committee (1996) *Clinical Audit in England*, HC 304, 31st report, 1995/6, London: The Stationery Office.

Public Accounts Committee (2002) *Inappropriate Adjustments to NHS Waiting Lists*, HC 517, 46th Report, 2001/2, London: The Stationery Office.

Public Accounts Committee (2006a) *The Refinancing of the Norfolk and Norwich PFI Hospital*, HC 694, 35th report, 2005/06, London: The Stationery Office.

Public Accounts Committee (2006b) *The NHS Cancer Plan: A Progress Report*, HC 791, 20th report, 2005/6, London: The Stationery Office.

Raftery, J. (2006) 'Review of NICE's Recommendations 1999-2005', *British Medical Journal*, vol 332, pp 1266-8.

Ranade, W. and Hudson, B. (2003) 'Conceptual Issues in Inter-Agency Collaboration', *Local Government Studies*, vol 29, no 3, pp 33-50.

Randall, E. (2001) *The European Union and Health Policy*, Basingstoke: Palgrave.

Rao, N. (2006) 'Introducing the New Government of London', *Local Government Studies*, vol 32, no 3, pp 215-21.

Rawnsley, A. (2001) *Servants of the People: The Inside Story of New Labour*, Harmondsworth: Penguin.

Redwood, J. (1994) *The Global Marketplace*, London: Harper Collins.

Reeve, C. (2004) *Nothing is Impossible: Reflections on a New Life*, New York, NY: Random House.

Regan, D. and Stewart, J. (1982) 'An Essay in the Government of Health: The Case for Local Authority Control', *Social Policy and Administration*, vol 16, no 1, pp 19-42.

Regen, E., Smith, J., Goodwin, N., McLeod, H. and Shapiro, J. (2001) *Passing on the Baton: Final Report of a National Evaluation of Primary Care Groups and Trusts*, Health Service Management Centre: University of Birmingham.

Rhodes, R. (1997) *Understanding Governance: Policy Networks, Governance, Reflexivity and Accountability*, Buckingham: Open University Press.

Rhodes, T. and Shaughnessy, R. (1990) 'Compulsory Screening: Advertising AIDS in Britain', *Policy and Politics*, vol 18, no 1, pp 55-61.

Richards, D. and Smith, M. (2002) *Governance and Public Policy in the UK*, Oxford: Oxford University Press.

Richards, D. and Smith, M. (2004) 'The Hybrid State; Labour's Response to the Challenge of Governance', in Ludlam, S. and Smith, M. (eds) *Governing as New Labour*, Basingstoke: Palgrave, pp 106-25.

Richards, P. (1972) *The Backbenchers*, London: Faber.

Richardson, J. (2000) 'Governments, Interest Groups and Policy Change', *Political Studies*, vol 48, pp 1006-25.

Richardson, J. and Jordan, G. (1979) *Governing Under Pressure*, Oxford: Martin Robertson.

Richardson, J. and Moon, J. (1984) 'The Politics of Unemployment in Britain', *Political Quarterly*, vol 55, pp 29-37.

Riddell, P. (2000) *Parliament Under Blair*, London: Politicos.

Ridley, F. and Jordan, G. (1998) *Protest Politics: Cause Groups and Campaigns*, Oxford: Oxford University Press.

Ritchie, J. (2000) *The Report of the Inquiry into Quality and Practice Within the National Health Service Arising from the Action of Rodney Ledward*, London: NHS Executive South East.

Rivett, G. (1998) *From Cradle to Grave: Fifty Years of the NHS*, London: King's Fund.

Robb, B. (1967) *Sans Everything*, London: Nelson.

Robinson, W. (2003) *Transnational Conflicts: Central America, Social Change and Globalisation*, London: Verso.

Roche, D. (2004) *PCTs: An Unfinished Agenda*, London: IPPR.

Rogers, A. and Pilgrim, D. (1991) 'Pulling down Churches: Accounting for the British Mental Health Users Movement', *Sociology of Health and Illness*, vol 13, no 2, pp 129-48.

Rogers A. and Pilgrim, D. (2001) *Mental Health Policy in Britain* (2nd edn), Basingstoke: Palgrave.

Rondinelli, D. (1981) 'Government Decentralisation in Comparative Perspective Theory and Practice in Developing Countries', *International Review of Administrative Science*, vol 47, pp 137-45.

Room, R. (2004) 'Disabling the Public Interest: Alcohol Strategies and Policies for England', *Addiction*, vol 99, no 9, pp 1083-99.

Rose, D. (1998) 'Television, Madness and Community Care', *Journal of Community and Applied Social Psychology*, vol 8, pp 213-28.

Rose, R. (1973) 'Comparing Public Policy: An Overview', *European Journal of Political Research*, vol 1, pp 67-94.

Rose, R. (1984) *Do Parties Make a Difference?* (2nd edn), London: Macmillan.

Rose, R. (1991) 'What is Lesson Drawing?', *Journal of Public Policy*, vol 11, no 1, pp 3-30.

Rose, R. and Davies, P. (1994) *Inheritance in Public Policy: Change without Choice in Britain*, New Haven, CT: Yale University Press.

Rosen, F. and Burns, J. (eds) (1983) *The Collected Works of Jeremy Bentham: Constitutional Code Vol I*, Oxford: Oxford University Press.

Ross, W. and Tomaney, J. (2001) 'Devolution and Health Policy in England', *Regional Studies*, vol 35, no 3, pp 265-70.

Royal College of Physicians (2006) *Falling Short: Organisation of Services for People who have a Fall*, www.rcplondon.ac.uk/news news.asp?PR_id=304, accessed 8 June 2006.

Royal Liverpool Children's Inquiry (2001) *The Report of the Royal Liverpool Children's Inquiry*, London: The Stationery Office.

Ruane, S. (2000) 'Acquiescence and Opposition: The Private Finance Initiative in the NHS', *Policy & Politics*, vol 28, no 3, pp 411-24.

Ruane, S. (2002) 'Public–Private Partnerships: The Case of the PFI', in Glendinning, C., Powell, M. and Rummery, K. (eds) *Partnerships, New Labour and the Governance of Welfare*, Bristol: The Policy Press, pp 199-212.

Ruane, S. (2005) 'The Future of Healthcare in the UK: Think Tanks and their Policy Prescriptions', in Powell, M., Bauld, L. and Clarke, K. (eds) *Social Policy Review 17*, Bristol: The Policy Press: pp 147-66.

Rush, M. (ed) (1990) *Parliament and Pressure Politics*, Oxford: Clarendon Press.

Rush, M. (2005) *Parliament Today*, Manchester: Manchester University Press.

Sabatier, P. (1987) 'Knowledge, Policy Orientated Learning and Policy Change', *Knowledge: Creation, Diffusion, Utilisation*, vol 8, no 4, pp 649-92.

Sabatier, P. (ed) (1999) *Theories of the Policy Process*, Boulder, CO: Westview.

Salter, B. (1994) 'The Politics of Community Care: Social Rights and Welfare Limits', *Policy & Politics*, vol 22, no 2, pp 119-31.

Salter, B. (1998) *The Politics of Change in the Health Service*, Basingstoke: Macmillan.

Salter, B. (2003) 'Patients and Doctors: Reformulating the UK Health Policy Community?', *Social Science and Medicine*, vol 57, no 5, pp 927-36.

Salter, B. (2004) *The New Politics of Medicine*, Basingstoke: Palgrave Macmillan.

Saltman, R., Bankhauskaite, V. and Vrangback, K. (eds) (2007) *Decentralisation in Healthcare*, Maidenhead: McGraw-Hill.

Saltman, R., Figueras, J. and Sakallerides, C. (eds) (1998) *Critical Challenges for Health Care Systems in Europe*, Buckingham: Open University Press.

Sampson, A. (2004) *Who Runs this Place? The Anatomy of Britain in the 21st Century*, London: John Murray.

Saywell, C., Beattie, L. and Henderson, L. (2000) 'Sexualised Illness: The Newsworthy Body in Media Representations of Breast Cancer', in Potts, L. (ed) *Ideologies of Breast Cancer: Feminist Perspectives*, Basingstoke: Macmillan, pp 37-62.

Schattschneider, E. (1960) *The Semi-Sovereign People*, New York, NY: Holt, Rinehart and Winston.

Scott, A. (1990) *Ideology and the New Social Movements*, London: Unwin Hyman.

Scottish Executive (2003) *Improving Health in Scotland: The Challenge*, Edinburgh: Scottish Executive.

Scottish Executive (2004) *Fair to All, Personal to Each: The Next Steps for NHS Scotland*, Edinburgh: Scottish Executive.

Seale, C. (2001) 'Sporting Cancer: Struggle Language in News Reports of People with Cancer', *Sociology of Health and Illness*, vol 23, no 3, pp 308-29.

Seale, C. (2002) *Media and Health*, London: Sage.

Seale, C. (2003) 'Health and the Media: An Overview', *Sociology of Health and Illness*, vol 25, no 6, pp 513-31.

Seale, C. (2005) 'Threatened Children: Media Representations of Childhood Cancer', in King, M. and Watson, K. (eds) *Representing Health: Discourses of Health and Illness in the Media*, Basingstoke: Palgrave, pp 94-114.

Seldon, A. (1994) 'Policy Making and Cabinet', in Kavanagh, D. and Seldon, A. (eds) *The Major Effect*, London: Macmillan, pp 154-66.

Seldon, A. (ed) (2001) *The Blair Effect*, Boston, MA: Little Brown.

Select Committee on Public Administration (2000) *Appointments to NHS Bodies*, London: The Stationery Office.

Select Committee on Public Administration (2002) *Ministerial Accountability and Parliamentary Questions*, HC 1086, 9th report, 2001/2, London: The Stationery Office.

Select Committee on Public Administration (2003) *On Target? Government by Measurement*, HC 62, 5th report, 2002/3, London: The Stationery Office.

Sexton, S. (2001) 'Trading Health Care Away', GATS, *Public Health and Privatisation Corner House Briefing 23*, www.thecornerhouse.org.uk, accessed 20 September 2006.

Shaw, E. (2004) 'What Matters is What Works: The Third Way and the Case of the Private Finance Initiative', in Leggett, W., Hale, S. and Martell, L. (eds) *The Third Way and Beyond: Criticisms, Futures and Alternatives*, Manchester: Manchester University Press.

Sheard, S. and Donaldson, L. (2006) *The Nation's Doctor: The Role of the Chief Medical Officer 1855-1998*, Oxford: Radcliffe.

Sheldon, T., Cullum, N., Dawson, D., Lankshear, A., Lowson, K., Watt, I., West, P., Wright, D. and Wright, J. (2004) 'What's the Evidence that NICE Guidance has been Implemented? Results from a National Evaluation using Time Series Analysis, Audit of Patients' Notes and Interviews', *British Medical Journal*, vol 329, p 999.

Shipman Inquiry, The (2001) *First Report*, London: The Stationery Office.

Shipman Inquiry, The (2004) *Fifth Report: Safeguarding Patients. Lessons from the Past – Proposals for the Future*, London: The Stationery Office.

SHM (2002) *NHS Beacon Programme Evaluation*, London: Modernisation Agency.

Short, C. (2005) *An Honourable Deception: New Labour, Iraq and the Misuse of Power*, London: Free Press.

Sibbald, B., Shen, J. and McBride, A. (2004) 'Changing the Skill Mix of the Healthcare Workforce', *Journal of Health Services Research and Policy*, vol 9, no 1, Supplement, S1-28.

Silk, P. and Walters, R. (1998) *How Parliament Works* (4th edn), London: Longman.

Simon, H. (1945) *Administrative Behaviour*, Glencoe: Free Press.

Simon, H. (1960) *The New Science of Management Decision*, Englewood Cliffs, CO: Prentice Hall.

Simpson, J. and Scott, T. (1997) 'Beyond the Call of Duty', *Health Service Journal*, 27 June, pp 28-30.

Smith, C. (1997) 'Putting Quality at the Heart of Health Care', Speech, 6 February.

Smith, J., Walshe, K. and Hunter, D. (2001) 'The Redisorganisation of the NHS', *British Medical Journal*, vol 323, pp 1262-3.

Smith, M. (1993) *Pressure, Power and Policy*, Brighton: Harvester Wheatsheaf.

Smith, M. (1999) *The Core Executive in Britain*, Basingstoke: Macmillan.

Smith, M., Richards, D. and Marsh, D. (2000) 'The Changing Role of Central Government Departments', in Rhodes, R. (ed) *Transforming British Government, vol 2: Changing Roles and Relationships*, Basingstoke: Macmillan, pp 146-63.

Smith, P. (2005) 'Performance Measurement in Healthcare: History, Challenges and Prospects', *Public Money and Management*, vol 25, no 4, pp 213-20.

Snape, S. (2003) 'Health and Local Government Partnerships: The Local Government Context', *Local Government Studies*, vol 29, no 3, pp 73-98.

SocietyGuardian (2000) 'The 15 most powerful people in health', 14 November, www.society.guardian.co.uk/health/story/0,789,397769,00.html, accessed 15 December 2004.

SOLACE (Society of Local Authority Chief Executives) (2001) *Healthy Living: The Role of Modern Local Authorities in Creating Healthy Communities*, London: SOLACE.

Sontag, S. (1991) *Illness as Metaphor: AIDS and its Metaphors*, London: Penguin.

Speers, T. and Lewis, J. (2004) 'Journalists and Jabs: Media Coverage of the MMR Vaccine', *Communication and Medicine*, vol 1, no 2, pp 171-82.

SPS (Sanitary and Phytosanitary Measures) (1994) *Agreement on the Application of Sanitary and Phytosanitary Measures*, Uruguay Round Agreement, www.wto.org/english/docs_e/legal_e/15sps_01_e.htm, accessed 14 December 2006.

SSI (Social Services Inspectorate) (2002) *Improving Older People's Services: Policy into Practice. The Second Phase of Inspections into Older People's Services*, London: DoH.

Starr, P. and Immergut, E. (1987) 'Health Care and the Boundaries of Politics', in Maier, C. (ed) *Changing Boundaries of the Political*, Cambridge: Cambridge University Press, pp 221-55.

Stephenson, P. (2003) 'Only 62 Targets Now', *Health Service Journal*, 8 February, p 8.

Stewart, J. (1958) *British Pressure Groups: Their Role in Relation to the House of Commons*, London: Greenwood.

Stewart, J. (2004) *Taking Stock: Scottish Welfare After Devolution*, Bristol: The Policy Press.

Stoker, G. (2004) 'New Localism, Progressive Politics and Democracy', in Gamble, A. and Wright, T. (eds) *Restating the State*, Oxford: Blackwell, pp 117-29.

Streeck, W. and Schmitter, P. (eds) (1985) *Private Interest Government: Beyond Market and State*, London: Sage.

Street, J. (1988) 'British Government Policy on AIDS', *Parliamentary Affairs*, vol 41, pp 490-508.

Strong, P. and Robinson, J. (1990) *The NHS: Under New Management*, Buckingham: Open University Press.

Sullivan, H. and Skelcher, C. (2002) *Working Across Boundaries: Collaboration in Public Services*, Basingstoke: Palgrave.

Sussex, J. and Goddard, M. (2002) 'Flexible Friends', *Health Service Journal*, 23 May, pp 28-9.

Talbot, C., Johnson, C. and Freestone, M. (2004) *Is Devolution Creating Diversity in Education and Health?: A Report on Health and Education Policy and Performance in Wales and Scotland*, Nottingham: Nottingham Policy Centre.

Tallis, R. (2004) *Hippocratic Oaths: Medicine and its Discontents*, London: Atlantic Books.

Tam, H. (1998) *Communitarianism: A New Agenda for Politics and Citizenship*, Basingstoke: Macmillan.

Tansey, G. and Worsley, T. (1995) *The Food System*, London: Earthscan.

Tarrow, S. (1998) *Power in Movement*, Cambridge: Cambridge University Press.

Taylor, M. (1999) 'Between Public and Private: Accountability in Voluntary Organisations', *Policy and Politics*, vol 27, no 1, pp 57-72.

Taylor, M. (2000) *Modernising Government: The Tension between Central Targets and Local Initiative*, London: IPPR.

Taylor, M. (2006) 'Communities in Partnership: Developing a Strategic Voice', *Social Policy and Society*, vol 5, no 2, pp 269-79.

TBT (Technical Barriers to Trade) (1994) *Agreement on Technical Barriers to Trade*, www.wto.org/english/tratop_e/tbt_e.htm, accessed 14 December 2006.

Terkildsen, N., Schnell, F. and Ling, C. (1998) 'Interest Groups, the Media and Policy Debate Formation: An Analysis of Message Structure, Rhetoric and Source Cues', *Political Communication*, vol 15, pp 45-61.

Tew, M. (1998) *Safer Childbirth? A Critical History of Maternity Care* (3rd edn), London: Free Association Books.

Thatcher, M. (1982) Speech to the Conservative Party Conference, Brighton, 8 October.

Thatcher, M. (1993) *The Downing Street Years*, London: Harper Collins.

Third Sector Commissioning Task Force (2006) *No Excuses. Embrace Partnership Now. Step towards Change!*, London: DoH.

Timmins, N. (1995) *The Five Giants: A Biography of the Welfare State*, London: Fontana.

Townsend, P. (2001) *Targeting Poor Health*, Cardiff: National Assembly for Wales.

Toynbee, P. and Walker, D. (2001) *Did Things Get Better?*, London: Penguin.

Treasury Committee (2001) *Treasury – Third Report*, HC 73, 2000/1, London: The Stationery Office.

Treaty Establishing a Constitution for Europe (2004) (http://europa.eu/constitution/en/lstoc1_en.htm).

Treaty of Rome (1957) (www.hri.org/docs/Rome57, accessed 14 December 2006).

Treaty on European Union (1992) *Official Journal of the European Communities*, C244, 31 August (http://.europa.eu.int/en/record/mt/top.html, accessed 19 March 2007).

TRIPS (Trade-related Aspects of Intellectual Property) (1994) *Trade Related Aspects of Intellectual Property, Annex 1c of Marrakech Agreement Establishing the World Trade Organisation*, www.wto.org.english/tratop_e/trips_e/t_agm0_e.htm, accessed 14 December 2006.

Truman, D. (1951) *The Governmental Process*, New York, NY: Knopf.

Tudor-Hart, J. (2004) 'Health Care or Health Trade?: A Historic Moment of Choice', *International Journal of Health Services*, vol 34, no 2, pp 245-54.

Tudor-Hart, J. (2006) *The Political Economy of Health Care: A Clinical Perspective*, Bristol: The Policy Press.

Turning Point (2004) *Turning 40*, London: Turning Point.

UN General Assembly (2000) *United Nations Millennium Declaration*, 55th Session, UN General Assembly A/Res/55/2,18 September 2000.

Van Herk, R., Klazinger, N., Schepers, R. and Casparie, A. (2001) 'Medical Audit: Threat or Opportunity for the Medical Profession', *Social Science and Medicine*, vol 53, pp 1721-2.

Waitzkin, H., Jasso-Aguilar, R., Landwehr, A. and Mountain, C. (2005) 'Global Trade, Public Health, and Health Services: Stakeholder's Constructions of the Key Issues', *Social Science and Medicine*, vol 61, pp 893-906.

Wales Audit Office (2006) *NHS Waiting Times: Follow up Report*, Cardiff: Wales Audit Office.

Walker, D. (2002) *In Praise of Centralism: A Critique of the New Localism*, London: Catalyst.

Wall, A. and Owen, B. (2002) *Health Policy* (2nd edn), London: Routledge.

Walshe, K. (2003) *Regulating Healthcare: A Prescription for Improvement*, Buckingham: Open University Press.

Walt, G. (1994) *Health Policy: An Introduction to Process and Power*, London: Zed Books.

Wanless, D. (2002) *Securing Our Future Health: Taking a Long-Term View. Final Report*, London: HM Treasury.

Wanless, D. (2003) *The Review of Health and Social Care in Wales*, Cardiff: Welsh Assembly.

Wanless, D. (2004) *Securing Health for the Whole Population*, London: HM Treasury.

Washer, P. (2004) 'Representation of SARS in the British Newspapers', *Social Science and Medicine*, vol 59, 2561-71.

Watney, S. (1997) *Policing Desire: Pornography, AIDS and the media* (3rd edn), London: Cassell.

Webb, P. (2000) *The Modern British Party System*, London: Sage.

Webster, C. (1988) *The Health Services Since the War*, vol 1, *Problems of Health Care. The National Health Service Before 1957*, London: HMSO.

Webster, C. (1996) *Government and Health Care*, vol 2, *The National Health Service 1958-79*, London: HMSO.

Webster, C. (1998) 'The BMA and the NHS', *British Medical Journal*, vol 317, pp 45-7.

Webster, C. (2002) *The National Health Service: A Political History* (2nd edn), Oxford: Oxford University Press.

Wellings, K. (1986) 'Help or Hype: An Analysis of Media Coverage of the 1983 "Pill Scare"', in Leathar, D., Hastings, G., O'Reilly, K. and Davies, J. (eds) *Health Education and the Media II*, Oxford: Pergamon Press, pp 109-16.

Wellings, K. (1988) 'Perceptions of Risk: Media Treatment of AIDS', in Aggleton, P. and Homans, H. (eds) *Social Aspects of AIDS*, London: Falmer, pp 83-105.

Wellings, K. and Kane, R. (1999) 'Trends in Teenage Pregnancy in England and Wales', *Journal of the Royal Society of Medicine*, vol 92, no 6, pp 277-82.

Welsh Assembly Government (2005) *Designed for Life*, Cardiff: National Assembly for Wales.

Whiteley, P. and Winyard, S. (1987) *Pressure for the Poor: The Poverty Lobby and Policy Making*, London: Methuen.

WHO (World Health Organisation) (1946) *Preamble to the Constitution of the World Health Organisation as adopted by the International Conference, New York 19 June - 22 July 1946* (Official Records of the World Health Organisation, no 2).

WHO (1981) *Global Health Strategy for Health for All by the Year 2000*, Geneva: WHO.

WHO (1998) *Health for All for the 21st Century*, Geneva: WHO.

WHO (2000) *The World Health Report: Health Systems*, Geneva: WHO.

WHO (World Health Organisation) Regional Office for Europe (1985) *Targets for Health for All: Targets in Support of the European Regional Strategy for Health for All*, Copenhagen: WHO.

WHO (World Health Organisation) Regional Office for Europe (1998) *Health 21: The Health for All Policy Framework for the 21st Century*, Copenhagen: WHO.

WHO and UNICEF (United Nations Children's Fund) (1978) *Declaration of Alma Ata*, Report of the International Conference on Primary Health Care, Geneva, WHO/UNICEF.

WHO and WTO (World Trade Organisation) (2002) *WTO Agreements and Public Health: A Joint Study by the WHO and WTO Secretariat*, WHO/WTO.

Wilkin, D., Coleman, A., Dowling, B. and Smith, K. (eds) (2002) *The National Tracker Survey of Primary Care Groups and Trusts 2001/2002: Taking Responsibility?*, Manchester: University of Manchester.

Williams, K. (1999) '"Dying of ignorance?" Journalists, News Sources and Media Reporting of HIV/AIDS', in Franklin, B. (ed) *Social Policy, the Media and Misrepresentation*, London: Routledge, pp 69-85.

Wilsford, D. (1991) *Doctors and the State: The Politics of Health Care in France and the United States*, London: Duke University Press.

Wilsford, D. (1994) 'Path Dependency, or why History Makes it Difficult but not Impossible to Reform Health Care Systems in a Big Way', *Journal of Public Policy*, vol 13, no 3, pp 251-83.

Wistow, G. and Harrison, S. (1998) 'Rationality and Rhetoric: The Contribution to Social Care Policy Making of Sir Roy Griffiths 1986-91', *Public Administration*, vol 76, no 4, pp 649-68.

Wolfenden Committee (1978) *The Future of Voluntary Organisations*, London: Croom Helm.

Wood, B. (2000) *Patient Power?: The Politics of Patients' Associations in Britain and America*, Buckingham: Open University Press.

Woods, K. (2002) 'Health Policy and the NHS in the UK 1997-2002', in Adams, J. and Robinson, P. (eds) *Devolution in Practice: Public Policy Differences within the UK*, London: IPPR.

Woods, K. (2004) 'Political Devolution and the Health Services in Great Britain', *International Journal of Health Services*, vol 34, no 2, pp 323-39.

Wright, O. (2003) 'Television Death Led to 14,000 Smear Tests', *The Times*, 23 February, p 5.

Wyatt, M. (2002) 'Partnership in Health and Social Care: The Implications of Government Guidance in the 1990s in England with particular reference to Voluntary Organisations', *Policy & Politics*, vol 30, no 2, pp 167-82.

Yamey, G. (2002a) 'Why Does the World Still Need WHO?', *British Medical Journal*, vol 325, pp 1294-8.

Yamey, G. (2002b) 'WHO's Management: Struggling to Reform a "Fossilised Bureaucracy"', *British Medical Journal*, vol 325, pp 1170-3.

You Gov/Sky News (2005) *Election Trends*, 4 May, London: You Gov.

Index

G

H

I

Q

R

S

T

U

V

W